Color Atlas of Applied Anatomy

Color Atlas of
Applied Anatomy

R.M.H. McMinn
M.D., Ph.D., F.R.C.S.
Emeritus Professor of Anatomy
Royal College of Surgeons of England and
University of London

R.T. Hutchings
Freelance Photographer
Formerly Chief Medical Laboratory Scientific Officer
Department of Anatomy
Institute of Basic Medical Sciences
Royal College of Surgeons of England

B.M. Logan
F.M.A.
Prosector
Department of Anatomy
Institute of Basic Medical Sciences
Royal College of Surgeons of England

Year Book Medical Publishers, Inc
35 East Wacker Drive, Chicago

To Margaret, Anne and Evelyn

Acknowledgements

By their comments and questions about anatomical problems, many students and colleagues have assisted in defining the kind of material that would be useful in this book, and we express our gratitude for the contribution they have made to it.

We are grateful to our artist Anne Hutchings, to our models, and to Dr K.M. Backhouse and the Master of the Hunterian Institute of the Royal College of Surgeons of England for permission to use facilities at the College.

Preface

This is a book about the anatomy of "how to get at things". Its scope ranges from such relatively simple items as which superficial veins are used for obtaining samples of blood to more complex procedures such as how the surgeon gains access to internal organs.

We must stress that this is a book about anatomy, not a how-to-do-it instruction manual of operative surgery or techniques. Although brief descriptions are given of the way various procedures and operations are carried out, the object is to explain the anatomical environment in which they take place and not to provide technical detail which is of interest only to the specialist. For this reason the dissections are not meant to provide an exact simulation of operations or other procedures but simply to illustrate possible pathways of anatomical approach, emphasising how the facts of anatomy can be used to display specific structures while leaving undisturbed important neighbouring items. Nor have we been concerned with pathology or the reasons *why* access to particular structures may be necessary. Diseased organs may have to be removed, broken bone ends plated together, severed peripheral nerves or vessels repaired or grafted – there are many reasons, but we repeat that this is essentially an anatomy book without too much diversion into other disciplines. Wherever possible, most of the principal items are covered on a double page spread, and in order not to disrupt this usually convenient arrangement this plan has been maintained even with the smaller photographic and textual items that may not completely fill the pages.

For medical and dental students and paramedical groups that have begun anatomical studies, it will add pertinent and practical interest to learning anatomy and will help to bridge the awkward gap that exists between academic anatomy and clinical practice. Most students will have to give injections and take samples of blood; many may never even see, let alone ever do, many of the items described, but all are surely interested in the anatomical principles of how things can be done to patients. Some of the procedures described may not be carried out very often even by the relevant specialists, but have been included as an aid to anatomical learning and understanding.

The book is principally a visual presentation and the text is not intended to give comprehensive coverage of every item discussed. But the Background notes include points relevant to the procedures described, and under the heading Hazards and Safeguards further emphasis is placed on those anatomical features that have special relevance.

For the postgraduate the book will serve as an anatomical refresher and a basis to which more specialised details can be added. Ever-increasing advances in technology are leading to new methods of investigation and treatment, and sound anatomical knowledge, ever the bedrock of *good* clinical practice, becomes more rather than less important. Although injury and disease can distort normal anatomy, the recognised standard pattern remains the fundamental guide.

We hope that undergraduates, postgraduates and other students of human anatomy will find this book to be a stimulating and medically relevant supplement to the more traditional teaching, by showing how anatomical facts are put to use in a practical context.

Contents

Head, Neck and Spine 10–51
Cervical lymph nodes 11
    Local excision 11
    Radical neck dissection 12
Internal jugular and brachiocephalic veins 14
Subclavian vein 16
    Infraclavicular venepuncture 16
    Supraclavicular venepuncture 16
Carotid arteries 17
    Approach to common carotid artery 18
    Approach to external and internal carotid arteries 18
Stellate ganglion 19
Submandibular gland 20
Larynx and trachea 21
    Laryngotomy 21
    Tracheostomy 21
Thyroid gland 22
Parathyroid glands 23
Tonsils and adenoids 24
    Tonsils 24
    Adenoids 25
Parotid gland 26
Maxillary sinus, maxillary artery and Vidian nerve 28
    Maxillary sinus 28
    Maxillary artery and Vidian nerve 28
Lacrimal sac 30
Orbit 30
Supra-orbital and supratrochlear nerves 31
Trigeminal ganglion 32
Maxillary nerve 34
    Extra-oral block 34
    Intra-oral block 34
Infra-orbital nerve 36
Infiltration anaesthesia of teeth 37
Posterior superior alveolar nerve 38
Nasopalatine and greater palatine nerves 39

Mandibular nerve 40
    Extra-oral block 40
    Intra-oral block 41
Inferior alveolar and lingual nerves 42
Mental and incisive nerves 43
Cranial cavity 44
    Burr holes 44
    Craniotomy 44
    Middle meningeal artery 45
Pituitary gland 46
    Transphenoidal approach 46
    Subfrontal approach 47
Subarachnoid and epidural spaces 48
    Cisternal puncture 48
    Lumbar puncture 49
    Epidural anaesthesia 49
Intervertebral disc 50

Upper Limb 52–93
Shoulder joint 52
    Anterior approach 52
    Posterior approach 54
    Supraspinatus tendon 55
    Puncture 57
Humerus 58
    Anterior approach 58
    Posterior approach 59
Elbow joint 60
    Medial and lateral approaches 60
    Posterior approach 61
    Anterior approach 62
    Puncture 63
Radius 64
Ulna 66

Wrist joint 68
    Posterior approach 69
    Puncture 69
Carpal bones 70
    Scaphoid 70
    Trapezium 70
Brachial plexus 70
    Supraclavicular approach 71
    Infraclavicular approach 71
    Supraclavicular block 72
    Axillary block 72
Subclavian and axillary arteries 73
    Approach to subclavian artery 74
    Approach to axillary artery 74
Musculocutaneous nerve 75
Brachial artery, median nerve and ulnar nerve in arm 77
    Approach in the arm 77
    Approach at the elbow 77
    Puncture of brachial artery 78
    Median nerve block at elbow 78
    Ulnar nerve block at elbow 78
Radial nerve in arm and forearm 80
    Approach in arm 81
    Approach at elbow 81
    Nerve block at elbow 82
    Nerve block at wrist 82
Radial artery 83
    Approach at wrist 83
    Puncture 83
Ulnar nerve and artery in forearm 84
    Approach at wrist 84
    Puncture of ulnar artery 84
    Ulnar nerve block at wrist 84
Median nerve in forearm and hand 86
    Approach in forearm 86
    Nerve block at wrist 87
    Approach in carpal tunnel 87
Hand spaces, synovial sheaths and digital nerves 88
    Dorsal subcutaneous and subaponeurotic spaces 88
    Palmar subaponeurotic space 89
    Midpalmar space 89
    Thenar space 89
    Web spaces 89
    Ulnar bursa 90
    Radial bursa 91
    Digital synovial sheaths 91
    Pulp spaces 92
    Subungual spaces 92
    Digital nerves 92
Superficial veins 93

Thorax 94–109
Thoracic wall 94
    Intercostal drainage 94
    Median sternotomy 94
    Anterolateral and posterolateral thoracotomy 94
    Thoraco-abdominal incision 95
Breast 96
Thymus 97
Heart 98
    External massage 99
    Internal massage 99
    Pericardial drainage 100
    Anterior approach 100
    Cardiopulmonary bypass 100
    Some open heart operations 101
    Other heart and great vessel operations 102
    Cardiac transplantation 103
Lungs 104
    Left pneumonectomy 104
    Right pneumonectomy 105
Oesophagus 106
    Cervical approach 107
    Thoracic approach 107
Thoracic sympathetic trunk 108
    Supraclavicular approach 108
    Transaxillary approach 108

Abdomen and Pelvis 110–165
Abdominal wall 110
    Midline and paramedian incisions 110
    Peritoneal drainage 110
    Subcostal, oblique and transverse muscle-cutting incisions 112
    Gridiron and lower transverse incisions 114
Inguinal hernia 116
Femoral hernia 117
Ductus (vas) deferens 118
Stomach 119
    Partial gastrectomy 119
    Vagotomy 121
Duodenum and pancreas 122
    Mobilisation of duodenum 124
    Approach to head of pancreas 125
Liver 126
    Left lobectomy 126
    Right lobectomy 127
    Needle biopsy 128
    Liver transplantation 129
Portal vein 130
Gallbladder and bile duct 130

Spleen 132
Suprarenal gland 134
Kidney 136
    Lumbar approach 138
    Needle biopsy 139
    Kidney transplantation 140
Abdominal aorta, inferior vena cava
        and ureter 142
    Inferior vena cava 142
    Ureter 143
    Aorta 143
Appendix 144
Colon 146
    Right hemicolectomy 146
    Transverse colectomy 147
    Left hemicolectomy 149
    Sigmoid colectomy 150
Rectum and anal canal 152
    Anterior resection 153
    Abdominoperineal resection 153
Male bladder, urethra and genital organs 154
    Catheterisation 155
    Retropubic, transvesical and transurethral
        approaches 156
    Testis 158
Female bladder, urethra and genital organs 158
    Approach to uterus, tube and ovary 160
Pudendal nerve 162
    Perineal block 162
    Vaginal block 162
Lumbar sympathetic trunk 164
    Sympathectomy 164
    Block 164
Coeliac plexus 165

Lower Limb 166–207
Hip joint 167
    Anterolateral approach 168
    Posterior approach 168
    Puncture 171
Femur 172
    Anterior approach 172
    Posterolateral approach 174
Knee joint 176
    Anteromedial approach 176
    Posterior approach 177
    Puncture 178
Tibia 178
    Anterior approach 178
    Posteromedial approach 179
    Posterolateral approach 180
Fibula 181

Ankle joint 182
    Anterior approach 182
    Puncture 183
    Posteromedial approach 184
    Posterolateral approach 185
Lumbar plexus 186
Sacral plexus 189
Sciatic nerve 190
    Gluteal approach 190
    Thigh approach 190
    Block 192
Femoral and lateral femoral cutaneous nerves 194
Obturator nerve 195
Femoral artery 197
    Triangle approach 197
    Canal approach 197
    Puncture 197
Popliteal artery 198
    Posterior approach 198
    Lateral approach 199
    Medial approach 201
Common peroneal, tibial and deep peroneal nerves 202
Posterior tibial artery 204
Sural nerve 205
Great saphenous vein 206

Intramuscular Injections 208–209
Deltoid 209
Gluteal 209
Vastus lateralis 209

Index 210

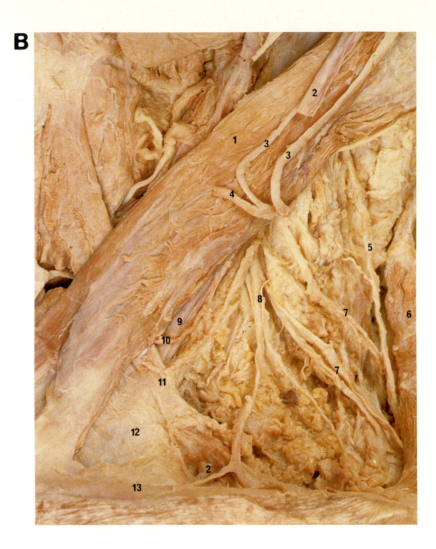

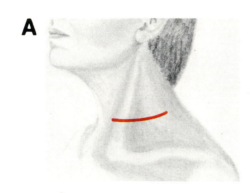

A
Incision line.

B
Lower part of the left posterior triangle. The accessory nerve must be preserved when dissecting out the fat that contains the lymph nodes.

1 Sternocleidomastoid
2 External jugular vein
3 Great auricular nerve (double)
4 Transverse cervical nerve
5 Accessory nerve
6 Trapezius
7 Cervical nerve to 6
8 Supraclavicular nerve
9 Internal jugular vein
10 Ansa cervicalis
11 Omohyoid
12 Investing layer of deep cervical fascia
13 Clavicle

HEAD, NECK AND SPINE
CERVICAL LYMPH NODES

Background

The lymph nodes of the neck consist of the deep cervical group, strung out along the internal jugular vein and carotid sheath (but outside the sheath), and various other groups mainly in the superficial tissues of the anterior and posterior triangles of the neck, and which all drain either directly or indirectly into the deep group. Among the nodes of the deep group are the jugulodigastric nodes, in the area between the internal jugular vein and the posterior belly of digastric, and the jugulo-omohyoid node overlying the tendon of the omohyoid muscle. They receive lymph from the tongue among other tissues, but the jugulodigastric group also receive tonsillar lymph and are frequently called tonsillar nodes. The superficial groups include submental and submandibular nodes near the lower border of the mandible, anterior cervical nodes along the anterior jugular vein and superficial cervical nodes along the external jugular vein. Deeper tissues drain to retropharyngeal nodes behind either side of the pharynx but in front of the prevertebral fascia, paratracheal nodes on either side of the trachea, and a midline group consisting of a single node or two in infrahyoid, prelaryngeal and pretracheal positions. Nodes in the head, called occipital, retroauricular (mastoid), parotid and buccal according to their positions, all drain to the deep cervical group.

Lymph nodes of the neck may need to be removed for tuberculous disease, where local excision of the affected nodes is all that is required, and for secondary cancerous spread, where an extensive excision must be carried out.

The local excision of tuberculous nodes is relatively simple, and involves dissection of the nodes with ligation of some veins to assist in access to some nodes. Damage to the (spinal) accessory nerve and internal jugular vein are the major hazards.

As part of the treatment for cancerous spread involving cervical nodes it may be necessary to remove the whole of the deep cervical chain with other nodes and tissues. This extensive operation of removing these nodes together with adjacent structures is commonly known as radical neck dissection. The object is not to remove small pieces of tissue one by one (which might lead to excessive contamination of the operation site by liberated cancer cells) but to remove nodes, veins, muscles and other tissues in one large mass or block. Apart from cervical nodes the block of tissue customarily removed includes (though subject to modification) the internal, external and anterior jugular veins, the lateral lobe of the thyroid gland, the submandibular gland and the lower pole of the parotid gland, together with sternocleidomastoid, the strap muscles and cutaneous branches of the cervical plexus. At the same time a number of important items must be preserved; these include the brachial plexus, the carotid vessels, the phrenic, facial, glossopharyngeal, vagus and hypoglossal nerves and the thoracic duct (or right lymphatic duct).

The general principle of the operation is to transect the lower end of sternocleidomastoid and the internal jugular vein and dissect upwards, gradually increasing the size of the block of tissue to be removed.

Local Excision

A skin incision (A) is made transversely along a skin crease at the appropriate level, and skin flaps including platysma are raised.

The external jugular vein is ligated and sternocleidomastoid retracted backwards to expose the deep cervical nodes adjacent to the internal jugular vein which is within the carotid sheath. If the upper nodes are to be removed the facial vein is ligated, and for nodes in the posterior triangle sternocleidomastoid can be retracted forwards without injury to the accessory nerve (B). The nodes are dissected out as required.

Hazards and Safeguards

The structure at greatest risk is the accessory nerve in the posterior triangle (B). It emerges from the posterior border of sternocleidomastoid and crosses the triangle embedded in the investing layer of deep cervical fascia that forms the roof of the triangle, to enter trapezius 5 cm above the clavicle. It can be distinguished from the cervical plexus branches to trapezius by the fact that it emerges from *within* the substance of sternocleidomastoid; the cervical plexus branches emerge *deep to* the muscle. Higher up the accessory nerve enters the anterior border of the muscle 3 cm below the mastoid process.

The hypoglossal nerve passes superficial to the posterior border of hyoglossus and then deep to mylohyoid, and must be avoided when removing nodes in the digastric triangle (as in C, page 13).

The phrenic nerve on scalenus anterior should not be at risk provided that dissection remains superficial to the prevertebral fascia that overlies the muscle and nerve (as in B, page 12).

Some infected nodes may be firmly adherent to the internal jugular vein and this thin-walled vessel may be torn easily.

Radical Neck Dissection

A double horizontal skin incision (A) is made; the upper incision extends from below the tip of the chin to the mastoid process but curving down to the level of the hyoid bone, and the lower is above the clavicle from the midline to the anterior border of trapezius. The skin (including platysma) between these incisions is raised as a bridge flap and retracted as required for working beneath it. (An alternative Y-shaped incision may give healing problems where the three stems meet.)

Sternocleidomastoid is detached from the sternum and clavicle so that the internal jugular vein which lies under cover of the muscle can be divided at its lower end. With its covering of carotid sheath the vein is dissected away from the common carotid artery and the vagus nerve.

Omohyoid is divided where it lies lateral to the internal jugular vein, and the adjacent fatty tissue in the lower part of the posterior triangle is dissected off the prevertebral fascia that forms the floor of the triangle. The superficial cervical vessels are transected to facilitate this part of the dissection.

The external jugular vein is divided, and the internal jugular vein and sternocleidomastoid are lifted forwards and upwards with the rest of the other freed tissues (B).

The lower ends of sternohyoid and sternothyroid are transected and the isthmus of the thyroid gland is divided, followed by division of the inferior thyroid vessels so that the lateral lobe can be mobilised from below upwards.

This whole mass of tissue – sternocleidomastoid, strap muscles, thyroid lobe, internal jugular vein, connective tissue and nodes – is peeled upwards, sacrificing all the cutaneous branches of the cervical plexus and the external and anterior jugular veins, but leaving intact the prevertebral fascia and brachial plexus, the carotid vessels, the phrenic, vagus and recurrent laryngeal nerves and the thoracic duct (or right lymphatic duct) (C). At the upper end of the operation field sternocleidomastoid and the internal jugular vein are divided as high as possible after removing the lower pole of the parotid gland. The marginal mandibular and cervical branches of the facial nerve are preserved.

The submandibular gland is then freed and the duct divided so that the gland and adjacent lymph nodes become part of the block dissection. Some lymph nodes are embedded within the gland, hence the need for its removal. The lingual and hypoglossal nerves must be left intact, but the facial vessels will require transection both above and below the gland (page 20).

The upper attachments of the strap muscles are removed and the accessory nerve is cut as it enters sternocleidomastoid. The whole block of tissue can now be removed.

Hazards and Safeguards

The above operation is an extensive procedure and can be subject to modification depending on the extent of disease. For example the thyroid gland and strap muscles may be preserved, or sometimes sternocleidomastoid and the accessory nerve entering trapezius can be left intact.

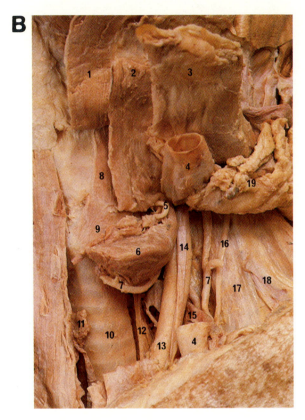

B
Left side of the neck. Sternocleidomastoid, the internal jugular vein and adjacent structures are being dissected out as a single tissue mass superficial to the prevertebral fascia, and turned upwards.

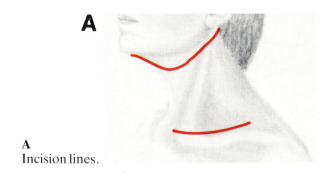

A
Incision lines.

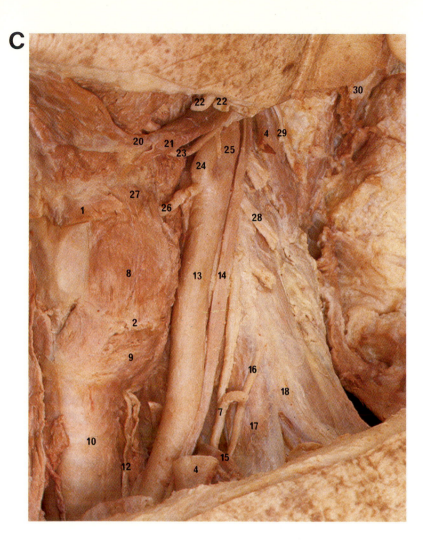

C

C

The completed dissection. The carotid vessels, thoracic duct, and the phrenic, vagus, recurrent laryngeal, internal laryngeal and hypoglossal nerves are preserved.

1   Sternohyoid
2   Sternothyroid
3   Sternocleidomastoid
4   Internal jugular vein
5   Superior thyroid artery
6   Lateral lobe of thyroid gland
7   Inferior thyroid artery
8   Thyrohyoid
9   Cricothyroid
10 Trachea
11 Isthmus of thyroid gland
12 Recurrent laryngeal nerve
13 Common carotid artery
14 Vagus nerve
15 Thoracic duct
16 Prevertebral fascia over phrenic nerve
17 Prevertebral fascia over scalenus anterior
18 Prevertebral fascia over brachial plexus
19 Fat and lymph nodes
20 Digastric tendon
21 Stylohyoid
22 Facial vessels
23 Hypoglossal nerve
24 External carotid artery
25 Internal carotid artery
26 Internal laryngeal nerve
27 Omohyoid
28 Third cervical ventral ramus
29 Accessory nerve
30 Parotid gland

The tearing of thin-walled veins is always an operative hazard, and on the left side the thoracic duct must not be damaged as it arches behind the carotid sheath at the level of the seventh cervical vertebra (but occasionally higher). The ascending cervical branch of the inferior thyroid artery adheres to the posterior wall of the carotid sheath and undue traction may tear the parent vessel or the thyrocervical trunk.

The lingual and hypoglossal nerves should be preserved when removing the submandibular gland; they lie superficial to hyoglossus but deep to mylohyoid (page 20). The marginal mandibular and cervical branches of the facial nerve should also be preserved when removing the lower pole of the parotid gland (page 27).

The brachial plexus and phrenic nerve are protected behind the prevertebral fascia but an unusually high subclavian vein may be hazardous in the lowest part of the dissection.

The upper end of the internal jugular vein can be identified deep to the posterior belly of digastric, with the accessory nerve usually superficial to the vein as the latter lies in front of the transverse process of the atlas.

Clearing the internal jugular vein from the region of the common carotid bifurcation may stimulate the carotid sinus or its nerve, causing a sudden but transient fall in blood pressure.

The sudden loss of venous outflow from the cranial cavity when the internal jugular vein is ligated may result in a temporary rise in intracranial and cerebrospinal fluid pressure, with headache, but normal pressures are usually restored within 24 hours.

Accidental damage to the common or internal carotid arteries must be repaired at once. If common carotid ligation is unavoidable there is a high risk of death or hemiplegia from cerebral ischaemia.

The sympathetic trunk is behind the common and internal carotid arteries, and the middle cervical ganglion or strands of the sympathetic trunk may be behind or in front of the inferior thyroid artery. Damage to the trunk will give rise to Horner's syndrome (page 19).

If the lateral lobe of the thyroid gland is being removed, the usual care must be taken to avoid injuring the recurrent laryngeal nerve (page 22).

INTERNAL JUGULAR AND BRACHIOCEPHALIC VEINS

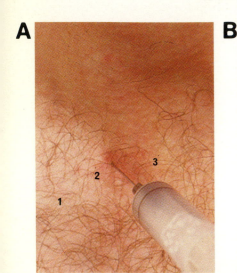

A

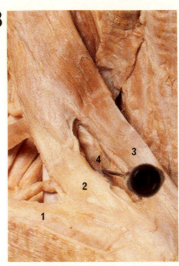

B

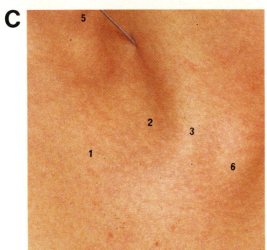

C

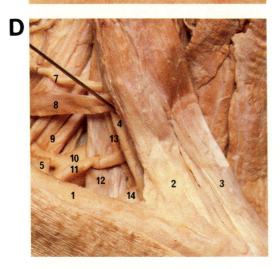

D

Background

The internal jugular vein runs down the neck within the carotid sheath to unite with the subclavian vein behind the sternoclavicular joint and form the brachiocephalic vein. The lower end of the internal jugular is behind the lateral edge of the small triangular interval between the sternal and clavicular heads of sternocleidomastoid; this muscle overlies the vein at higher levels. In the lower neck the tendon of omohyoid is a guide to the position of the internal jugular: the tendon overlies the vein superficially. The right brachiocephalic vein passes straight down and is joined by its fellow (which has crossed obliquely behind the lower part of the manubrium of the sternum) at the lower border of the first costal cartilage to form the superior vena cava.

For measurements of central venous pressure the venous catheter can be threaded into the right atrium or superior vena cava via the right internal jugular or brachiocephalic veins (instead of using the subclavian vein – page 16). These veins can also be used for obtaining venous blood in the rare event of not being able to use (or find!) subcutaneous limb veins.

Venepuncture

For entering the internal jugular vein, the triangular gap between the sternal and clavicular heads of sternocleidomastoid is palpated above the medial end of the clavicle and the *needle* inserted *backwards* and slightly laterally (A & B). For introducing a *catheter* here, the direction is *downwards* and slightly laterally towards the first costal cartilage.

An alternative site for internal jugular puncture is 3 cm above the clavicle at the posterior border of sternocleidomastoid, in the direction of the jugular notch (C & D).

For entering the brachiocephalic vein, the needle or catheter is introduced at the angle between the clavicle and sternocleido-mastoid in the direction of the sternal angle (between the manubrium and body of the sternum) (E & F).

A

Puncture of the right internal jugular vein between the two heads of sternocleidomastoid, with the needle directed backwards and slightly laterally.

B

Dissection of A.

C

Puncture of the right internal jugular vein at the posterior border of sternocleidomastoid, with the needle directed towards the jugular notch of the sternum.

D

Dissection of C.

Hazards and Safeguards

The veins are large and relatively easy to enter but are thin-walled. The internal carotid artery, phrenic nerve and brachial plexus are at risk if penetration is too deep.

If the left brachiocephalic vein has to be used there is a possibility of damage to the thoracic duct.

As with subclavian puncture (page 16), the patient should be in the head-down position to reduce the risk of embolism.

E
Puncture of the right brachiocephalic vein, with the needle directed towards the sternal angle.

F
Dissection of E.

1 Clavicle
2 Clavicular head of sternocleidomastoid
3 Sternal head of sternocleidomastoid
4 Internal jugular vein
5 External jugular vein
6 Jugular notch
7 Superficial cervical artery
8 Omohyoid
9 Brachial plexus
10 Subclavian artery
11 Suprascapular artery
12 Scalenus anterior
13 Phrenic nerve
14 Subclavian vein
15 Brachiocephalic vein

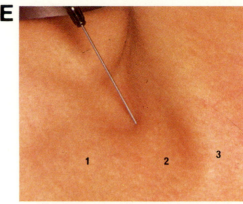

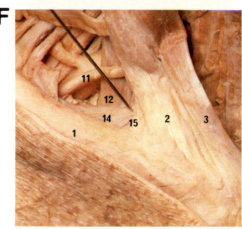

SUBCLAVIAN VEIN

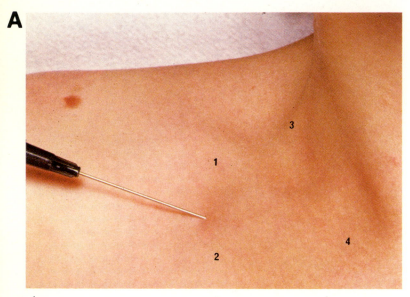

A

Infraclavicular puncture of the subclavian vein, from below the midpoint of the clavicle on a line directed to just above the jugular notch.

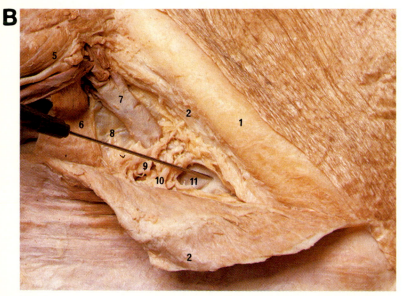

B

Dissection of A. Part of pectoralis major is detached from the clavicle and the clavipectoral fascia divided to show the subclavian vein deep to it and passing under cover of the clavicle.

Background

The subclavian vein begins as the continuation of the axillary vein at the outer border of the first rib, crossing it in a shallow groove in front of scalenus anterior, which separates the vein from the subclavian artery that is behind the muscle and at a higher level. The vein lies behind the clavicle and unites with the internal jugular vein behind the sternoclavicular joint to form the brachio-cephalic vein, with the thoracic duct (on the left) or right lymphatic duct joining the angle of the union. The external jugular vein runs into the subclavian lateral to scalenus anterior. The apex of the lung, covered by cervical pleura and more superficially by the suprapleural membrane, is behind the medial third of the clavicle and so behind the subclavian vein.

Measurements of central venous pressure can be obtained by introducing a venous catheter into the right atrium or superior vena cava. This may be done by pushing the catheter through from a right cubital fossa vein (page 93), but it may be necessary to use the subclavian or the internal jugular veins (page 14). The subclavian vein can be entered either below or above the clavicle, the infraclavicular route being more popular.

Infraclavicular Venepuncture

From a point 2 cm below the midpoint of the clavicle a needle is introduced along a line directed to just above the jugular notch of the manubrium of the sternum (A). Contact is made with the clavicle at the junction of its middle and medial thirds, and a loss of resistance should be felt as the needle pierces the clavipectoral fascia, to enter the vein just behind the fascia (B). The catheter is then threaded through the lumen of the needle and pushed onwards into the brachiocephalic vein and then further still to enter the superior vena cava.

Supraclavicular Venepuncture

A needle is inserted through the skin 2 cm above the clavicle at the junction of its medial and middle thirds (almost at the lateral border of sternocleidomastoid). The needle is directed medially and downwards (C & D) to enter the subclavian vein behind the sternoclavicular joint. The catheter is then threaded through into the superior vena cava.

Hazards and Safeguards

The greatest danger is penetration of the cervical pleura, producing pneumothorax or haemothorax. A reflux of venous blood into the syringe indicates when the needle is properly placed in the vein.

The procedure should be carried out with the patient in the head-down (Trendelenburg) position, to reduce the risk of air embolism.

C
Supraclavicular puncture of the subclavian vein, from above the junction of the medial and middle thirds of the clavicle on a line directed towards the sternoclavicular joint.

D
Dissection of C. The vein crosses the first rib in front of scalenus anterior; the subclavian artery is behind the muscle and in front of the suprapleural membrane.

1   Clavicle
2   Pectoralis major
3   External jugular vein
4   Clavicular head
    of sternocleidomas
5   Deltoid
6   Pectoralis minor
7   Cephalic vein
8   Clavipectoral fascia
9   Thoraco-acromial
    vessels
10 Lateral pectoral nerve
11 Subclavian vein
12 Subclavian artery
13 Suprascapular artery
14 Scalenus anterior
15 Sternoclavicular joint

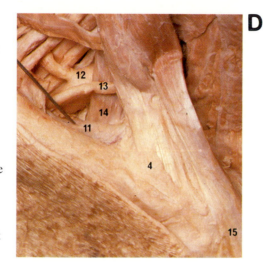

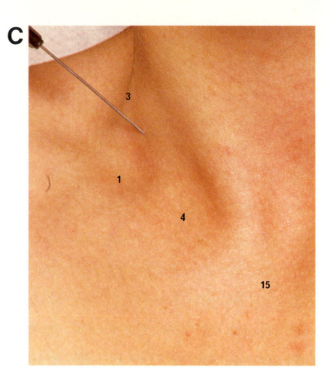

CAROTID ARTERIES

Background
The left common carotid artery is a direct branch from the aortic arch but the right arises from the brachiocephalic artery. In the lower neck the common carotid is within the carotid sheath, beside the trachea and larynx, with the internal jugular vein lateral to it and the vagus nerve deeply placed between the vessels. The sympathetic trunk is behind the artery and outside the sheath, which is overlapped superficially by the infrahyoid muscles and sternocleidomastoid. The bifurcation of the common carotid into the external and internal branches is usually stated to be level with the upper border of the thyroid cartilage (or upper part of the fourth cervical vertebra) but it is frequently higher, near the tip of the greater horn of the hyoid bone. Above the division the external carotid lies medial to the internal carotid and can be distinguished instantly from the internal by having branches; the internal carotid has no branches in the neck.

For opening the carotids to remove diseased intima (carotid endarterectomy) the vessels can be exposed by retracting sterno-cleidomastoid and opening the carotid sheath.

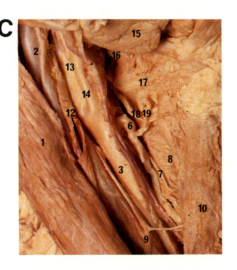

B

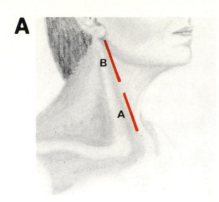

A
Incision line for common carotid artery (A) and external and internal carotids (B).

B
Lower right side of the neck, with sternocleidomastoid retracted backwards to reveal the carotid sheath which is incised to display the common carotid artery.

C
Upper right side of the neck, with sternocleido-mastoid retracted backwards to reveal the carotid sheath which is incised to display the bifur-cation of the common carotid artery.

1	Sternocleidomastoid	**11**	Sternothyroid
2	Internal jugular vein	**12**	Cut end of facial vein
3	Common carotid artery	**13**	Internal carotid artery
4	Cut edge of carotid sheath	**14**	External carotid artery
5	Superior thyroid vein	**15**	Submandibular gland
6	Superior thyroid artery	**16**	Hypoglossal nerve
7	External laryngeal nerve	**17**	Greater horn of hyoid
8	Inferior constrictor of pharynx	**18**	Internal laryngeal nerve
9	Ansa cervicalis	**19**	Superior laryngeal artery
10	Omohyoid		

Approach to Common Carotid Artery

With the head turned to the opposite side, a skin incision 6 cm long is made along the anterior border of sternocleidomastoid, the centre of the incision being 6 cm above the clavicle (A).

The investing layer of deep cervical fascia is incised in the same line, and sternocleidomastoid and the strap muscles freed from the underlying carotid sheath. The sternocleidomastoid branch of the superior thyroid artery will require to be ligated.

The carotid sheath is incised longitudinally above omohyoid to expose the common carotid artery, from which the internal jugular vein is dissected free and retracted medially (B).

Approach to External and Internal Carotid Arteries

A skin incision is made along the anterior border of sternocleido-mastoid from just above the angle of the mandible and downwards for about 9 cm (A). The incision is deepened to include platysma.

The anterior margin of sternocleidomastoid is defined and retracted backwards.

The facial vein is divided before it enters the internal jugular vein, and the carotid sheath is incised longitudinally to expose the bifurcation of the common carotid artery into the external and internal branches (C).

Hazards and Safeguards

The thin-walled internal jugular vein is lateral to the common and internal carotid arteries, and thyroid veins may drain into it near omohyoid and below the facial vein.

The vagus nerve lies deeply between the internal jugular vein and the common or internal carotid arteries, within the carotid sheath.

The sympathetic trunk (with the superior cervical ganglion at the level of the second and third cervical vertebrae) lies behind the common or internal carotid arteries, outside the carotid sheath.

Just above the greater horn of the hyoid bone, the hypoglossal nerve crosses the carotid vessels and the loop of the lingual artery superficially, after giving off the superior root of the ansa cervicalis which is embedded in the anterior wall of the carotid sheath.

The internal and external branches of the superior laryngeal nerve lie medial to the external carotid artery.

The external carotid can be distinguished from the internal because it gives off branches; the internal and common carotids do not. At the bifurcation of the common carotid the internal carotid is rather confusingly *lateral* to the external carotid.

STELLATE GANGLION

Background

The stellate ganglion (properly known as the cervicothoracic ganglion) is the composite name given to the fused inferior cervical and first thoracic sympathetic ganglia. The inferior cervical ganglion lies in front of the ventral ramus of the eighth cervical nerve and behind the vertebral vessels. The first thoracic ganglion is in front of the head of the first rib and behind the pleura. If a fused stellate ganglion is present it is roughly between these two individual ganglia positions – between the base of the transverse process of the seventh cervical vertebra and the head of the first rib, immediately behind the apex of the pleura and separated from it by the suprapleural membrane (Sibson's fascia). The transverse process of the seventh cervical vertebra is on a level 3 cm above the sternoclavicular joint and is palpable here between the trachea medially and sternocleidomastoid and the common carotid artery laterally.

Blockade of the stellate ganglion can be achieved by local anaesthetic with the needle introduced through the front of the lower neck so that the solution gravitates down to the ganglion.

Stellate Ganglion Block

With the neck extended, the index and middle fingers palpate the interval between the trachea and the lower end of sternocleidomastoid, gently displacing the common carotid artery laterally with the muscle (D).

The needle is inserted vertically backwards in the line of the palpating fingers 3 cm above the sternoclavicular joint until it strikes the transverse process of the seventh cervical vertebra. It is then withdrawn for 0.5 cm and the injection made after the usual aspiration test.

The development of Horner's syndrome whose most obvious features are constriction of the pupil (myosis) and drooping of the upper eyelid (ptosis) indicates successful injection.

Hazards and Safeguards

The needle must be withdrawn slightly after striking the transverse process since the solution must gravitate down in front of the prevertebral fascia, not behind it (E).

The needle at this level is above the dome of the pleura but pneumothorax is always a hazard.

Aspiration must ensure that the needle is not in a vessel or dural nerve sheath. The accidental injection of anaesthetic into the vertebral artery, which is a possibility with a needle placed too deeply, will cause convulsions.

A temporary hoarseness of the voice may occur if the recurrent laryngeal nerve is affected by the solution gravitating down between the trachea and oesophagus.

1 Sternocleidomastoid
2 Cricoid cartilage
3 Trachea
4 Jugular notch
5 Top of sternoclavicular joint
6 Common carotid artery
   and cut edge of sheath
7 Branches of ansa cervicalis
8 Superior thyroid vessels
9 Sternothyroid
10 Sternohyoid
11 Sympathetic trunk
12 Inferior thyroid artery
13 Prevertebral fascia
14 Isthmus of thyroid gland

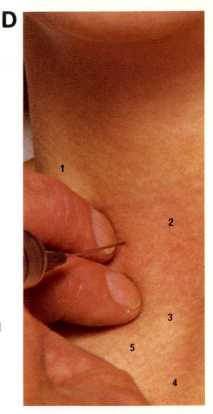

D
Right stellate ganglion block, from the front and slightly left. The needle is introduced 3 cm above the sternoclavicular joint between sternocleidomastoid and the trachea towards the seventh cervical transverse process. The *needle* remains well above the level of the ganglion; the *solution* gravitates down to it.

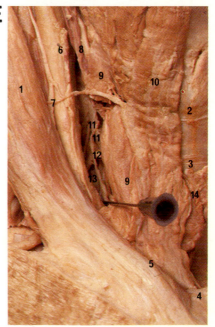

E
Dissection of D, from the front and right. The investing layer of deep cervical fascia and omohyoid are removed. Strands of the sympathetic trunk run both behind and in front of the inferior thyroid artery.

SUBMANDIBULAR GLAND

Background

The submandibular gland lies in the digastric triangle below the mandible, most of it superficial to mylohyoid but with a small deep part passing forwards underneath the posterior free border of that muscle. The gland overlaps the two bellies of digastric and has a capsule derived from the investing layer of deep cervical fascia, but this capsule is much thinner than the one surrounding the parotid gland. The facial vein and the cervical branch of the facial nerve cross the gland superficially while the facial artery enters the triangle deep to the posterior belly of digastric and grooves the posterior and upper surface of the gland before passing on to the face. Submandibular lymph nodes lie round about the gland, and some are embedded within it. The posterior part of the gland lies on hyoglossus which is in the floor of the digastric triangle behind mylohyoid. The hypoglossal nerve enters the triangle deep to the posterior belly of digastric and runs above the greater horn of the hyoid bone between the gland and hyoglossus and then goes deep to mylohyoid. The lingual artery runs above the greater horn but passes deep to hyoglossus. The submandibular duct and the lingual nerve are also found on hyoglossus; the nerve (with the submandibular ganglion attached) hooks under the duct from lateral to medial as they both run forward deep to mylohyoid.

The gland may have to be removed because of calculous disease (stones) or tumours.

B

Right submandibular gland, with skin, platysma and cervical fascia removed. The gland is being dissected out and pulled down from its bed, leaving the lingual nerve and lingual artery (obscured by the nerve in this view) and the hypoglossal nerve intact. In this specimen the mandibular branch of the facial nerve arises from the cervical branch which has been dissected out when removing skin and platysma. The gland's deep part which is pulled out from behind mylohyoid is here very small.

A

Incision line.

Approach

A skin incision (A) is made about 5 cm below and parallel to the lower border of the mandible, beginning at the angle and passing forwards. The incision includes platysma, and skin flaps including platysma are raised.

The superficial surface of the gland is exposed from within its capsule, preserving the cervical branch of the facial nerve.

The facial vein is divided above and below the gland and the facial artery is also ligated in two places – where it emerges on to the face from the upper part of the gland, and where it runs deep to the gland, below and behind it – so that a length of each vessel is eventually removed with the gland.

The gland is pulled down to expose the lingual nerve and the submandibular duct (B). The nerve with the ganglion attached is freed from connective tissue that adheres to the gland, and the duct is divided as it lies on hyoglossus.

The deep part of the gland deep to mylohyoid is dissected out and the whole gland can then be removed.

Hazards and Safeguards

The marginal mandibular branch of the facial nerve normally runs just *above* the lower border of the mandible, but 20% pass down off the face to run *below* the mandible for a variable distance before passing up on to the face again. The skin incision is made well below the mandible to avoid damaging the nerve which lies in the subcutaneous tissue between the skin and platysma and so is included in the upper skin flap if platysma is included. The cervical branch of the facial nerve is always superficial to the gland and is similarly avoided if platysma is raised with the skin flap.

Segments of the facial artery and vein are usually removed with the gland since attempts to dissect them off the gland may lead to troublesome bleeding.

The lingual artery passes deep to hyoglossus and should not be disturbed.

The lingual and hypoglossal nerves are at risk and unless infiltrated by tumour tissue should be preserved.

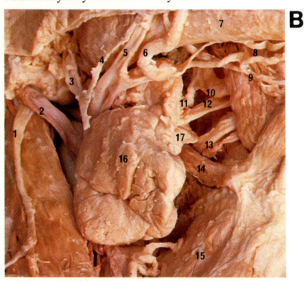

1	Great auricular nerve on sternocleidomastoid	**8**	Submental vessels
		9	Mylohyoid and nerve
2	Anterior division of retromandibular vein	**10**	Lingual nerve
		11	Submandibular ganglion
3	Cervical branch of facial nerve	**12**	Submandibular duct
		13	Hypoglossal nerve and vena comitans
4	Marginal mandibular n.	**14**	Posterior belly of digastric
5	Facial vein	**15**	Thyrohyoid
6	Facial artery	**16**	Superficial part of gland
7	Mandible	**17**	Deep part of gland

LARYNX AND TRACHEA

Background

For the relief of respiratory obstruction at vocal cord level, it may be necessary to make an artificial opening in the cervical part of the respiratory tract below this level – in the lower larynx or upper trachea. The laryngeal prominence (Adam's apple) of the thyroid cartilage is an easily identifiable landmark, and about 3 cm lower the next firm structure in the midline is the cricoid cartilage, below which the trachea continues into the thorax behind the jugular (suprasternal) notch. The cricothyroid membrane stretches between the cricoid and the lower border of the thyroid cartilage, and below the cricoid the cricotracheal membrane joins the cricoid to the first cartilaginous ring of the trachea. The isthmus of the thyroid gland overlies the second, third and fourth tracheal rings, with the lateral lobes of the thyroid gland on each side where it is overlapped by sternohyoid, sternothyroid and sternocleidomastoid, and with inferior thyroid veins coursing down over the lower rings. The anterior jugular veins run vertically a centimetre or two from the midline.

An emergency opening in the larynx (laryngotomy) can be made through the cricothyroid membrane. To make an artificial opening in the cervical part of the trachea (tracheostomy), the isthmus of the thyroid gland is divided and a small circle of anterior tracheal wall removed so that a tracheostomy tube can be inserted. Tracheostomy should not be confused with tracheotomy, which implies only incising the trachea without removing any part of it (Greek: *stoma*, a mouth or opening; *tome*, a cut or incision). Tracheostomy should be carried out as an elective procedure in a properly equipped operating theatre; the need for whipping out a penknife for a dramatic emergency incision is exceptionally rare, and laryngotomy is usually considered preferable to tracheotomy.

Approach for Laryngotomy

The laryngeal prominence and cricoid cartilage are palpated.

A short transverse incision is made (or a wide needle inserted) in the midline between the cricoid and the lower border of the thyroid cartilage (C). The knife or needle passes through the skin, the investing and pretracheal layers of deep cervical fascia, the central part of the cricothyroid membrane (D) and the mucous membrane of the larynx. In this emergency stab procedure there is no attempt to dissect structures by layer.

Approach for Tracheostomy

The cricoid cartilage is palpated.

A skin incision (C) is made transversely in a convenient skin crease about 2 cm below the lower border of the cricoid and deepened to include the deep cervical fascia. The skin flaps above and below are raised to expose the anterior jugular veins and the sternohyoid and sternothyroid muscles.

The interval between the two sternohyoids is opened up and the two sternothyroids that lie slightly deeper are retracted laterally.

The isthmus of the thyroid gland is defined (D) and divided vertically to expose the front of the trachea.

A transverse incision is made in the tracheal wall between the second and third rings and converted into a circular opening by

C
Incision lines for laryngotomy (L) and tracheostomy (T).

D
Midline of the neck. Part of the investing layer of deep cervical fascia is removed (on the left of the picture) but the pretracheal layer, which forms the capsule for the thyroid gland, is incised to display the larynx. The transverse line indicates the position of the incision in the cricothyroid membrane for laryngotomy. For tracheostomy the isthmus of the thyroid gland is divided vertically so that a circular area of the underlying anterior tracheal wall can be excised. In this specimen the anterior jugular veins are unusually large.

1. Investing layer of deep cervical fascia
2. Pretracheal fascia
3. Laryngeal prominence
4. Lower border of thyroid cartilage
5. Cricothyroid membrane
6. Cricoid cartilage
7. Cricothyroid
8. Anterior jugular vein
9. Isthmus of thyroid gland
10. Inferior thyroid veins over trachea
11. Anastomosis between anterior jugular veins
12. Jugular notch
13. Sternocleidomastoid
14. Sternohyoid

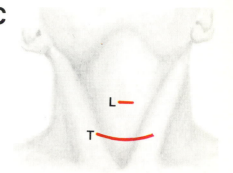

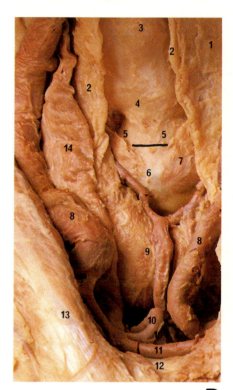

removing parts of adjacent rings so that a hole about 1 cm in diameter is produced. The tracheostomy tube is then inserted.

Hazards and Safeguards

Haemorrhage from the isthmus and inferior thyroid veins is the main danger in tracheostomy but should be easily avoided in an elective procedure.

THYROID GLAND

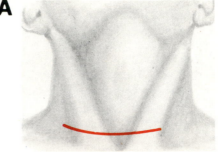

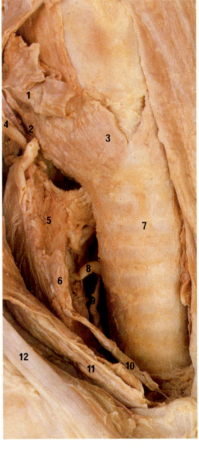

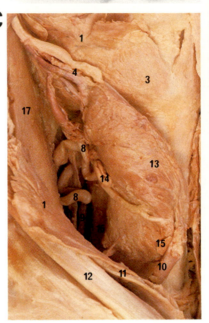

Background

The thyroid gland lies in the front of the neck, within its own capsule derived from the pretracheal fascia, with the isthmus on the second to fourth cartilaginous rings of the trachea. Each lateral lobe is overlapped by sternohyoid, sternothyroid and sternocleido-mastoid, and the carotid sheath is behind each lobe. Medially are the larynx and trachea, pharynx and oesophagus, the inferior constrictor of the pharynx and cricothyroid, and the external and recurrent laryngeal nerves. The external laryngeal nerve runs downwards just behind the superior thyroid artery to supply cricothyroid, and is relatively unimportant compared to the recurrent laryngeal nerve which may be behind, in front of, or in between branches of, the inferior thyroid artery and which supplies all the other intrinsic muscles of the larynx, thus being responsible for moving the vocal cord on its own side. The parathyroid glands are at the back of each lobe.

The commonest operation on the thyroid gland is partial thyroidectomy for diffuse enlargement (simple goitre) or thyrotoxicosis (toxic goitre). Cancerous lesions may require total thyroidectomy. A method for partial thyroidectomy is described here; the operation involves removal of most of both lobes and the isthmus, leaving the posterior part of each lobe and the parathyroid glands in situ at the side of the trachea. Being fairly superficial the approach to the gland from the front of the neck is straightforward; the major hazard in all thyroid surgery is the recurrent laryngeal nerve.

Approach

A skin incision (A) is made transversely but slightly curved downwards about 2.5 cm above the jugular notch, extending as far laterally as the lateral borders of both sternocleidomastoids. The incision includes platysma, and skin flaps are raised as high as the laryngeal prominence and as low as the jugular notch.

A vertical incision is made in the investing layer of deep cervical fascia in the midline and the gap between the sternohyoids (above) and the slightly deeper sternothyroids (below) is opened up to expose the trachea and the isthmus (B).

The sternohyoids and sternothyroids are retracted laterally, or they can be divided near their *upper* ends (so avoiding their nerve supplies from the ansa cervicalis) to provide adequate exposure of the lateral lobes.

The superior and middle thyroid veins (up to three, draining laterally to the internal jugular vein) of one lobe are ligated and the upper pole of the lobe is drawn downwards after ligating the superior thyroid artery.

The inferior thyroid artery is followed as it arches medially beneath the lateral border of the lobe from behind the common carotid artery, and then the recurrent laryngeal nerve is identified. The artery and its branches are ligated either lateral to the nerve or at the surface of the lobe, and the inferior thyroid veins are also divided as they lie in front of the trachea.

A

Incision line.

B

Right side of the front of the neck, with division of the isthmus of the thyroid gland and lateral retraction of the right lateral lobe. Sternothyroid is divided and the ends turned back; at operation it may be sufficient simply to retract it. The most important structure to be identified is the recurrent laryngeal nerve.

C

Right side of the front of the neck, with the right lateral lobe of the thyroid gland retracted medially and turned over to show the parathyroid glands on the posterior surface of the lateral lobe.

1	Sternothyroid	10	Inferior thyroid vein
2	External laryngeal nerve	11	Sternohyoid
3	Cricothyroid	12	Sternocleidomastoid
4	Superior thyroid vessels	13	Posterior surface of
5	Lateral lobe		lateral lobe
6	Isthmus	14	Superior parathyroid gland
7	Trachea	15	Inferior parathyroid gland
8	Inferior thyroid artery	16	Oesophagus
9	Recurrent laryngeal nerve	17	Common carotid artery

The opposite lateral lobe is mobilised in the same way.

The required portion of a lobe is removed, dissecting it off from the trachea and transecting the isthmus. The required part of the other lobe and the rest of the isthmus are then removed.

Hazards and Safeguards

The greatest danger in thyroid operations is damage to the recurrent laryngeal nerve, resulting in paralysis of the vocal cord on that side. Its relationship to the inferior thyroid artery is variable; on the left the nerve is more likely to be behind the artery, while on the right it is more likely to be behind or between branches of the artery, but it must always be carefully sought. It passes upwards approximately in the groove between the trachea and oesophagus, to lie immediately behind the cricothyroid joint and also behind a condensation of connective tissue (sometimes known as the ligament of Berry) that connects the lobe to the side of the cricoid cartilage and the first two or three tracheal rings, and enters the larynx by passing deep to the inferior constrictor of the pharynx.

A small vein that runs on the anterior surface of the nerve may assist in its identification, and at operation the nerve is commonly seen to take a knee-shaped bend as it passes under the inferior constrictor (but in cadaver dissections the bend is usually straightened out).

The nerve often divides into two on a level with the upper border of the thyroid isthmus.

In less than 1% of subjects the nerve on the right side is not recurrent; it runs medial to the lateral lobe on the inferior constrictor (like the external laryngeal nerve) and is at risk when mobilising the upper pole.

The external laryngeal nerve lies posterior to the superior thyroid artery in contact with the inferior constrictor and cricothyroid. It is not likely to be damaged if the artery is ligated at the very tip of the upper pole. Damage to it does not usually produce any detectable effect; if there is slight hoarseness of the voice it soon recovers (due to hypertrophy of the opposite cricothyroid).

Bleeding from the various veins may be troublesome and tears of the thin internal jugular vein must be avoided.

On the left the thoracic duct (or right lymphatic duct on the right) arches laterally behind the carotid sheath before entering the junction of the internal jugular and subclavian veins. It usually rises as high as the seventh cervical vertebra, i.e. one vertebral level lower than the arch of the inferior thyroid artery but occasionally the two may be very close.

Enlarged lobes may stretch the strap muscles, and it is important to define properly the plane deep to sternothyroid and sternohyoid for exposure of the lateral lobe.

The parathyroid glands must be left with the remaining part of each lobe.

PARATHYROID GLANDS

Background

The parathyroid glands normally lie behind the lateral lobes of the thyroid gland but within the thyroid capsule. The superior gland on each side is usually on a level with the junction of the upper and middle thirds of the lateral lobe; the inferior is behind the lower pole near the angle between the inferior thyroid artery and the recurrent laryngeal nerve. Both upper and lower glands are supplied by the inferior thyroid artery. Although normally four in number (in 90% of subjects) there may be more or less.

The glands may have to be tackled surgically because of tumours or excessive secretion (hyperparathyroidism). Individual tumours are removed; for hyperparathyroidism all four glands can be removed and fragments of one of them implanted into the brachioradialis muscle of one arm (some parathyroid secretion is essential to life, and if hyperparathyroidism recurs in the implant it is easier to remove tissue from an arm than from the neck). Alternatively three whole glands and one half of the fourth can be removed.

Approach

The thyroid gland and its lobes are exposed as described for thyroidectomy (page 22).

Each lobe is retracted forward so that the posterior surface can be inspected and the parathyroids identified (C). They are brownish-yellow in colour, and this should help to distinguish them from fat and thyroid tissue. In case of difficulty the upper and lower branches of the inferior thyroid artery should be identified on the posterior surface of the lobe, and when traced upwards and downwards respectively should lead to the glands, which have a very small branch entering them – another feature that helps to distinguish them from a lobule of fat. The glands of each pair are not necessarily on the same level on each side. Each gland is dissected out and removed as required.

Hazards and Safeguards

The recurrent laryngeal nerve must be preserved from injury as carefully as in thyroidectomy.

If the glands cannot be found in their expected sites, any aberrant branches of the inferior thyroid artery should be followed. It may be necessary to explore the mediastinum, especially in the region of the thymus.

TONSILS AND ADENOIDS

Background

The (palatine) tonsil (A) lies in the tonsillar sinus (commonly called the tonsillar fossa) of the oral part of the pharynx, between the palatogolossal fold in front and the palatopharyngeal fold behind (these folds form "the pillars of the fauces"). It has upper and lower poles, a medial surface covered by mucous membrane indented by the tonsillar crypts (and near its upper margin by the larger intratonsillar cleft) and supplied by the tonsillar branch of the glossopharyngeal nerve and lesser palatine nerves (from the maxillary nerve via the pterygopalatine ganglion), and a lateral surface covered by the tonsillar capsule and set against the bed of the tonsillar fossa which is formed by the superior constrictor of the pharynx. This muscle separates the tonsil from the facial artery and two of its branches – the tonsillar artery which pierces the constrictor after passing over the upper border of styloglossus and is the main arterial supply, and the ascending palatine which also sends a small branch into the tonsil. Other tonsillar vessels are derived from the lingual and ascending pharyngeal arteries. Tonsillar veins form a plexus round the capsule and pierce the superior constrictor to enter the pharyngeal plexus, but some enter the external palatine (paratonsillar) vein which runs down from the soft palate and across the upper part of the tonsillar bed before going through the constrictor. The glossopharyngeal nerve crosses the outer surface of the lower part of the bed, running obliquely downwards and forwards to pass below the superior constrictor and enter the tongue. Lymph drains to the jugulodigastric group of deep cervical nodes (page 11).

The pharyngeal tonsil (A), known as adenoids when enlarged, is an aggregation of lymphoid follicles in the mucous membrane of the posterior wall of the nasopharynx at the junction with the roof. It is obscured anteriorly by the soft palate and is only visible through the mouth if a mirror is used to look up behind the soft palate.

Although not removed as frequently as in past decades, removal of the tonsils (tonsillectomy) and adenoids (adenoidectomy) remain among the commonest of all surgical operations. Being approached through the mouth, access is easy.

Approach to the Tonsil

The patient lies with the operating table tilted in the head-down position so that the upper pole of the tonsil is the lower one as seen in this position.

Through the opened mouth the tonsil is easily seen between the palatoglossal and palatopharyngeal arches (pillars of the fauces). It is dissected away from the tonsillar bed by cutting through the mucous membrane at the margins of the arches, beginning at the upper pole and working towards the lower, and keeping close to the tonsillar capsule. The attachment to the tonsillar bed is by fairly loose tissue but there is a denser triangular fold of connective tissue near the lower pole.

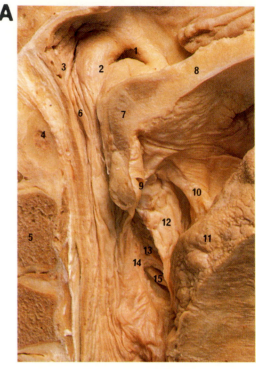

A

A
Left side of a median sagittal section of the head. As in most dissecting room cadavers, the lymphoid tissue of the pharyngeal and palatine tonsils is not prominent, but the openings of crypts on the upper part of the posterior wall of the nasopharynx clearly indicate the position of the pharyngeal tonsil. The palatine tonsil, between the palatoglossal and palatopharyngeal folds in the oral part of the pharynx, is in process of being removed by incision along its posterior border. It is being lifted off the underlying superior constrictor muscle, and the glossopharyngeal nerve is seen deep to the lower border of the muscle.

1 Opening of auditory tube
2 Salpingopharyngeal fold
3 Pharyngeal tonsil
4 Anterior arch of atlas
5 Body of axis
6 Nasopharynx
7 Soft palate
8 Hard palate
9 Uvula
10 Palatoglossal fold
11 Tongue
12 Palatine tonsil
13 Superior constrictor of pharynx
14 Palatopharyngeal fold
15 Glossopharyngeal nerve

Hazards and Safeguards

Haemorrhage is usually easily controlled but the paratonsillar vein running between the upper part of the capsule and the superior constrictor may prove troublesome.

Any lack of care inside the mouth may cause some injury to the soft palate or uvula, the tongue or the teeth, but more serious damage is only likely if the pharyngeal wall is perforated.

If the lower part of the tonsillar bed is penetrated, the glosso-pharyngeal nerve (A) is at risk (it can be deliberately approached here, beneath the lower border of the superior constrictor).

The tonsillar and ascending palatine arteries run upwards on the outer surface of the superior constrictor, and if the facial artery is unduly tortuous it may form a loop deep to the tonsillar bed.

The internal carotid artery is normally well out of harm's way, being 2.5 cm posterior and lateral to the tonsillar bed with fat and loose connective tissue separating it from the pharynx, but an abnormally curled internal carotid has been known to be cut by coming into contact with the pharyngeal wall.

Approach to the Adenoids

With the head in the same position as for tonsillectomy, the adenoids are palpated by a finger passed under the soft palate. The lymphoid mass is directed into an adenoid curette which is specially designed to cut off the enclosed tissue as the instrument is swept down the pharyngeal wall.

Hazards and Safeguards

Improper use of the curette may cause the mucous membrane to be shredded off in strips rather than cutting off the lymphoid mass cleanly. Accidental damage to the uvula and soft palate must be avoided.

Haemorrhage is usually easily controlled; if it persists it may indicate incomplete lymphoid removal which prevents the constriction of cut vessels.

Mucosal damage near the auditory tube may lead to scarring and interference with tubal function.

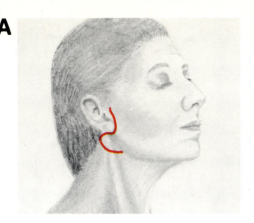

A

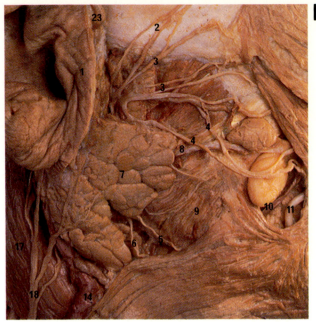

B

PAROTID GLAND

Background

The parotid gland fills in an irregular space between three pieces of bone and their attached muscles – the mastoid process with sterno-cleidomastoid and the posterior belly of digastric, the ramus of the mandible with masseter and the medial pterygoid, and the styloid process with stylohyoid, stylopharyngeus and styloglossus. The gland has a tough capsule derived from the investing layer of deep cervical fascia. The facial nerve is embedded within the gland, together with the retromandibular vein, external carotid artery and its two terminal branches (maxillary and superficial temporal), lymph nodes, and filaments from the auriculotemporal nerve which convey secretomotor fibres to the gland. The main embedded structures – nerve, vein and arteries – lie in that order from superficial to deep, i.e. the nerve is the most superficial. The gland is sometimes referred to as having superficial and deep parts, superficial and deep to the nerve, as though the nerve was clasped in a parotid sandwich, but glandular tissue fuses all round the nerve branches. The nerve enters the gland deeply and posteriorly just after leaving the stylomastoid foramen, and when in the substance of the gland divides into two branches which in turn give rise to the five branches (or rather groups of branches, for they are not all single) that fan out from the anterior margin of the gland (B).

Tumours of the gland or infections due to stones are the usual reasons for surgical operations on it, and any procedure should preserve as far as possible the facial nerve and its branches. Superficial parotidectomy means removing the part that is super-ficial to the nerve, while in total parotidectomy the whole gland is removed. The operations are essentially exercises in dissecting out the facial nerve after identifying it posteriorly and then following it forwards.

Approach

An approximately S-shaped skin incision (A) is made from in front of the ear, backwards to the mastoid process, and downwards and forwards below the angle of the mandible to the external jugular vein. The incision includes platysma.

The anterior border of sternocleidomastoid is followed up to the mastoid process, and the gland retracted forwards to expose the posterior belly of digastric and stylohyoid and the cartilage of the external acoustic meatus. An anterior branch of the great auricular nerve may need to be cut.

The trunk of the facial nerve is approached along a plane in front of the anterior margin of the cartilaginous part of the meatus, above stylohyoid and the posterior belly of digastric. The stylo-mastoid branch of the posterior auricular artery is slightly more superficial than the nerve and is a guide to the proximity of the nerve. The cartilage of the meatus in this region has a slight projection that conveniently points to the nerve (C).

The nerve is carefully followed forwards to all its branches, dissecting off all the glandular tissue that lies superficially.

At the anterior margin of the gland the parotid duct is dissected forwards to the anterior border of masseter and divided here. The operation thus far constitutes superficial parotidectomy.

To continue for total parotidectomy, the facial nerve and its branches are dissected clear of the underlying glandular tissue (D) and the external carotid artery and retromandibular vein are divided near the upper border of stylohyoid. The styloid process may require to be fractured and the stylomandibular ligament divided. The maxillary and superficial temporal arteries and their accompanying veins are divided at the upper pole of the gland, and gland tissue can be removed above or below the nerve trunk or between its two main branches, whichever is more convenient.

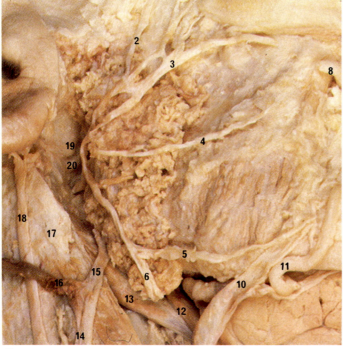

C

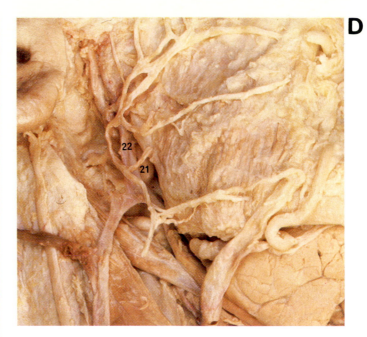

D

1 Tragus	
2 Temporal	
3 Zygomatic	branches of facial nerve
4 Buccal	
5 Marginal mandibular	
6 Cervical	
7 Parotid gland	
8 Parotid duct	**16** Posterior auricular vein
9 Masseter	**17** Sternocleidomastoid
10 Facial vein	**18** Great auricular nerve
11 Facial artery	**19** Projection on meatal cartilage
12 Stylohyoid	**20** Stem of facial nerve
13 Posterior belly of digastric	**21** External carotid artery
14 External jugular vein	**22** Retromandibular vein
15 Posterior division of 22	**23** Superficial temporal artery

A

Incision line.

B

Right parotid gland, after removal of the capsule and some of the upper part of the gland, with the branches of the facial nerve fanning out from the gland over the face.

C

The gland after removal of the superficial part, i.e. the part superficial to *and behind* the facial nerve. A small projection of the meatal cartilage at its junction with the bony part of the external acoustic meatus points towards the stem of the facial nerve.

D

Complete removal of the gland. Here the retromandibular vein and external carotid artery have been preserved to show their positions within the gland – nerve, vein, artery from superficial to deep. At operation they are removed with the gland.

Hazards and Safeguards

The branches of the nerve within the gland lie immediately superficial to the main veins, and the superficial part of the gland is superficial to what has been called the 'faciovenous plane'. It is possible to identify this plane by following the external jugular vein upwards to lead to the posterior division of the retromandibular vein within the gland.

All the facial nerve branches become more and more superficial as they are traced towards the anterior margin of the gland. The upper division of the main trunk usually gives origin to the temporal, zygomatic and buccal branches which are often double; the lower division provides the marginal mandibular and cervical branches and often the lower of the buccal branches. The cervical branch is the least important, supplying only platysma, but it may arise low down outside the gland from a common stem with the marginal mandibular branch (as in B on page 20); if the cervical branch has to be cut it must be positively identified as such to avoid severing the marginal mandibular by mistake. This latter nerve supplies muscles round the lip and paralysis produces an unsightly deformity.

The external carotid artery enters the posteromedial surface of the gland after giving off the posterior auricular branch that runs backwards along the upper border of the posterior belly of digastric. The internal carotid artery lies deeper and must not be mistaken for the external; unlike the external, the internal carotid does not give any branches in the neck.

MAXILLARY SINUS, MAXILLARY ARTERY AND VIDIAN NERVE

Background

The maxillary sinus (maxillary antrum) varies in size depending on the degree to which it extends into the zygomatic and alveolar processes of the maxilla. The infra-orbital canal causes a bulge at the junction of the roof and anterior wall, and the anterior superior alveolar nerve runs in a canal in the anterior wall near its medial margin. The nasolacrimal canal runs on the medial side of the upper medial wall to open into the inferior meatus of the nose. The opening of the sinus into the nose is high up on the medial wall, in the semilunar hiatus of the middle meatus. The lateral part of the posterior wall is penetrated about halfway down by the posterior superior alveolar nerve and vessels.

The sinus can be washed out by making an artificial opening with a trocar introduced through the nostril into the inferior meatus and pushed through the fairly thin bone of the medial wall just above the hard palate, but for more extensive procedures the sinus can be entered from the front by lifting the upper lip and removing bone from the anterior wall (Caldwell-Luc procedure). This route, described below, is also used for the initial stages of access to the maxillary artery and the nerve of the pterygoid canal as they lie in the pterygopalatine fossa behind the maxilla; bone is removed from the posterior wall of the sinus to enter the fossa.

The pterygopalatine fossa is the space between the posterior wall of the maxilla and the anterior surface of the pterygoid process of the sphenoid bone. Laterally it opens into the infratemporal fossa through the pterygomaxillary fissure. Its medial wall is the perpendicular plate of the palatine bone, at the upper end of which is the sphenopalatine foramen leading into the nasal cavity. The maxillary artery enters the fossa through the pterygomaxillary fissure and leaves through the sphenopalatine foramen, changing its name to sphenopalatine artery and becoming the main supply to the mucous membrane of the nose. The maxillary nerve enters the back of the fossa through the foramen rotundum and immediately turns laterally, lying just above the maxillary artery and giving off zygomatic and posterior superior alveolar branches. It then turns forward again to enter the inferior orbital fissure and become the infra-orbital nerve. The nerve of the pterygoid canal (Vidian nerve) enters the fossa through its own canal whose opening is about 8 mm *below and medial* to the foramen rotundum (A and B). The nerve runs into the back of the pterygopalatine ganglion which is immediately in front of the canal opening, and there is a stout connexion between the ganglion and the maxillary nerve. Various nasal, palatine, orbital and pharyngeal branches leave the ganglion which houses the parasympathetic cell bodies whose axons pass to the lacrimal gland and also to glands in the nose, palate and pharynx.

The maxillary artery may have to be ligated in the fossa to stop persistent epistaxis (nose-bleeding). The nerve of the pterygoid canal, which clinicians still commonly call the Vidian nerve, can be severed from its connexion with the pterygopalatine ganglion (Vidian neurectomy) to arrest intractable rhinorrhoea (excessive nasal secretion); nasal glands are under cholinergic control, and

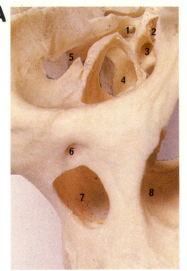

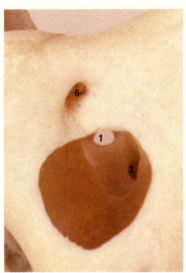

interruption of the parasympathetic fibres to the ganglion by cutting the nerve as it leaves its canal will break the secretomotor pathway. These are uncommon specialized procedures but are included here as interesting and intricate examples of applied anatomy.

Approach to the Maxillary Sinus

With the upper lip retracted upwards and the angle of the mouth retracted laterally, an incision is made in the mucous membrane beginning 1 cm from the midline and 1 cm above the gingival margin and continuing laterally for about 4 cm.

The mucous membrane and periosteum are raised to expose the bone that forms the anterior wall of the sinus, and a round area of bone about 1.5–2 cm in diameter is removed (A and B). The underlying mucous membrane of the sinus is then incised so that the sinus can be entered.

Hazards and Safeguards

The upper extent of bone removal should stop 0.5 cm below the infra-orbital foramen (which is 0.5 cm below the infra-orbital margin) to avoid damaging the infra-orbital nerve.

The lower extent of bone removal should not reach the floor of the sinus to avoid the apices of the teeth and their nerves.

Approach to the Maxillary Artery and Vidian Nerve

The maxillary sinus is entered as described above.

The mucous membrane over the posterior wall of the sinus is removed, and an elliptical area of bone of the posterior wall is gently nibbled away.

The underlying periosteum is incised in a cruciate manner so that maxillary artery and its branches in the pterygopalatine fossa can be dissected out from the fat of the fossa and identified (C). The main artery can be ligated at an appropriate point.

To sever the connexion of the nerve of the pterygoid canal with the pterygopalatine ganglion, the thicker bone at the medial margin of the opening that has been made in the back of the sinus is chiselled away to expose the more medial part of the fossa.

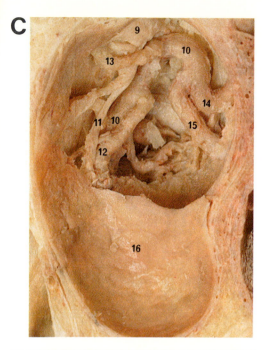

C

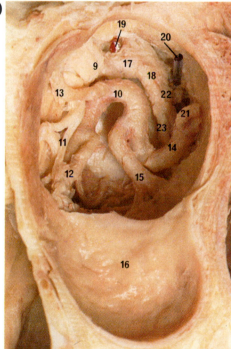

D

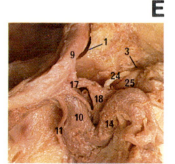

E

1	Foramen rotundum
2	Sphenoidal sinus
3	Pterygoid canal
4	Pterygoid process seen through opening in posterior wall of maxillary sinus
5	Inferior orbital fissure
6	Infra-orbital foramen
7	Opening in anterior wall of sinus
8	Nasal cavity
9	Maxillary nerve
10	Maxillary artery
11	Posterior superior alveolar nerve
12	Posterior superior alveolar artery
13	Infra-orbital artery
14	Sphenopalatine artery
15	Greater palatine artery
16	Lower part of posterior wall of sinus
17	Connexion between 9 and 18
18	Pterygopalatine ganglion
19	Marker in 1
20	Marker in 3
21	Posterior superior nasal artery
22	Posterior superior nasal nerve
23	Greater palatine nerve
24	Nerve of 3
25	Artery of 3

A

Right side of the skull, from above and in front, with bone removed to show the opening made in the anterior wall of the maxilla to give access to the sinus, and the opening made in the posterior wall of the sinus to reach the pterygopalatine fossa, into which open the foramen rotundum and the pterygoid canal.

The main artery is divided as it passes to the sphenopalatine foramen so that the connexion between the maxillary nerve and pterygopalatine ganglion can be displayed and followed to the ganglion which is behind the artery (D). The ganglion lies right in front of the mouth of the pterygoid canal, and a very small knife can be passed behind the ganglion to cut the nerve of the pterygoid canal (E) from it.

Hazards and Safeguards

The initial opening in the posterior wall of the sinus to expose the maxillary artery must not be made too far medially as the bone at the posteromedial angle of the sinus is thick. The removal of the thin bone in the middle of the back of the sinus will enable the artery to be seen but not the pterygopalatine ganglion and the mouth of the pterygoid canal. To display these it is necessary to remove the thicker bone towards the posteromedial angle of the sinus.

In the pterygopalatine fossa the maxillary nerve lies just above the highest part of the rather tortuous maxillary artery (C).

The artery and its branches in general lie anterior to the nerve and its branches.

The pterygopalatine ganglion does not have the rounded appearance expected of a ganglion; rather it must be recognized as being the region where the medial end of the connexion to the maxillary nerve divides into palatine and nasal branches – the palatine passing vertically downwards and the nasal medially (D).

Cutting the nerve of the pterygoid canal not only deprives the nasal glands of their secretomotor fibres (which is the object of the operation) but also denervates the lacrimal gland, and eye drops may be required for corneal and conjunctival protection.

B

The opening in the posterior wall of the right maxillary sinus, viewed by looking backwards and upwards through the anterior maxillary opening, showing the apertures of the foramen rotundum and pterygoid canal (enlarged to the same magnification as C, D and E).

C

Dissection of the right maxillary artery in the pterygopalatine fossa (magnified ×4), through the opening in the posterior wall of the maxillary sinus.

D

As in C, with the maxillary artery displaced downwards by cutting the sphenopalatine and posterior superior nasal branches, to show the maxillary nerve and its connexion with the pterygopalatine ganglion which overlies the aperture of the pterygoid canal. A red marker is in the foramen rotundum and a blue one in the pterygoid canal.

E

Dissection of the right pterygopalatine fossa, from above and in front, with bone removed to show the nerve of the pterygoid canal joining the back of the pterygopalatine ganglion. At the same magnification as D and E.

A

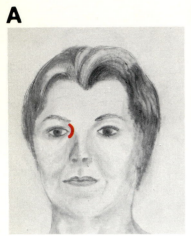

B

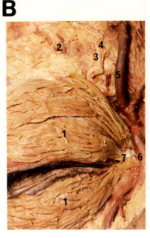

C

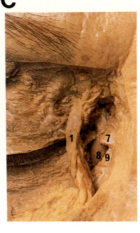

1	Orbicularis oculi	16	Infra-orbital margin
2	Supra-orbital vessels	17	Posterior lacrimal crest
	and nerve (not dissected)	18	Fossa for lacrimal sac
3	Supratrochlear artery	19	Infra-orbital foramen
4	Supratrochlear nerve	20	Inferior oblique
5	Supratrochlear vein	21	Lacrimal nerve and vessels
6	Angular vein	22	Superior ophthalmic vein
7	Medial palpebral ligament	23	Lateral rectus
8	Lacrimal sac	24	Optic nerve
9	Anterior lacrimal crest	25	Superior rectus
10	Supra-orbital margin	26	Levator palpebrae
11	Supra-orbital notch		superioris
12	Frontal notch	27	Frontal nerve
13	Optic canal	28	Eyeball
14	Superior orbital fissure	29	Supra-orbital nerve
15	Inferior orbital fissure		

LACRIMAL SAC

Background

The lacrimal sac, which is the upper blind end of the nasolacrimal duct, lies in its fossa at the front of the medial wall of the orbit (D). The fossa is formed by the lacrimal grooves of the lacrimal bone and of the frontal process of the maxilla, and the bones here separate the orbit from the nasal cavity. The anterior and posterior lacrimal crests mark the corresponding boundaries of the composite groove. The medial palpebral ligament is attached to the anterior lacrimal crest and so lies in front of the sac. Lacrimal secretion drains into the sac through the lacrimal canaliculi, one near the medial end of each eyelid.

When the nasolacrimal duct becomes blocked (e.g. by a flap of mucous membrane or a stone), it may be necessary to make an artificial communication between the lacrimal sac and the nasal cavity (dacryocystorrhinostomy, commonly known for short as a DCR). This allows tear secretion to escape into the nose instead of being dammed back and causing excessive watering of the eye. The sac is approached by cutting through the medial palpebral ligament and a hole is made in the bone of the fossa for the sac so that an anastomosis can be made between the sac and the mucous membrane of the nose.

Approach

A skin incision (A) is made about 8 mm medial to the inner canthus.

Orbicularis oculi (B) is detached from the anterior lacrimal crest and reflected laterally followed by division of the medial palpebral ligament which is reflected to expose the lacrimal sac (C).

The periosteum along the anterior lacrimal crest is incised and an anterior periosteal flap raised off the frontal process of the maxilla for a few millimetres.

A posterior periosteal flap is raised laterally off the floor of the fossa, carrying the lacrimal sac with it.

The bone of the anterior lacrimal crest and lacrimal fossa is removed, leaving intact the underlying nasal mucous membrane. The lacrimal sac and nasal mucosa can then be anastomosed after making a short vertical incision in each.

Hazards and Safeguards

The angular vein (and perhaps one of its small tributaries) crosses the medial palpebral ligament and is the structure most likely to be troublesome in approaching the lacrimal sac.

The lower border of the medial palpebral ligament is free but the upper border blends with the lacrimal fascia that lies anterior to the sac.

ORBIT

Background

The orbital cavity is 5 cm deep, with the eye occupying the anterior 2.5 cm and the optic nerve and the other nerves and vessels fanning forwards from the apex (at the back) but predominantly concentrated towards the centre and the medial side. At the front the lacrimal gland is at the upper lateral angle, the trochlea for the superior oblique at the upper medial angle, and the nasolacrimal duct at the lower medial angle. The lower lateral angle is free of important structures, containing only intra-orbital fat.

Retrobulbar injection of anaesthetic solution enables a number of operations on orbital contents to be carried out, e.g. operations on the rectus muscles for strabismus (squint) or even removal of the eye. The object in retrobulbar anaesthesia is to introduce the solution behind the eye, and the route is along the inferolateral aspect of the orbit (D) through the orbital fat; this path offers the least danger of damaging orbital contents.

Retrobulbar Injection

The inferolateral margin of the orbit is palpated.

The patient turns the eye upwards and inwards, and the needle is inserted through the skin (or, to avoid going through the skin, through the lower conjunctival fornix) just above the inferolateral margin (E) and directed below the level of the eye towards the back of the orbit for 3.5 cm. The injection is made after frequent attempts at aspiration to ensure that the needle is not in a vessel.

A

Incision line.

B

Right orbit, after removal of skin, showing the medial palpebral ligament and angular vein (which is the beginning of the facial vein). The vein here is large and obscures the underlying angular artery (which is the terminal part of the facial artery).

C

Right orbit, after reflecting orbicularis oculi laterally and transecting the medial palpebral ligament to reveal the lacrimal sac. The next stage of the operation is to perforate the bone of the sac's fossa, open the sac and anastomose it to an opening made in the nasal mucosa.

D

Right bony orbit, showing the needle position for retrobulbar injection.

E

Retrobulbar injection of the right orbit. The needle passes upwards and inwards from the inferolateral angle towards the back of the orbital cavity, and is at first lateral to the inferior oblique muscle.

F

Right orbit from above, after removal of the orbital fat, showing the needle tip near the back of the lateral part of the orbit.

G

Right supra-orbital nerve block, above the supra-orbital margin.

Hazards and Safeguards

The needle should pass through orbital fat only, and any undue resistance suggests that the needle is penetrating muscle or periosteum, or even the eye or the optic nerve, in which case it must be partially withdrawn and redirected.

The turning of the eye upwards and outwards helps to take the inferior oblique (E) farther from the path of the needle.

Introducing the needle for 3.5 cm means that the tip stops 1.5 cm short of the apex (F) and so does not damage the concentration of structures entering through the superior orbital fissure.

Haemorrhage from orbital vessels usually becomes apparent as subconjunctival haemorrhage, which may appear over any part of the eye and not just inferolaterally.

SUPRA-ORBITAL AND SUPRATROCHLEAR NERVES

Background

After emerging from the cavernous sinus the ophthalmic nerve enters the orbit and divides into its three main branches – lacrimal, frontal and nasociliary. The frontal nerve divides into a large supra-orbital (lateral) and a small supratrochlear (medial) branch which leave the orbit through the supra-orbital notch (or foramen) and frontal notch respectively to supply part of the scalp.

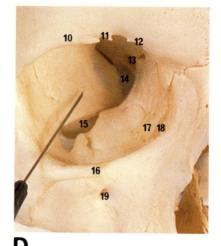

D

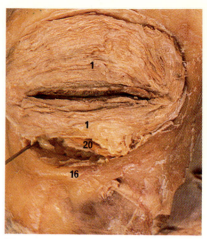

E

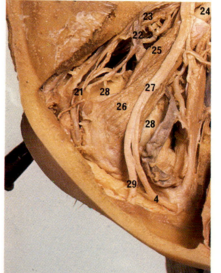

F

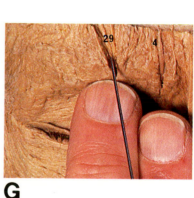

G

Due to its proximity to the optic nerve within the orbit the ophthalmic nerve trunk itself is not a candidate for blockade, but its branches will be affected by retrobulbar injection of the orbit (page 31). However the supra-orbital and supratrochlear branches may be infiltrated above the supra-orbital margin to produce anterior scalp anaesthesia.

Approach for Nerve Blocks

The centres of two fingers placed vertically beside the midline at the level of the supra-orbital margin will indicate the position on this margin of the frontal and supra-orbital notches (G).

The needle is inserted just above the margin to infiltrate the tissues in each of these areas.

Hazards and Safeguards

The usual aspiration check must ensure that the needle is not in the vessels that accompany each of the nerves.

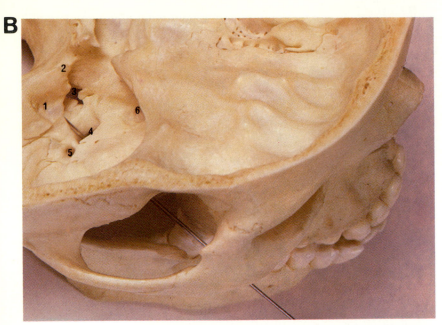

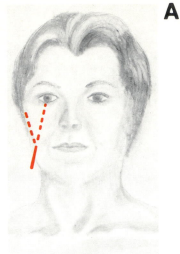

B

A

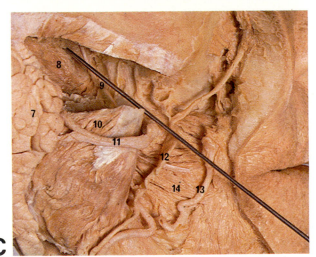

C

1	Trigeminal impression	**17**	Neck of mandible
2	Apex of petrous temporal	**18**	Mandibular notch
3	Foramen lacerum	**19**	Coronoid process
4	Foramen ovale	**20**	Trigeminal ganglion on 1
5	Foramen spinosum	**21**	Ophthalmic nerve in superior
6	Foramen rotundum		orbital fissure
7	Parotid gland	**22**	Maxillary nerve in 6
8	Lateral pterygoid	**23**	Mandibular nerve in 4
9	Buccal nerve	**24**	Middle meningeal artery in 5
10	Masseter	**25**	Lesser petrosal nerve
11	Parotid duct	**26**	Greater petrosal nerve
12	Facial vein	**27**	Inferior alveolar nerve
13	Facial artery	**28**	Lingual nerve
14	Buccinator	**29**	Medial pterygoid
15	Zygomatic arch	**30**	Mandible
16	Lateral pterygoid plate		

TRIGEMINAL GANGLION

The trigeminal ganglion lies in a pocket of dura mater in the trigeminal impression, situated on the anterior surface of the apex of the petrous temporal bone that forms the posterior wall of the middle cranial fossa. The cavernous sinus, with the ophthalmic and maxillary branches of the trigeminal nerve entering it and also containing the internal carotid artery and the oculomotor, trochlear and abducent nerves, lies anteromedial to the ganglion, and the foramen ovale with the mandibular and lesser petrosal nerves entering it is in front of and slightly lateral to the ganglion. The motor root of the trigeminal nerve and greater petrosal nerve on its way to the foramen lacerum, are below the ganglion, while above and in front is the temporal lobe of the brain. The trigeminal ganglion corresponds to the dorsal root ganglion of a spinal nerve

and contains the cell bodies of all the afferent fibres in the three branches of the nerve with the sole exception of those of the fibres concerned with proprioception (whose cell bodies are in the mesencephalic nucleus in the midbrain).

To alleviate intractable pain in the distribution of the nerve (e.g. trigeminal neuralgia) it is possible to produce prolonged anaesthesia by injection or electrocoagulation of the ganglion, and this can be done by passing the needle upwards through the foramen ovale, either from the front lateral to the mouth (B) or from the side below the zygomatic arch (D).

Approach for Ganglionic Block

A skin wheal of local anaesthetic is raised 3 cm lateral to the angle of the mouth (A).

A long needle is inserted through the wheal in the direction of the pupil with the eye looking straight ahead and to a point level with the midpoint of the zygomatic arch when viewed from the side (A).

At a depth of 7.5 cm from the site of the needle insertion the tip should strike the bony roof of the infratemporal fossa (C). Under radiological guidance the needle is then educated through the foramen ovale until the tip is seen to lie in the region of the ganglion (B). The occurrence of paraesthesia in the distribution of the three main branches suggests proper placement.

An alternative approach is from the side of the face (D and E) just below the zygomatic arch and 2 cm in front of the posterior border of the condyle of the mandible (compare with the approach to the mandibular nerve, page 40).

Hazards and Safeguards

In the approach from the front the needle must be kept lateral to the buccinator (C) and not be allowed to enter the mouth medially.

Aspiration before injection is essential to ensure that the needle is not in a vessel or the cavernous sinus, and that cerebrospinal fluid is not being withdrawn because the needle has entered the subarachnoid space below the temporal lobe or the trigeminal cave of dura and arachnoid mater behind and below the posterior part of the ganglion. The inadvertent injection of anaesthetic solution into cerebrospinal fluid will result in unconsciousness and paralysis of a variable number of cranial nerves.

The ganglion is a very flat structure (E), not bulbous like most ganglia, and the needle going through the foramen ovale must be kept close to the downward and laterally-sloping bone of the trigeminal impression.

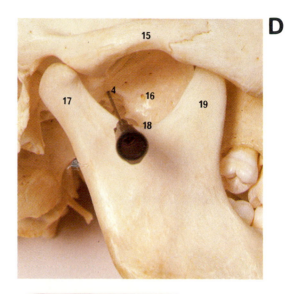

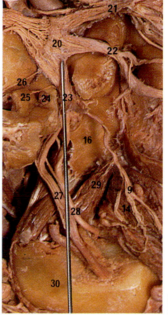

A
Anterior approach to the trigeminal ganglion, from 3 cm lateral to the angle of the mouth in the direction of the pupil.

B
Right side of the skull, from above and the right, with the needle approaching the trigeminal impression through the foramen ovale.

C
Right side of the face, with part of the mandible and masseter removed, showing the needle passing lateral to buccinator and through the infratemporal fossa and lateral pterygoid to reach the foramen ovale.

D
Right side of the skull, showing the lateral approach to the foramen ovale.

E
Right side of the face, from the right and above, with much of the base of the skull and mandible removed. After passing through temporalis, masseter and the lateral pterygoid (all removed), the needle is seen lying against the trigeminal ganglion after entering the foramen ovale. Because of the flatness of the ganglion, the needle must be kept as close as possible to the bone of the trigeminal impression.

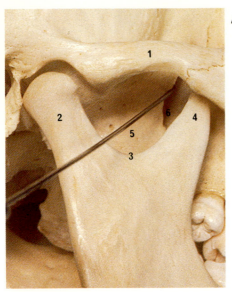

A

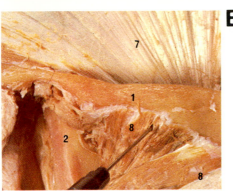

B

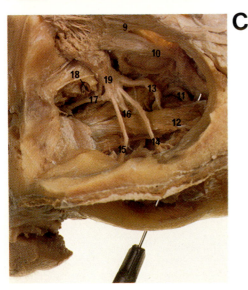

C

MAXILLARY NERVE

Background

After leaving the cavernous sinus the maxillary nerve passes forwards through the foramen rotundum to enter the pterygopalatine fossa where it turns laterally to run into the inferior orbital fissure where it changes its name to the infra-orbital nerve. This passes forwards again to enter the infra-orbital groove and canal.

Infiltration anaesthesia of the upper teeth is by far the commonest example of any form of nerve blockade involving branches of the maxillary nerve (page 37), but it is also possible to block the main nerve by extra-oral or intra-oral routes. The extra-oral approach is through the side of the face below the zygomatic arch, entering the pterygopalatine fossa through the pterygo-maxillary fissure in front of the lateral pterygoid plate (A). In the intra-oral approach the pterygopalatine fossa is entered from below through the greater palatine canal at the side of the hard palate (D).

Approach for Extra-oral Block

From a point 3 cm in front of the posterior border of the neck of the mandible the needle is passed slightly forwards and upwards (at an angle of 115° to both the horizontal and coronal planes) (B).

The needle passes through masseter, temporalis and the mandibular notch into the infratemporal fossa and through the lateral pterygoid; at a depth of 5 cm it should touch the anterior border of the pterygoid process. It is then manoeuvred forwards to reach the pterygomaxillary fissure (A) and passed 5 mm deeper into the pterygopalatine fossa (C) where the injection is made after aspiration to ensure that the needle is not in a vessel.

Hazards and Safeguards

Apart from the many small branches of the maxillary artery, the needle can hardly avoid the pterygoid venous plexus. After withdrawal of the needle a haematoma may occur and this may spread through the inferior orbital fissure to give a 'black eye'.

Diffusion of anaesthetic solution into the orbit could possibly affect the optic nerve and cause a transient blindness of which the patient should be warned.

Approach for Intra-oral Block

The mucous membrane at the opening of the greater palatine foramen is anaesthetised by inserting the needle (as for greater palatine nerve block, page 39) in an upward and lateral direction midway between the gingival margin and the midline of the palate, level with the second molar tooth (D).

The needle is then directed upwards into the greater palatine canal and advanced for 3 cm so that the tip comes to lie in the region of the maxillary nerve in the pterygopalatine fossa (E), just lateral to the sphenopalatine foramen.

Hazards and Safeguards

Any undue resistance to the needle as it passes up the greater palatine canal suggests that it is entering periosteum, and this must be avoided. It is helpful to bend the needle near its hub before starting the passage up the canal.

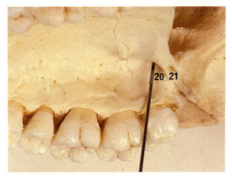

D

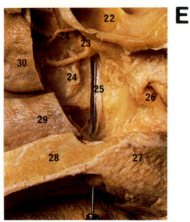

E

A
Right side of the skull, with the needle entering the pterygopalatine fossa through the pterygomaxillary fissure.

B
Right side of the face, with the needle entering masseter below the zygomatic arch, to pass through temporalis into the infratemporal fossa and then the pterygopalatine fossa.

C
Right infratemporal fossa, from above, after removal of the floor of the lateral part of the middle cranial fossa. The needle passes through the lateral pterygoid and into the pterygopalatine fossa to reach the maxillary nerve.

D
Right side of the hard palate, with the needle entering the greater palatine foramen.

E
Right half of a median sagittal section of the head, with part of lateral wall of the nasal cavity removed and the greater palatine canal opened up. The upper end of the canal (lateral to the sphenopalatine foramen) opens into the pterygopalatine fossa where the maxillary nerve lies.

1	Zygomatic arch
2	Neck of mandible
3	Mandibular notch
4	Coronoid process
5	Lateral pterygoid plate
6	Pterygomaxillary fissure
7	Temporalis
8	Masseter
9	Ophthalmic nerve
10	Maxillary nerve in foramen rotundum
11	Maxillary artery
12	Lateral pterygoid
13	Buccal nerve
14	Deep temporal nerve (to 7)
15	Nerve to 8
16	Nerve to 12
17	Auriculotemporal nerve
18	Middle meningeal artery in foramen spinosum
19	Mandibular nerve in foramen ovale
20	Greater palatine foramen
21	Lesser palatine foramen
22	Sphenoidal sinus
23	Sphenopalatine foramen and artery
24	Posterior superior nasal vessels and nerve
25	Greater palatine nerve in canal
26	Opening of auditory tube
27	Soft palate
28	Hard palate
29	Inferior concha
30	Middle concha

INFRA-ORBITAL NERVE

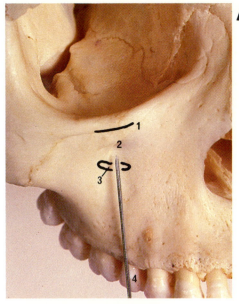

Background

After traversing the inferior orbital fissure and the infra-orbital groove and canal, the infra-orbital nerve emerges on the face through the infra-orbital foramen and divides into palpebral, nasal and labial branches. While passing through the maxilla it has given off middle and anterior superior alveolar branches. The infra-orbital foramen lies 0.5 cm below the infra-orbital margin in the line of the second premolar tooth and in the same vertical plane as the pupil of the eye when looking straight ahead. The attachment of levator labii superioris is just above the foramen and that of levator anguli oris just below it.

The nerve can be blocked by injecting upwards through the vestibule of the mouth and infiltrating the tissues at the opening of the foramen (A). Apart from the skin anaesthesia from eyelid to upper lip, the incisor, canine and premolar teeth will be affected, together with the labial side of the alveolus.

Approach for Nerve Block

With the middle finger of the operator's hand on the skin over the foramen the upper lip is retracted upwards by the index finger and thumb.

The needle is inserted upwards in the line of the second premolar tooth to pass through the mucous membrane just lateral to the top of the sulcus, i.e. more lateral than for infiltration anaesthesia of the upper teeth, and continue upwards towards the foramen (B).

The finger on the overlying skin will detect when the injection is being made at the foramen, and finger pressure applied when the correct position is reached will help the solution to enter the foramen.

Hazards and Safeguards

The solution must enter the interval between levator labii superioris above the foramen and levator anguli oris below it (B). If undue resistance to the needle is felt it has probably entered levator anguli and so is too low down in the canine fossa.

A

Right infra-orbital foramen. The approach is along the line of the second premolar tooth.

B

Right side of the face, showing the needle tip at the level of the infra-orbital nerve as it emerges from its foramen.

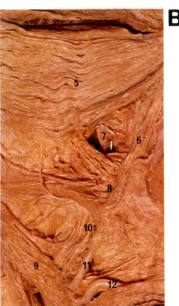

1 Origin of levator labii superioris
2 Infra-orbital foramen
3 Origin of levator anguli oris
4 Second premolar tooth
5 Orbicularis oculi
6 Levator labii superioris
7 Infra-orbital nerve
8 Zygomaticus minor
9 Zygomaticus major
10 Levator anguli oris
11 Facial artery
12 Superior labial artery

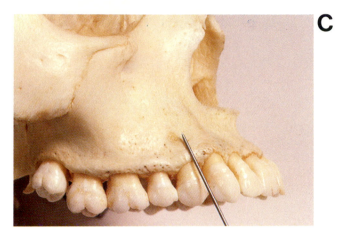

C

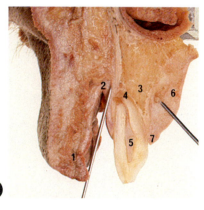

D

1 Lip
2 Buccal fold
3 Alveolar process of maxilla
4 Apex of tooth
5 Pulp cavity
6 Mucoperiosteum of hard palate
7 Gingival margin

INFILTRATION ANAESTHESIA OF UPPER TEETH

Background

The superior alveolar branches of the maxillary and infra-orbital nerves unite above the tooth roots within the maxilla to form the superior dental plexus which supplies the pulp cavities of the upper teeth and the tissues on the buccal (outer) surface of the jaw. The greater palatine and nasopalatine nerves (also from the maxillary nerve, after passing through the pterygopalatine ganglion) supply the palatal (inner) aspect of the jaw. The bone of the alveolar part of the maxilla that bears the teeth is relatively porous, and local anaesthetic solution deposited in the region of an upper jaw tooth (infiltration anaesthesia) will readily diffuse into the bone. Infiltration of the buccal aspect of the jaw will allow painless drilling of upper teeth, but painless extraction will require anaesthesia of the palatal aspect as well.

Approach

For infiltration anaesthesia on the buccal aspect of the jaw the needle is inserted into or just below the buccal fold (where the mucous membrane is reflected from the jaw to the cheek) opposite the appropriate tooth, and the tip is directed upwards to the level where the apex of the tooth root is considered to lie (C and D).

For infiltration on the palatal aspect the needle is inserted midway between the gingival margin and the midline of the palate opposite the appropriate tooth (D).

Aspiration must ensure that the needle is not in a vessel.

Hazards and Safeguards

The needle point must not be allowed to penetrate the periosteum and strip it off the bone; this causes pain at the time and residual pain when the anaesthesia has worn off.

C

Right maxilla. The needle is directed to the level of the apex of the appropriate tooth – here, the first premolar.

D

Vertical section through the right first premolar tooth. On the buccal aspect the needle lies adjacent to the periosteum near the tooth apex, having passed through the mucous membrane of the buccal fold. On the palatal side, the injection is midway between the midline of the palate and the gingival margin; the needle tip should again lie adjacent to the periosteum of the appropriate tooth.

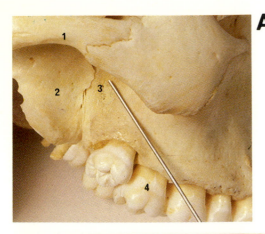

A

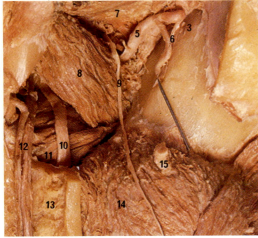

B

POSTERIOR SUPERIOR ALVEOLAR NERVE

Background

The posterior superior alveolar nerve arises from the maxillary nerve in the pterygopalatine fossa. It runs down in contact with the infratemporal (posterior) surface of the maxilla which it pierces about halfway down to lie under the mucous membrane of the maxillary sinus and take part in the superior dental plexus, usually supplying the three molar teeth except for the mesiobuccal root of the first molar. It is accompanied by corresponding branches of the maxillary vessels.

Because of the ease of infiltration anaesthesia of the upper teeth (page 37) it is rarely necessary to block the posterior superior alveolar nerve itself, but this can be done through the vestibule of the mouth by advancing the needle upwards along the posterior surface of the maxilla (A).

Approach for Nerve Block

The needle is inserted through the buccal fold level with the second molar tooth, in a direction upwards and backwards at an angle of 45° to the vertical and occlusal planes.

The needle is advanced for 2 cm, keeping as close to the maxillary periosteum as possible. At this level the tip should be in the region where the nerve pierces the bone (B), and the injection is made here after aspiration. (Advancing the needle for 3 cm is an alternative method for maxillary nerve block – page 34.)

Hazards and Safeguards

If the needle is not kept as close to the maxilla as possible, the pterygoid venous plexus or the lateral pterygoid muscle may be entered.

1	Zygomatic arch	12	Inferior alveolar nerve and vessels
2	Lateral pterygoid plate	13	Mandible
3	Posterior wall of maxilla	14	Buccinator
4	Second molar tooth	15	Parotid duct
5	Maxillary artery	16	Incisive fossa
6	Posterior superior alveolar	17	Right central incisor tooth
	nerve and vessels	18	Greater palatine foramen
7	Upper head of lateral pterygoid	19	Mucoperiosteum of hard palate
8	Lower head of lateral pterygoid	20	Greater palatine nerve forming
9	Buccal nerve		plexus with nasopalatine nerve
10	Lingual nerve	21	Incisive foramen
11	Medial pterygoid		

C

Front of the hard palate and the incisive fossa; the incisive *foramina* are not seen as they lie deeper in the fossa. For dental anaesthesia the needle does not enter the fossa.

D

As in C, but for more extensive procedures the needle enters the fossa along the line of the central incisor tooth.

E

Right side of the hard palate, from the left and below. For greater palatine nerve block the needle does not enter the foramen.

F

Right side of the hard palate, from the left and below, showing infiltration of the greater palatine nerve.

A

Right side of the skull, from the right and slightly below, indicating how the needle enters the mucous membrane level with the second molar tooth and passes upwards and backwards at 45°.

B

Right side of the face, with part of the zygomatic arch and mandible removed. The needle pierces buccinator and the tip lies where the posterior superior alveolar vessels and nerve pierce the posterior wall of the maxilla.

NASOPALATINE AND GREATER PALATINE NERVES

Background

The nasopalatine nerve is a branch from the pterygopalatine ganglion that enters the nose through the sphenopalatine foramen, crosses the roof of the nose and then runs obliquely downwards and forwards under the mucous membrane of the nasal septum, lying in a groove on the vomer. It passes through the incisive foramen to the incisive fossa and then enters the roof of the mouth to supply the hard palate and palatal alveolus in the region of the incisor and canine teeth of its own side.

In nasopalatine nerve block the object is to block the nerve just after it emerges from the incisive fossa (C). The teeth affected will be the incisors of its own side and probably the canine also (see below).

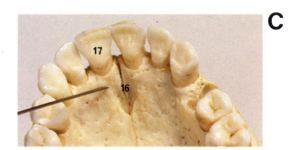

The greater palatine nerve leaves the pterygopalatine ganglion in the pterygopalatine fossa and runs down in the greater palatine canal to emerge through the greater palatine foramen, which lies at the level of the second molar tooth about 1 cm above the gingival margin. The nerve passes forwards in a groove on the under surface of the bony palate at the junction of the alveolar and palatal processes of the maxilla, probably reaching as far forward as the canine tooth and forming a plexus with the nasopalatine nerve. The accompanying anterior end of the greater palatine artery passes upwards through the incisive fossa and foramen to anastomose on the nasal septum with the sphenopalatine artery.

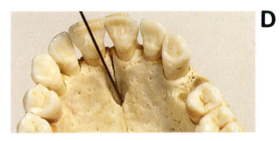

For greater palatine nerve block the object is to anaesthetise the nerve just in front of its foramen. The block should produce anaesthesia as far forward as the first premolar tooth; the canine is in the region of cross-innervation between greater palatine and nasopalatine nerves, and the effect of these nerve blocks on this tooth can vary.

Approach for Greater Palatine Nerve Block

The needle is inserted in an upward and lateral direction level with the second molar tooth, midway between the gingival margin and the midline of the palate; it is directed to just in front of the expected position of the foramen (E and F), and the injection made after aspiration.

Approach for Nasopalatine Nerve Block

The injection is made in an upward and slightly medial direction just lateral to the midline above the gingival margin.

For procedures involving the adjacent bone of the maxilla, the needle can be pushed up into the incisive canal for 1 cm in a line parallel with the long axis of the central incisor tooth (D).

Hazards and Safeguards

The midline tissue over the incisive fossa into which the incisive foramina open is very sensitive, and a slightly lateral injection is less painful.

For greater palatine block, if the needle is placed too far back or into the foramen, the anaesthetic solution may affect the lesser palatine nerves and so produce anaesthesia in the soft palate and tonsillar area. This is often found to be an unpleasant sensation.

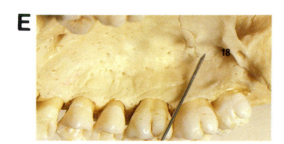

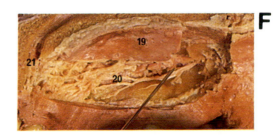

MANDIBULAR NERVE

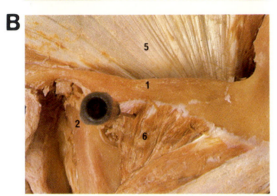

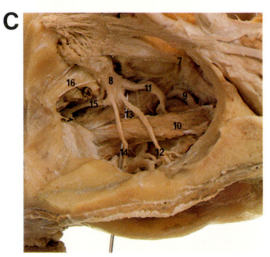

Background

The mandibular nerve leaves the skull through the foramen ovale which is immediately behind the lateral pterygoid plate. Below the foramen the nerve breaks up into its various branches. Of these the inferior alveolar, lingual and buccal are the ones commonly blocked through the mouth for various dental procedures in the lower jaw (page 42). If the whole nerve is to be anaesthetised it can be done through the side of the face (extra-oral approach) below the zygomatic arch, reaching the foramen ovale behind the lateral pterygoid plate (A). An intra-oral method is also possible, with the object of placing the anaesthetic solution in front of the neck of the mandible (D) so that solution gravitates between the pterygoid muscles and so affects at least the three branches of dental importance.

Approach for Extra-oral Block

From a point 2 cm in front of the neck of the mandible and immediately below the zygomatic arch, the needle is introduced in a slightly forward and downward direction.

The needle passes through masseter, temporalis and the mandibular notch (B) into the infratemproal fossa and through the lateral pterygoid; at a depth of about 4.5 cm the tip should contact the lateral pterygoid plate. Short in-and-out movements direct the needle backwards until it slips off the plate, and the tip now lies adjacent to the nerve (C). Paraesthesia may be produced in the distribution of the nerve and the injection is made after the usual aspiration test.

(In approaching the trigeminal ganglion by this route – page 32 – the needle is advanced 1 cm deeper through the foramen ovale.)

Hazards and Safeguards

Vessels in the infratemporal fossa may be perforated, and so may the middle meningeal vessels if the needle is too far back; the foramen spinosum through which they pass is just posterior to the foramen ovale.

If the needle is advanced too deeply when behind the lateral pterygoid plate it may enter the lateral wall of the pharynx.

A
Right side of the skull, viewed slightly from below, with the needle directed slightly downwards and forwards below the zygomatic arch to the back of the lateral pterygoid plate, behind which lies the foramen ovale.

B
Right side of the face, with the needle entering masseter below the zygomatic arch to pass through the infratemporal fossa and reach the lateral pterygoid plate.

C

Right infratemporal fossa, from above after removal of the floor of the lateral part of the middle cranial fossa. The needle passes through the lateral pterygoid to lie adjacent to the mandibular nerve as it divides into its various branches. The lingual and inferior alveolar nerves are not seen in this view as they are deep to the muscular branches and deep to the lateral pterygoid muscle.

D

Right side of the skull, with the needle introduced from the front so that the tip lies beneath the foramen ovale.

E

Right infratemporal fossa, with fat and part of the mandible removed. Injection into the space between the pterygoid muscles enables the anaesthetic solution to percolate through the fat and infiltrate the major branches of the mandibular nerve.

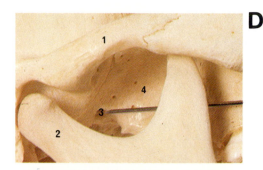

D

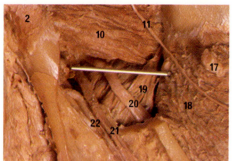

E

Approach for Intra-oral Block

The mouth is opened widely to bring the head of the mandible forward out of the mandibular fossa, and the intertragic notch behind the head of the mandible is palpated by a fingertip overlying the skin in front of the external acoustic meatus.

The needle is introduced through the mucous membrane of the mouth medial to the ramus of the mandible and the temporalis tendon – similar to the needle insertion for inferior alveolar block (page 42) but at a slightly higher level – and directed towards the palpating fingertip behind the head of the mandible. The neck of the mandible is contacted about 2.5 cm from the mucous membrane entry point (D and E); the needle is withdrawn slightly, an aspiration check carried out and the injection made.

Hazards and Safeguards

Since the needle passes through the infratemporal fossa containing the maxillary artery and its many branches as well as the extensive pterygoid plexus of veins, aspiration is especially important before injection. The needle tip should be in the loose fatty tissue between the pterygoid muscles, often known clinically as the pterygomandibular space, so that the anaesthetic solution can percolate to the mandibular nerve branches that traverse the space.

1	Zygomatic arch
2	Neck of mandible
3	Foramen ovale
4	Lateral pterygoid plate
5	Temporalis
6	Masseter
7	Maxillary nerve in foramen rotundum
8	Mandibular nerve in 3
9	Maxillary artery
10	Lateral pterygoid
11	Buccal nerve
12	Deep temporal nerve
13	Nerve to 10
14	Nerve to 6
15	Auriculotemporal nerve
16	Middle meningeal artery in foramen spinosum
17	Parotid duct
18	Buccinator
19	Medial pterygoid
20	Lingual nerve
21	Inferior alveolar nerve
22	Inferior alveolar artery

INFERIOR ALVEOLAR AND LINGUAL NERVES

Background

From their origins just below the foramen ovale as the largest branches of the mandibular nerve, the inferior alveolar and lingual nerves pass down between the lateral and medial pterygoid muscles. The inferior alveolar nerve enters the mandibular foramen, giving off the nerve to mylohyoid as it does so, and lying at this point immediately lateral to the medial pterygoid and to the spheno-mandibular ligament which is attached to the lingula and overlaps the opening of the foramen. Within the mandible it supplies all the teeth of its own side, and gives off the mental nerve which comes to the surface of the bone through the mental foramen (page 43). The lingual nerve is joined by the chorda tympani which runs into it from above and behind 1–2 cm below the skull. As it emerges between the two pterygoid muscles the lingual nerve is about 1 cm in front of the inferior alveolar nerve and medial to it. It crosses the medial surface of the medial pterygoid and passes under the lower border of the superior constrictor of the pharynx to enter the mouth, lying in contact with the periosteum of the mandible below and behind the third molar tooth. Running forwards on the side of the tongue it hooks under the submandibular duct from the lateral to the medial side while on the surface of hyoglossus. It is the sensory nerve of the anterior two-thirds of the tongue, the adjacent floor of the mouth and the lingual aspect of the mandible.

Since the bone of much of the mandible that bears the teeth is less porous than the maxilla, infiltration anaesthesia is only effective for the anterior teeth (incisors and premolars). For anaesthetising the molars, inferior alveolar nerve block is necessary. This is achieved by introducing the solution into the area between the ramus of the mandible laterally and the lingula with the attached sphenomandibular ligament medially, so that it can affect the nerve at the opening of the mandibular foramen (A). The lingual nerve which is anteromedial to the inferior alveolar can be anaesthetised at the same time.

Approach for Nerve Blocks

Through the open mouth the anterior border of the ramus of the mandible (often called the coronoid notch because of its slight concavity) and the ridge of mucous membrane overlying the ptery-gomandibular raphe are identified.

With the barrel of the syringe lying over the opposite premolar teeth, the needle is inserted into the mucous membrane 1 cm above the level of the occlusal surface of the third molar tooth and immediately lateral to the pterygomandibular ridge.

The needle then pierces the buccinator and about 0.5 cm deeper it lies lateral to the lingual nerve (on the surface of the medial pterygoid) (B) which can be anaesthetised by injection here.

After insertion for a further 1 cm the tip lies above the lingula (C) where the main injection is made. Aspiration must ensure that the needle is not in a vessel.

In prognathous or edentulous patients the mandibular foramen is a few millimetres higher than normal and so the injection must be at a higher level.

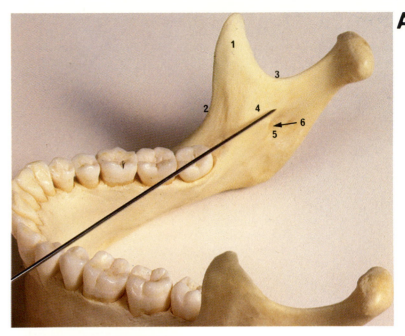

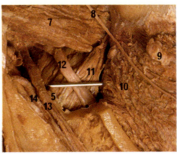

1	Coronoid process
2	Coronoid notch
3	Mandibular notch
4	Ramus of mandible
5	Lingula
6	Mandibular foramen
7	Lateral pterygoid
8	Buccal nerve
9	Parotid duct
10	Buccinator
11	Medial pterygoid

Hazards and Safeguards

If the needle tip is too far lateral it may enter the temporalis insertion (C) or come into contact with the internal oblique ridge of the mandible.

If the needle tip is too far medial it may enter the medial pterygoid (B and C) and so lie medial to the sphenomandibular ligament which will divert the solution away from the mouth of the mandibular foramen.

If the needle passes too far back it may enter the parotid gland (C) and part or all of the facial nerve may be paralysed.

The inferior alveolar vessels lie deeper and close to the companion nerve just before entering the mandibular foramen (B and C).

An inferior alveolar nerve block will normally anaesthetise all the teeth of that side of the mandible as far as the midline, although there may be some cross-innervation of the central incisor from the opposite side.

A

The mandible, from above and the left, showing the line of approach to the right inferior alveolar nerve above the opening of the mandibular foramen. The correct line is from the premolar region of the opposite side.

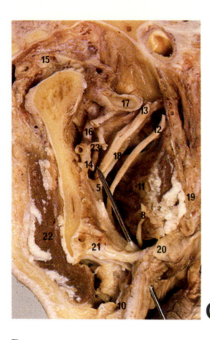

12 Lingual nerve
13 Inferior alveolar nerve
14 Inferior alveolar artery
15 Parotid gland
16 Maxillary artery
17 Styloid process
18 Sphenomandibular ligament
19 Superior constrictor of pharynx
20 Pterygomandibular raphe
21 Temporalis
22 Masseter
23 Inferior alveolar vein
24 Second premolar tooth
25 Mental foramen
26 Depressor anguli oris
27 Depressor labii inferioris
28 Mental nerve and vessels

B

Right infratemporal fossa, with fat and part of the mandible removed. The tip of the needle lies adjacent to the inferior alveolar nerve above the opening of the mandibular foramen.

C

Horizontal section of the right side of the head, about 1 cm above the opening of the mandibular foramen and looking down on to it. The fat of the pterygomandibular space (between the ramus of the mandible and the pterygoid muscles) is removed. The needle tip lies in the 'funnel' formed by the mandible laterally and the lingula with the attached sphenomandibular ligament medially so that injected anaesthetic solution gravitates down into the foramen. The inferior alveolar artery is behind the nerve.

D

Right side of the mandible, with the needle directed into the mental foramen from above and behind, along the line of the second premolar tooth.

E

Lower right side of the face, with fibres of depressor anguli oris separated to show the needle tip entering the mental foramen. In this specimen some fibres of depressor labii inferioris extend to below the foramen; usually they stop in front of it, with only depressor anguli immediately below it.

MENTAL AND INCISIVE NERVES

Background

The mental nerve, a terminal branch of the inferior alveolar, emerges on to the face through the mental foramen which is in the mandible usually just below the apex of the second premolar tooth (and in approximately the same vertical plane as the infra-orbital foramen and the supra-orbital notch). The opening of the foramen faces backwards and upwards (D). In the edentulous mandible where there has been resorption of the alveolar part of the bone the foramen (and the canal leading to it) are very near its upper margin. The attachment of depressor labii inferioris is in front of the foramen and that of depressor anguli oris just below it (D). The nerve supplies the lower lip and the adjacent mucous membrane and skin of the chin.

The incisive nerve, the other terminal branch of the inferior alveolar, continues forwards within the mandible and supplies the first premolar, canine and the two incisor teeth.

Local anaesthetic injected through the mucous membrane of the mouth into the opening of the mental foramen will anaesthetise the mental and incisive nerves and therefore the first premolar, canine and incisor teeth, the lower lip and adjacent skin.

Approach for Nerve Blocks

Through the open mouth and with the angle of the mouth retracted, the needle is inserted downwards and forwards through the mucous membrane in the depth of the sulcus between the cheek and mandible adjacent to the second premolar tooth. After a small mucosal injection the needle is advanced into the opening of the foramen (E) and the injection made.

Hazards and Safeguards

Since the opening of the foramen faces *backwards* the needle must approach it from above and behind so that the tip can enter the opening and allow the solution to flow through it and affect the incisive nerve as well as the mental. Injection too far forward or too low will enter muscle (E).

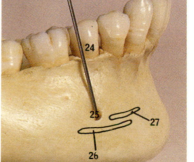

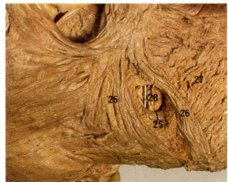

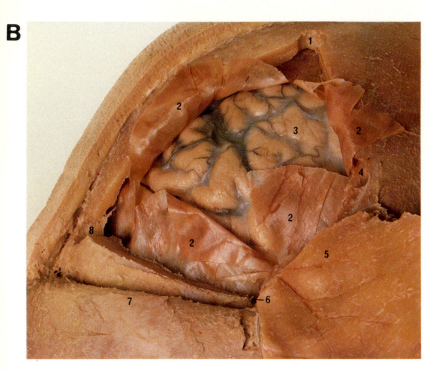

B

CRANIAL CAVITY

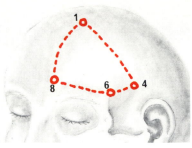

A

1 Posterior medial burr hole
2 Dura mater
3 Arachnoid overlying frontal lobe
4 Posterior frontal burr hole

5 Bone flap turned down
6 Lateral frontal burr hole
7 Scalp flap turned down
8 Anterior medial burr hole
9 Frontal bone
10 Parietal bone
11 Squamous part of temporal bone
12 Greater wing of sphenoid bone
13 Zygomatic arch
14 Frontal branch of middle meningeal artery and vein
15 Parietal branch of middle meningeal artery and vein
16 Pterion
17 Temporalis
18 Superficial temporal vessels and auriculotemporal nerve

Background

To gain access to the cranial cavity through the vault of the skull, holes can be made and flaps cut in the bone after appropriate incisions in the overlying scalp, avoiding the major vessels and nerves. There are three main groups of vessels and nerves in the scalp: at the front, the supra-orbital vessels and nerve, passing up from the supra-orbital margin 3 cm from the midline; at the side, the superficial temporal vessels and auriculo-temporal nerve, crossing the root of the zygomatic arch in front of the tragus of the ear; and at the back, the occipital vessels passing up from the back of the mastoid process with the greater occipital nerve entering the scalp 3–4 cm medial to the artery.

Most of the bone of the skull vault consists of inner and outer layers (tables) of compact bone with an intervening layer of cancellous bone, the diploë, that contains bone marrow. The outer table is thicker than the inner; where the side of the skull is formed largely by the squamous part of the temporal bone, the bone is thin and single-layered with no diploë.

Access through the skull vault is obtained by burr holes, trephine and bone flaps. Burr holes (up to 15 mm in diameter) are made by drilling and so obviously destroy small areas of bone. A trephine removes a round disc of bone which can be replaced and can be up to 5 cm in diameter. For wider access, roughly rectangular flaps of bone can be removed (craniotomy) by making several burr holes and then cutting the bone between adjacent holes. These flaps can also be replaced (by stitching their pericranium to that of the surrounding skull). The choice and position of these modes of approach obviously depends on the position and size of the feature being dealt with (e.g. extradural haemorrhage, aneurysm, brain abscess or tumour). Some examples are given below.

Scalp incisions should avoid where possible the major arteries and nerves. Short linear incisions are sufficient for burr holes and trephining but for craniotomy flaps an appropriate scalp flap is required. The incisions for such flaps are usually based on the anatomy of the three main groups of vessels and nerves, although the profuse anastomosis between scalp vessels gives plenty of scope for variations if required.

Burr Holes

After shaving and cleaning the chosen area, an incision 3 cm long is made in the scalp (and through the temporalis muscle if appropriate) down to the bone. Near the vertex incisions are made in the sagittal plane (anteroposteriorly) but near the base of the skull they are made coronally (vertically). The pericranium is incised in the same line and scraped to each side.

The burr hole is made first with a skull perforator until the inner table of the skull is just perforated, and then a special burr or drill is used to enlarge the hole.

The underlying dura can be inspected, and in the case of extradural haemorrhage blood clot can be removed and bleeding vessels dealt with. If necessary the hole can be enlarged by nibbling away the edge with bone forceps.

If the dura is to be opened it is picked up with a sharp hook and incised, avoiding any obvious vessels.

Hazards and Safeguards

Drilling must obviously be carried out with great care to avoid sudden penetration into the brain, and progress checked frequently.

The dura should not be separated from the bone round the margin of the hole; this helps to prevent bleeding from extradural veins. Bleeding from bone is controlled by plugging with bone wax.

If burr holes are required near the median sagittal plane they are placed 3 cm from the midline to avoid the superior sagittal sinus. Those at the front of the skull may involve the frontal sinus but any opening can be repaired with a graft of dura mater or pericranium.

Craniotomy

The scalp incisions are made semicircular or rectangular.

The bone flaps are made by cutting burr holes (usually four or five) and then cutting the bone between adjacent holes with a Gigli saw (a type of serrated wire that is threaded from one hole to another using a guide beneath the intervening bone. Where possible the bone flap is left hinged on a part of the temporalis muscle.

To give a specific example, an anterior craniotomy flap (as might be used for the subfrontal approach to the pituitary gland – page 47), involves making four burr holes under the scalp flap.

The scalp flap is approximately semicircular, from the midline to the front of the ear, arching upwards over the chosen positions for the burr holes. The flap is turned down as far as the supra-orbital margin.

For the cranial flap, the anterior medial burr hole is made above the frontal sinus (previously visualized radiologically) and the posterior medial hole several centimetres behind it and 3 cm from the midline. The lateral frontal hole is behind the zygomatic process of the frontal bone and level with the floor of the anterior cranial fossa, and the posterior frontal hole is made some distance above it but not as high as the posterior medial hole.

The Gigli saw is used to cut the bone between the holes, except for the bone between the two holes at the base of the flap which is fairly thin and can be cut with bone forceps until the bridge of bone remaining is small enough to be broken. The part of temporalis attached to the flap is left intact.

The bone flap is raised by separating it from the underlying dura and it is hinged down on its temporalis flap.

The dura is picked up with a sharp hook and incised, often in a cruciate manner, avoiding obvious blood vessels.

Hazards and Safeguards

As for burr holes.

A
Position of a left anterior craniotomy flap.

B
Anterior part of the left side of the cranial cavity. The dura is being reflected after turning down the scalp and bone flaps.

C
Left side of the skull, showing the area of pterion – where parts of the frontal, parietal, temporal and sphenoid bones make an H-shaped suture pattern.

D
Left side of the head, showing the frontal and parietal branches of the middle meningeal vessels overlying the dura. A burr hole at pterion will give access to the frontal branch.

MIDDLE MENINGEAL ARTERY

Background

After entering the skull through the foramen spinosum, the middle meningeal artery runs laterally and slightly forwards on the floor of the middle cranial fossa between the bone and the dura and divides into two branches. The frontal (anterior) branch passes upwards over the inner aspect of pterion (C) (the H-shaped sutural area between the frontal, parietal, temporal and sphenoid bones) and then backwards, giving off branches including one that approximately overlies the central sulcus of the cerebral hemisphere (but still in an extradural position; the artery supplies dura and bone, not brain). The parietal (posterior) branch runs backwards approximately along the line of the lateral sulcus. Veins accompany the artery and its branches and are responsible for the grooves on the bones.

The anterior branch is the one most commonly ruptured by head injuries and fractures of the skull, and it may be necesssary to open the skull to arrest bleeding and evacuate blood clot that collects extradurally to cause pressure symptoms.

Approach

A burr hole to overlie the frontal branch of the middle meningeal artery (D) is made 3 cm above the middle of the zygomatic arch. The vessel is identified, increasing the size of the hole if necessary, bleeding is controlled and blood clot removed.

Hazards and Safeguards

The middle meningeal vessels in the region of pterion are frequently embedded in a tunnel of bone rather than lying in a groove, and this increases the risk of haemorrhage in head injuries.

If the artery cannot be found at pterion the dura must be followed down under the temporal lobe.

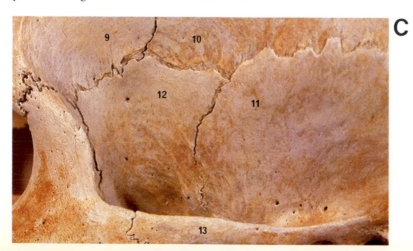

C

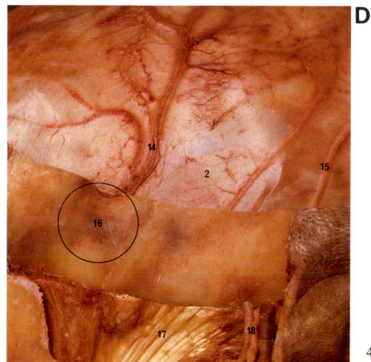

D

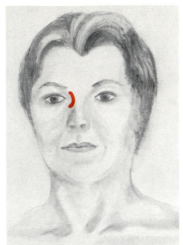

A

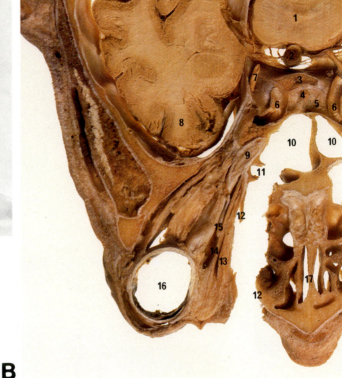

B

PITUITARY GLAND

Background

The pituitary gland lies in the pituitary fossa (sella turcica), indenting the upper surface of the body of the sphenoid bone which contains the two sphenoidal air sinuses. The dura mater in the fossa contains the intercavernous (venous) sinus, consisting of a number of anastomotic connections between the cavernous sinuses which lie on either side of the gland and body of the sphenoid. The most anterior part of a large sphenoidal sinus is immediately adjacent anterolaterally to the optic nerve and the most posterior ethmoidal air cell.

It is possible to approach the gland through the anterior cranial fossa by elevating the frontal lobe of the brain (subfrontal approach) but it is more common to use a route through the sphenoidal sinuses (transphenoidal approach), reaching these through the medial wall of one orbit by breaking through the air cells of the ethmoidal sinus.

Transphenoidal Approach

A skin incision (A) is made along the medial margin of the right orbit (for a right-handed operator) and deepened down to the periosteum.

The skin and periosteum are reflected laterally off the frontal and nasal bones and the maxilla. The trochlea of the superior oblique is detached and the periosteal elevation continued backwards along the medial wall of the orbit as far as the anterior ethmoidal vessels, with lateral displacement of the orbital contents. The anterior ethmoidal vessels are ligated as they pass through their foramen.

The ethmoidal sinus is entered through the exposed anterior part of the lamina papyracea (lateral wall of the ethmoid labyrinth), and the partitions between the air cells broken away in a backward direction but keeping the roof and medial wall of the sinus intact, as well as the posterior part of the lateral wall (B).

The uppermost part of the right nasal cavity is entered and the anterior wall of the right sphenoidal sinus can then be seen. The

midline of the body of the sphenoid is identified by the presence of the sphenoidal rostrum which joins the upper posterior part of the nasal septum.

The anterior wall of the body of the sphenoid is opened centrally (by removing part of the rostrum) and towards the right side, so entering the (right) sphenoidal sinus.

The septum between the right and left sphenoidal sinuses is removed so that a hole can be made in the central part of the anterior wall of the pituitary fossa. The hole is enlarged to expose more widely the dura mater of the fossa, which is then incised to reveal the gland.

Hazards and Safeguards

The septum dividing the right and left sphenoidal sinuses must not be used as a guide to the midline, as it is usually off-centre. The midline is indicated by the upper posterior part of the nasal septum and the rostrum of the sphenoid, and this is where the body of the bone is opened.

The intercavernous sinus may cause troublesome bleeding when the dura of the pituitary fossa is incised. When the gland is removed a flow of cerebrospinal fluid helps to flush out the fossa. Bleeding and the escape of cerebrospinal fluid are controlled by plugging the fossa with a graft of muscle removed from the lateral side of the thigh.

The (right) optic nerve may be damaged by improper retraction of the orbital contents.

Accidental entry into the left cavernous sinus (from a right-sided approach) may injure the oculomotor nerve or the internal carotid artery.

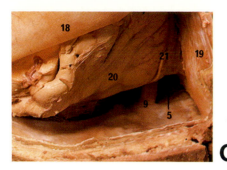

C

A
Incision line.

B
Cross section of the right half of the head, through the upper part of the pituitary fossa, showing the transphenoidal route to the pituitary gland. After entering the right sphenoidal sinus through the ethmoidal air cells, the septum between the two sphenoidal sinuses is removed so that the gland can be approached through the anterior wall of the pituitary fossa (posterior wall of the sinuses).

C
Right side of the cranial cavity, from the front and the right, indicating the subfrontal route to the pituitary gland with elevation of the frontal lobe of the brain.

Subfrontal Approach
For a right-handed operator the approach is under the right cerebral hemisphere.

An anterior craniotomy flap using four burr holes is cut and hinged on the anterior part of temporalis (as on page 44, B, but on the right side).

The dura is incised and the frontal lobe elevated to display the olfactory bulb and tract (C). The tract is divided behind the bulb to prevent accidental avulsion of the bulb from the cribriform plate.

The tract is followed backwards to the posterior margin of the lesser wing of the sphenoid, and the optic nerve identified as it enters the optic canal.

The pituitary stalk is identified piercing the diaphragma sellae which is incised to enter the pituitary fossa. Further steps depend on the type of operation being performed (e.g. removal of a tumour or removal of the gland itself – hypophysectomy).

Hazards and Safeguards
The olfactory tract is severed from the olfactory bulb because accidental avulsion of the bulb can produce troublesome haemorrhage from ethmoidal vessels at the cribriform plate.

The internal carotid artery of both sides as well as both optic nerves must be identified and preserved if dissecting out tumour tissue.

1 Pons
2 Basilar artery
3 Dorsum sellae
4 Pituitary stalk
5 Diaphragma sellae
6 Internal carotid artery
7 Oculomotor nerve
8 Temporal lobe
9 Optic nerve
10 Sphenoidal sinus
11 Posterior ethmoidal air cell
12 Lateral wall of ethmoidal sinus
13 Periosteum of orbit
14 Medial rectus
15 Nasociliary nerve
16 Eyeball
17 Nasal septum
18 Dura mater
19 Falx cerebri
20 Under surface of frontal lobe
21 Cut end of olfactory tract

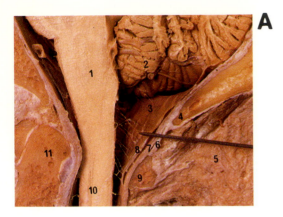

A

SUBARACHNOID AND EPIDURAL SPACES

Background

The subarachnoid space which contains cerebrospinal fluid is situated between the arachnoid which is in apposition to the dura mater and the pia mater which adheres to the surface of the brain, spinal cord and the emerging cranial and spinal nerves. The cranial part of the subarachnoid space is inside the skull and is continuous with the spinal part through the foramen magnum. The extradural space in the skull is normally non-existent, since the outer (endosteal) layer of cranial dura mater is in fact the periosteum of the inside of the skull; only if this periosteum becomes lifted off the bone (e.g. by a middle meningeal haemorrhage) can a cranial extradural space be said to exist.

In the vertebral column, the extradural space is in the vertebral canal, outside the spinal dura mater and bounded by the posterior surfaces of the vertebral bodies and the vertebral arches (pedicles and laminae). The dural sheaths containing the ventral and dorsal nerve roots run through the space to reach their respective intervertebral foramina, and the rest of the space is occupied by fatty tissue and the internal vertebral venous plexus. This spinal extradural space is frequently known as the epidural space – the terms are synonymous – especially with respect to anaesthesia (see below).

The cerebrospinal fluid manufactured by the choroid plexus of the third ventricles and the body and inferior horn of the lateral ventricles passes through the aqueduct of the midbrain into the fourth ventricle where it is supplemented by further fluid produced by the separate choroid plexus of that ventricle. This combined product escapes from the ventricular system through the three foramina in the roof of the fourth ventricle – the median aperture (foramen of Magendie) and the two lateral apertures (foramina of Luschka) – to enter the cranial subarachnoid space. Over the cerebral hemispheres the arachnoid and pia mater are close and the subarachnoid space is narrow, but in certain areas where the brain surface is more irregular, the arachnoid bridges larger parts of the space forming cisterns (cisternae). One of the largest of these is the cerebellomedullary cistern, commonly known as the cisterna magna, situated in the angle between the cerebellum and medulla oblongata. This cistern is accessible to a needle introduced from behind beneath the skull to the foramen magnum (A), and a sample of cerebrospinal fluid can be obtained from here (cisternal puncture) if for some reason (such as a blockage of the space in the thoracic region) the much more common lumbar puncture (see below) cannot be performed.

Although subject to some variation, the spinal cord in the adult normally ends at the level of the disc between the first and second lumbar vertebrae, but the subarachnoid space continues until the second piece of the sacrum. Between these two levels the subarachnoid space contains the filum terminale (which is not a neural element but an unimportant thread of pia mater), and the highly important cauda equina, consisting of the dorsal and ventral roots of the lumbar, sacral and coccygeal nerves. The lumbar part of the subarachnoid space is the common site for obtaining specimens of cerebrospinal fluid (lumbar puncture); a needle introduced between the spines of the third and fourth lumbar vertebrae is not in danger of damaging the spinal cord because this has ended higher up, and the relatively small nerve roots of the cauda equina offer no resistance to a penetrating needle tip and are simply pushed aside (B).

The same site as for lumbar puncture can also be used for spinal (intradural) anaesthesia – introducing anaesthetic solution into the lumbar part of the subarachnoid space so that it diffuses into the nerve roots. Epidural anaesthesia, commonly used in obstetrics, involves placing the anaesthetic solution in the epidural (extradural) space, using a similar route between lumbar spines but leaving the needle tip or epidural catheter outside the dura without penetrating into the subarachnoid space (C). The anaesthetic effect is due to the solution gravitating around the dural sheaths of the lumbar and sacral nerves and diffusing into them.

Cisternal Puncture

The neck is flexed with the chin on to the manubrium of the sternum.

After local anaesthesia of the skin, the needle is inserted in the midline level with the tips of the mastoid processes and between the external occipital protuberance and the spine of the axis, and advanced forwards and upwards to the under surface of the occipital bone at the foramen magnum. After penetrating skin and fascia the needle passes through the ligamentum nuchae (the cervical equivalent of the supraspinous and interspinous ligaments in the lower parts of the vertebral column), and at the margin of the foramen magnum will penetrate the posterior atlanto-occipital membrane and the dura and arachnoid (A) at a level of 4.5–5.5 cm from the skin surface.

Hazards and Safeguards

The needle must not be inserted more than 6 cm from the skin surface to avoid injury to the medulla.

The needle must remain in the midline to avoid the vertebral arteries which enter the foramen magnum at each side 1.5 cm from the midline.

A

Right half of a median sagittal section of the head, illustrating cisternal puncture. The medulla may be injured if the needle is advanced more than 6 cm from the skin surface.

B

Right half of a median sagittal section of part of the lumbar vertebral column, illustrating lumbar puncture. The needle is in the subarachnoid space, among the nerve roots of the cauda equina; they are not damaged as they offer no resistance to the needle. (In a patient the lumbar spine will be more flexed than it is here.)

C

As B, but with the needle in the epidural space, without penetrating the dura. The fatty tissue and the internal vertebral venous plexus of the space are removed to show the dura clearly; the veins of the plexus are a potential hazard to a penetrating needle.

Lumbar Puncture

With the patient lying on one side with the knees up to the chest to flex the lower part of the vertebral column, the fourth lumbar spine is identified on a line drawn between the highest points of the iliac crests, and the third spine then palpated above it.

After local anaesthesia of the skin, the lumbar puncture needle is inserted in the midline between the third and fourth lumbar spines (B), pointing slightly upwards in the direction of the umbilicus. The needle passes through the supraspinous and interspinous ligaments, through or between ligamenta flava into the epidural space, and then through the dura and arachnoid, when a certain amount of 'give' is usually felt. The stylet of the needle is withdrawn to see whether cerebrospinal fluid will escape, indicating a successful puncture.

Hazards and Safeguards

If the needle contacts bone (vertebral spine or lamina), it must be withdrawn to subcutaneous level and then advanced at a slightly different angle. The space between the fourth and fifth lumbar spines can also be used.

If the needle enters and stays in part of the internal vertebral venous plexus, pure blood will emerge from the needle. This is particularly likely if the needle is pushed too far and penetrates the anterior surface of the dura. Cerebrospinal fluid that is merely blood-stained at first and then runs clear implies only minor damage to a vessel before proper entry into the subarachnoid space.

Extreme penetration could possibly damage an intervertebral disc.

Epidural Anaesthesia

The procedure is similar to that for lumbar puncture, but the choice of space is not critical; that between the second and third lumbar spines is often used, counting up from the fourth spine as the landmark.

The needle is advanced to pass through or between ligamenta flava but not to penetrate the dura (C).

An alternative approach to the epidural space, from below into the sacral hiatus between the sacral cornua (which are palpable) is now rarely used.

Hazards and Safeguards

If the needle is advanced too far the dura will be penetrated and cerebrospinal fluid will flow from the needle. A needle correctly placed in the epidural space will not deliver cerebrospinal fluid, and a test injection of a small amount of air or solution will meet with no resistance; if the tip remains within a ligamentum flavum or interspinous tissue there will be resistance to such injection.

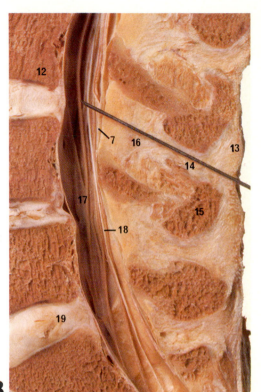

1	Medulla oblongata
2	Cerebellum
3	Cisterna magna
4	Margin of foramen magnum
5	Ligamentum nuchae
6	Posterior atlanto-occipital membrane
7	Dura mater
8	Arachnoid mater
9	Posterior arch of atlas
10	Spinal cord
11	Dens of axis
12	Body of third lumbar vertebra
13	Supraspinous ligament
14	Interspinous ligament
15	Spine of fourth lumbar vertebra
16	Ligamentum flavum
17	Cauda equina
18	Filum terminale
19	Lumbosacral disc
20	Epidural space

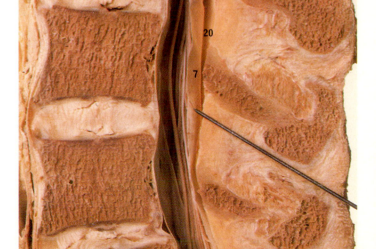

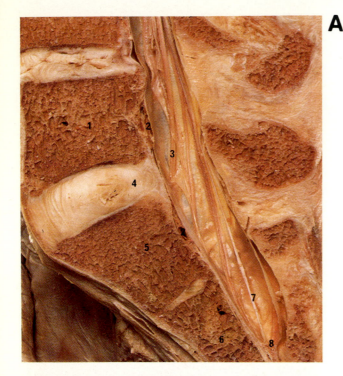

A

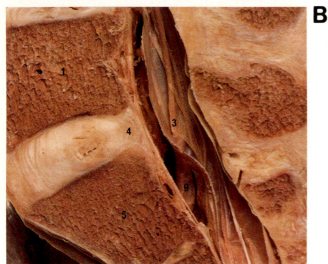

B

INTERVERTEBRAL DISC

Background

The bodies of adjacent vertebrae (from the third cervical to the first piece of the sacrum) are connected by intervertebral discs which consist of a nucleus pulposus surrounded by the annulus fibrosus. The back of each disc forms the lower part of the anterior boundary of an intervertebral foramen, the upper part of that boundary being the vertebral body below the level of the attachment of its pedicle, which forms the upper margin of the foramen. The pedicle of the vertebra below is at the lower margin of the foramen, while the zygapophyseal joint (facet joint) between the superior and inferior articular processes of adjacent vertebrae forms the posterior boundary of the foramen. The spinal nerve emerges from the foramen immediately beneath the pedicle at its upper margin, e.g. the fifth lumbar nerve emerges beneath the pedicle of the fifth lumbar vertebra, but the meningeal sheath containing the dorsal and ventral nerve roots (that are going to unite immediately distal to the ganglion of the dorsal root to form the spinal nerve itself) crosses over the back of the disc numbered one above the vertebra, e.g. the sheath containing the fifth lumbar nerve roots lies behind the fourth lumbar disc – the disc below the fourth vertebra (A and B). When there is a prolapse (backward protrusion) of the nucleus pulposus ('slipped disc'), the projecting material may irritate the dural sheath behind it (since protrusion usually occurs towards the side of the back of a disc and not in the midline). Thus the fourth lumbar disc may cause pressure on the fifth lumbar nerve roots, *not* the fourth nerve roots because they do not normally reach as low as the fourth disc. Disc protrusion occurs most commonly in the lower lumbar region, especially in the fifth lumbar (lumbosacral) disc, so that the nerve roots involved are those of the first sacral nerve.

It may be necessary to remove the protruded part of a disc. This is done, as described below, by opening into the vertebral canal from behind by removing the ligamentum flavum between the laminae of adjacent vertebral arches, together with part of a lamina (laminotomy) or a whole lamina (laminectomy) depending on the amount of access required.

Approach

The patient lies on the unaffected side with the spine in flexion and with a lateral convexity upwards (to open up the intervertebral foramina as much as possible).

A vertical skin incision (C) is made at the side of the lower lumbar spines and deepened through the posterior layer of lumbar fascia.

Erector spinae (sacrospinalis) is separated from the lumbar spines and from the intervening interspinous ligament and laminae, and retracted laterally.

The required ligamentum flavum is incised and cut away with part or all of adjacent laminae as necessary to expose the extradural space (D, E and F). The dura with the sheath containing nerve roots and the posterior part of the disc can then be defined by clearing the extradural fat, and the protruded part of the disc is removed.

Hazards and Safeguards

Great care must be taken to avoid damaging the dura and the contained nerve roots. The ligamentum flavum must be very carefully incised since the dura may lie very close. The ligamentum itself may be as much as 5 mm thick.

Haemorrhage from the posterior branches of lumbar arteries in erector spinae and from epidural veins cannot be avoided.

If the disc is entered to remove degenerate fragments, the anterior part of the annulus must be left intact to avoid damaging the inferior vena cava or aorta.

A

Right half of a median sagittal section of the lumbosacral region of the vertebral column, showing nerve roots of the cauda equina within the subarachnoid space. Note that as the first sacral nerve roots leave the main space to enter their own meningeal sheath they pass behind the fifth lumbar (lumbosacral) disc.

B

As A, with the meninges reflected backwards to show the meningeal sheath of the first sacral nerve roots.

C

Incision line.

D

Right halves of the lower three lumbar vertebrae, for comparison with E and F.

E

Right side of the lumbar vertebral column, from behind, showing partial removal of two adjacent laminae to display a meningeal nerve sheath.

F

Similar to E but with complete removal of laminae.

1 Fifth lumbar vertebral body
2 Internal vertebral venous plexus
3 First sacral nerve roots
4 Lumbosacral disc
5 First piece of sacrum
6 Second piece of sacrum
7 Filum terminale
8 Lower end of subarachnoid space
9 Meningeal sheath for first sacral nerve roots
10 Lamina of third lumbar vertebra
11 Zygapophyseal joint
12 Dura mater
13 Meningeal sheath for fourth lumbar nerve roots
14 Lumbar fascia over erector spinae
15 Fourth lumbar vertebral body
16 Fourth lumbar disc
17 Meningeal sheath for fifth lumbar nerve roots

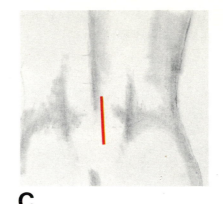

C

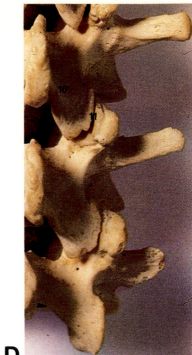

D

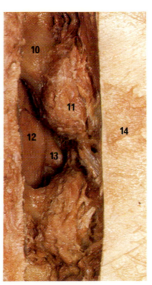

E

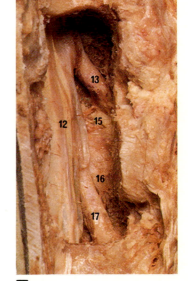

F

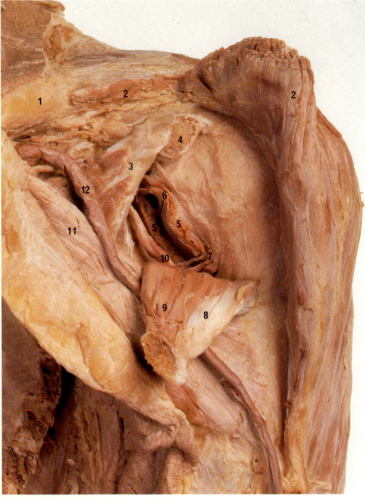

B

A

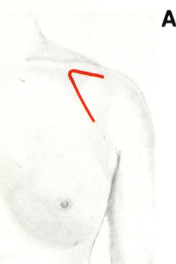

SHOULDER JOINT

Background

The capsule of the shoulder joint is surrounded by what are commonly called the rotator cuff muscles – supraspinatus above, subscapularis in front, and infraspinatus and teres minor behind. The lateral part of supraspinatus is under cover of the coraco-acromial ligament with part of the subdeltoid (subacromial) bursa intervening between the ligament and the muscle. The long head of biceps emerges from the capsule of the joint to lie in the inter-tubercular groove, and pectoralis major crosses the front of the joint and the groove to become attached to the lateral lip of the groove. Deltoid lies superficially over the front, side and back of the joint with the cephalic vein in the deltopectoral groove between deltoid and pectoralis major. The axillary (circumflex) nerve passes from front to back immediately beneath the lowest part of the capsule.

The approach to the joint can be from the front or back. At the front the deltopectoral groove is opened up and subscapularis is transected to reveal the front of the capsule. At the back trapezius is detached from the scapula before cutting teres minor and if necessary infraspinatus to expose the back of the capsule.

Anterior Approach

A skin incision (A) is made along the deltopectoral groove and continued laterally from the upper end of the groove along the line of the clavicle as far as the acromioclavicular joint.

The groove between deltoid and pectoralis major is opened up and deltoid detached from the clavicle (B), ligating tributaries of the cephalic vein. (Alternatively deltoid can be split along a line about 1cm from its medial border, leaving the cephalic vein undisturbed in the groove.)

Either of the above muscle separations will expose the tip of the coracoid process. The tip is detached together with its attached muscles (coracobrachialis and the short head of biceps) (B) and retracted medially.

The humerus is rotated laterally to stretch and define sub-scapularis which is divided 2.5cm from its insertion and the cut ends are turned back to expose the joint capsule (B, C and D).

Hazards and Safeguards

The cephalic vein lies in the deltopectoral groove; it pierces the clavipectoral fascia between pectoralis minor and the clavicle, as do the thoraco-acromial vessels, the lateral pectoral nerve and some lymphatic channels. The fascia is not disturbed but some vascular branches may need ligation.

Before the tip of the coracoid process is detached with coraco-brachialis and the short head of biceps, the medial and lateral borders of this muscle mass must be defined; the attachment of pectoralis minor is posterior to coracobrachialis and is not removed.

The musculocutaneous nerve enters coracobrachialis and must not be damaged when the tip of the coracoid and the attached muscle mass is retracted (B).

The anterior circumflex humeral vessels run along the lower border of subscapularis. The veins often form a plexus and are a guide to the lower border of the muscle.

A

Incision line.

B

Left shoulder, from the front. Deltoid has been detached from the front of the clavicle and turned outwards, and the tip of the coracoid process, with coracobrachialis and the short head of biceps still attached, has been cut off and turned downwards (at operation it is retracted medially). The underlying subscapularis has been cut vertically to display the capsule which can then be incised. The musculocutaneous nerve must not be damaged when displacing coracobrachialis. The anterior circumflex humeral vessels are a guide to the lower border of subscapularis; in this specimen two venae commitantes run with the artery but they often form a plexus.

C

Horizontal section through the left shoulder, from above.

D

The same section illustrating the line of approach to the joint from the front.

1 Clavicle
2 Deltoid
3 Pectoralis minor
4 Coracoid process
5 Subscapularis
6 Capsule
7 Anterior circumflex humeral vessels
8 Short head of biceps
9 Coracobrachialis
10 Musculocutaneous nerve
11 Pectoralis major
12 Cephalic vein
13 Glenoid fossa
14 Glenoid labrum
15 Head of humerus
16 Greater tuberosity
17 Tendon of long head of biceps in intertubercular groove
18 Lesser tuberosity
19 Lateral cord of brachial plexus
20 Axillary artery

C

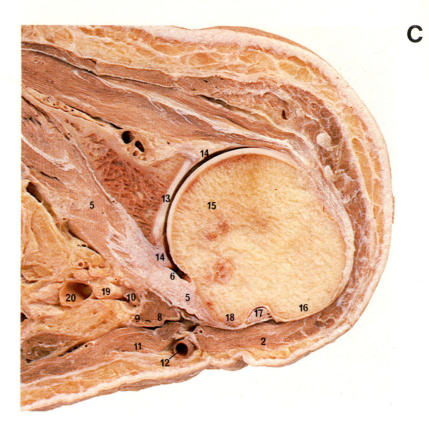

D

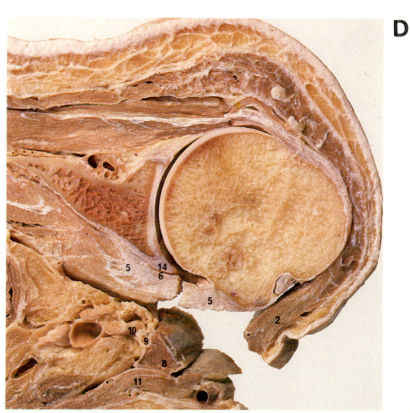

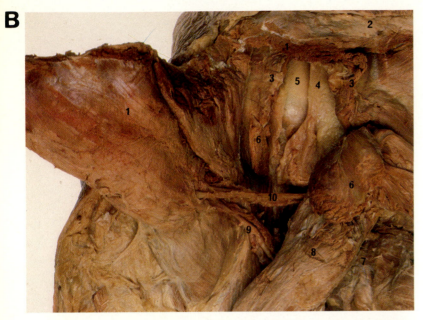

B

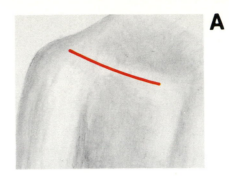

A

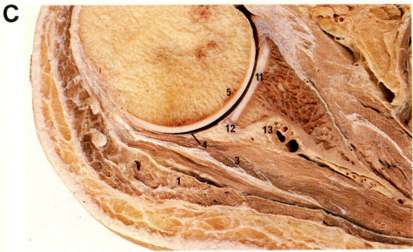

C

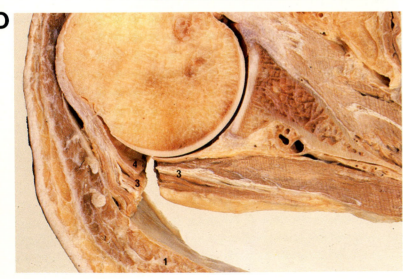

D

Posterior Approach

A skin incision (A) is made along the spine of the scapula.

Deltoid is detached from the spine and from the lateral edge of the acromion.

The tendons of infraspinatus and teres minor are exposed, and teres minor is incised vertically 2.5 cm from its insertion, so exposing the joint capsule which can then be opened (B, C and D). If necessary infraspinatus can also be incised.

Hazards and Safeguards

The posterior circumflex humeral vessels and the axillary nerve lie below the joint capsule, passing backwards through the quadrilateral space (bounded above by teres minor, below by teres major, medially by the long head of triceps and laterally by the humerus). The nerve normally lies horizontally at a level 5–6 cm below the acromion (B). It must not be damaged when cutting teres minor or retracting deltoid.

If infraspinatus is incised the proximal end should not be retracted too forcibly, to avoid damaging the suprascapular nerve that enters its deep surface after curving round the base of the scapular spine.

A

Incision line for posterior approach to the shoulder joint.

B

Left shoulder, from behind. Deltoid has been detached from the lower lip of the spine of the scapula and from part of the acromion, and turned outwards. Too much displacement could damage the axillary nerve and the posterior circumflex humeral vessels which pass behind the humerus immediately below the capsule of the joint to enter deltoid. The cut ends of infraspinatus and teres minor are turned back and the capsule is incised to expose the head of the humerus.

C

Horizontal section through the left shoulder, from above.

D

The same section illustrating the approach to the joint from behind.

SUPRASPINATUS TENDON

Background

Supraspinatus arises from the supraspinous fossa of the scapula and its tendon passes over the top of the shoulder joint capsule to be inserted partly into the capsule but mostly into the uppermost facet of the greater tuberosity of the humerus. The subdeltoid (subacromial) bursa lies immediately above the lateral part of the muscle, intervening between the muscle and the coraco-acromial ligament medially and the deltoid laterally.

One of the well-recognized injuries in the shoulder region is a tear of the supraspinatus tendon, and for repair it can be approached from above by incising trapezius and cutting through the acromion behind the acromioclavicular joint.

Approach

A skin incision (E) is made above and parallel to the upper border of the spine of the scapula, and continued laterally over the middle of the acromion.

The trapezius is cut just above the scapular spine and the fascia over supraspinatus incised to expose the more medial part of the muscle.

The lateral part of supraspinatus and its tendon are brought into view by splitting the acromion in the line of the skin incision. The anterior portion of the acromion (still attached to the clavicle at the acromioclavicular joint) can be moved forward with the clavicle by splitting the deltoid vertically (F) in the continuing line of the acromial incision and opening the underlying subacromial (sub-deltoid) bursa. The supraspinatus tendon lies beneath the bursa.

Hazards and Safeguards

The axillary nerve must not be damaged when cutting and retracting the deltoid. It passes behind the surgical neck of the humerus and lies horizontally 5–6 cm below the tip of the acromion (F), so that when splitting the deltoid vertically the cut must not extend as low as this.

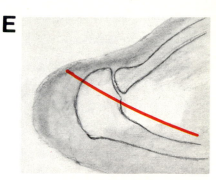

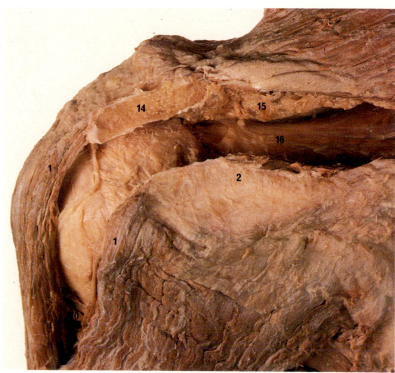

1 Deltoid
2 Spine of scapula
3 Infraspinatus
4 Capsule
5 Head of humerus
6 Teres minor
7 Teres major
8 Long head of triceps
9 Posterior circumflex humeral vessels
10 Axillary nerve
11 Glenoid fossa
12 Glenoid labrum
13 Suprascapular nerve and vessels
14 Acromion
15 Trapezius
16 Supraspinatus

E
Incision line for the approach to supraspinatus.

F
Left shoulder, from above and behind. Deltoid and the acromion are split in the line of the skin incision and trapezius is cut above the spine of the scapula, allowing the lateral part of supraspinatus to be exposed. Too much backward retraction of deltoid may damage the axillary nerve which passes horizontally behind the humerus 5–6 cm below the acromion.

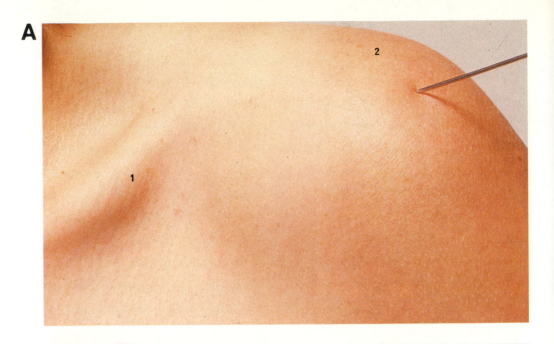

A

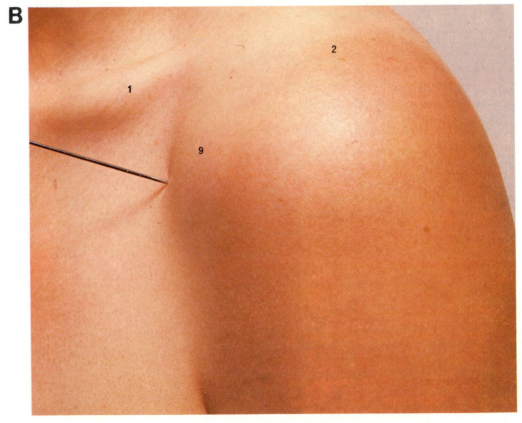

B

Puncture of the Shoulder Joint

Various routes for aspiration or injection are described, from the front, side or back. The simplest is probably from the side below the acromion (A), with the needle directed slightly downwards to pass through deltoid, the subacromial bursa and the supraspinatus tendon before penetrating the capsule (C).

The more posterior approach is from below the junction of the acromion with the spine of the scapula, directed towards the coracoid, while from the front (B) the needle is introduced through the deltopectoral groove below and medial to the tip of the coracoid process, passing backwards and laterally at an angle of about 30° through the coracobrachialis-biceps origin and subscapularis into the capsule.

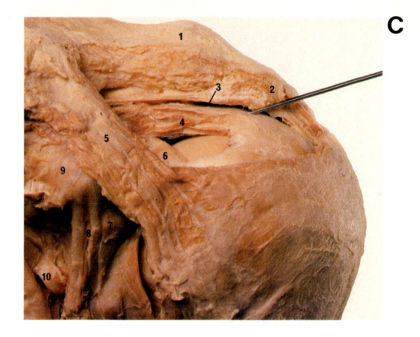

C

A
Puncture of the left shoulder joint, from the side. The needle passes medially beneath the acromion.

B
Puncture from the front. The needle passes downwards and laterally, below and lateral to the coracoid process.

C
Left shoulder, for comparison with A. The needle passes through subacromial bursa and supraspinatus before entering the joint. If approached from the front as in B, the needle would pass through the origin of coracobrachialis and the short head of biceps from the coracoid process (lateral to the brachial plexus) and then through subscapularis.

1 Clavicle
2 Acromion
3 Subacromial bursa
4 Supraspinatus
5 Deltoid
6 Long head of biceps
7 Short head of biceps
8 Coracobrachialis
9 Coracoid process
10 Musculocutaneous nerve

B

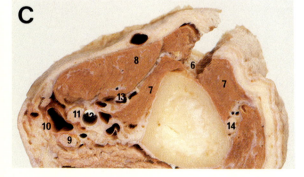

A

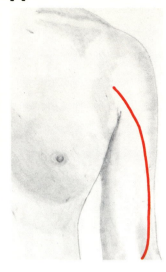

1 Pectoralis major
2 Cephalic vein
   (displaced medially)
3 Capsule
4 Tendon of long head
   of biceps
5 Deltoid
6 Anterior surface
   of humerus
7 Brachialis
8 Biceps
9 Ulnar nerve
10 Basilic vein
11 Median nerve
12 Brachial artery
13 Musculocutaneous nerve
14 Radial nerve
15 Lateral head of triceps
16 Medial head of triceps
17 Teres major
18 Long head of triceps
19 Nerve to 18
20 Nerve to 15
21 Profunda brachii artery
22 Nerve to 16
23 Branch of 21
24 Posterior surface
    of humerus

HUMERUS

Background

At the upper end of the shaft of the humerus, pectoralis major, latissimus dorsi and teres major gain attachment to the lateral lip, floor and medial lip respectively of the intertubercular groove. The large deltoid insertion is into the lateral part of the shaft half way down, with the smaller coracobrachialis in a similar position on the medial side. Much of the front of the shaft is covered by brachialis with biceps in front of it and the brachial vessels and the median nerve under cover of the medial border of biceps. The ulnar nerve which in the upper part of the arm is on the medial side of this neurovascular bundle pierces the medial intermuscular septum to enter the posterior compartment and reach the back of the medial epicondyle. Triceps is the only muscle of the posterior compartment, with the radial nerve and the profunda vessels spiralling behind the shaft from the medial to the lateral side and then piercing the lateral intermuscular septum to run down in the anterior compartment in front of brachialis, becoming covered lower down by brachioradialis which has its origin from the lateral supracondylar line.

The front of the upper part of the shaft can be exposed by opening up the deltopectoral groove, while lower down brachialis can be split vertically along its anterolateral side, so keeping away from the brachial vessels and the median and ulnar nerves that lie more medially. The lower end of the shaft can be visualized by opening up the interval between brachialis and brachioradialis. The back of the shaft is exposed by cutting through triceps, taking particular care to avoid damaging the radial nerve and its branches to that muscle.

Anterior Approach

The skin incision (A) follows the deltopectoral groove to the deltoid insertion and then passes along the lateral border of biceps, curling towards the middle of the cubital fossa at the lower end.

A

Incision line for anterior approach.

B

Left arm, from the front. The upper part of the shaft of the humerus is displayed between the medial border of deltoid and the insertion of pectoralis major into the lateral lip of the intertubercular groove. Lower down, brachialis is incised vertically but obliquely towards the midline of the shaft, and the cut edges are separated with the periosteum to expose the bone.

C

Cross section below the middle of the left arm, from below, with brachialis split down to the humerus. The cut through the muscle is made obliquely from the lateral side towards the centre of the shaft, to keep as far away as possible from the brachial artery and median nerve. The radial nerve must be remembered when stripping the periosteum from the lateral side of the lower part of the shaft.

The cephalic vein is retracted medially and the medial fibres of deltoid are detached from the clavicle so that the flap of muscle can be turned laterally. The shaft of the humerus can now be followed to the deltoid insertion (B).

The lower part of the shaft is exposed by incising brachialis longitudinally at the lateral border of biceps. The incision in brachialis is made *obliquely* to reach the bone in the middle of the shaft which can then be exposed by peeling back the periosteum on each side (B and C). Flexing the elbow facilitates the exposure.

The lowest part of the front of the shaft can be approached between brachioradialis which is retracted laterally and brachialis which is retracted medially.

Hazards and Safeguards

Tributaries of the cephalic vein converge on it in the deltopectoral groove.

The lateral cutaneous nerve of the forearm (the continuation of the musculocutaneous nerve) becomes superficial at the lower lateral border of biceps where the muscle fibres give place to tendon.

The obliqueness of the cut through brachialis ensures that the brachial artery and median nerve are well away from the incision line (C).

The radial nerve is protected by being first behind the humerus and then behind the lateral part of brachialis, but it is very close to the bone and must be remembered when stripping the periosteum backwards on the lateral side.

Posterior Approach

A skin incision (D) is made vertically in the midline from below the acromion to the olecranon.

The long and lateral heads of triceps are separated, carefully avoiding in the upper part of the separation the underlying radial nerve and profunda brachii vessels. The incision which is through muscle fibres in the upper part is continued down into the tendinous part, then the medial (deep) head of triceps is split in the midline down to the periosteum (E and F).

Hazards and Safeguards

The radial nerve and profunda vessels cross the upper extremity of the medial head of triceps (under cover of the long and lateral heads), and pass obliquely downwards from the medial to the lateral side of the humerus, before piercing the lateral inter-muscular septum to enter the flexor compartment. The nerve gives four branches to triceps (E), not three as might be expected: the medial head receives two branches. In order from above down the motor nerves go to the long head, medial head, lateral head and medial head. The incision in the medial head is made between the two nerves to that head; nerves to the long and medial heads will therefore lie medial to the incision line, and nerves to the lateral and medial heads to the lateral side.

The ulnar nerve and brachial vessels will be seen above the medial side of the medial head of triceps if the long head is retracted medially.

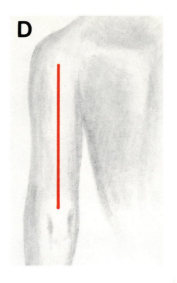

D

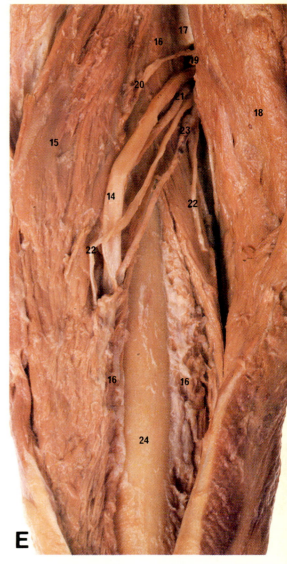

D
Incision line for posterior approach.

E
Left arm, from behind. The long and lateral heads of triceps are separated and the medial head is split vertically to expose the shaft of the humerus.

E

F
Cross section of the middle of the left arm, orientated for comparison with E, showing the exposure of the shaft through triceps.

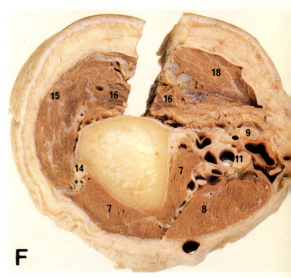

F

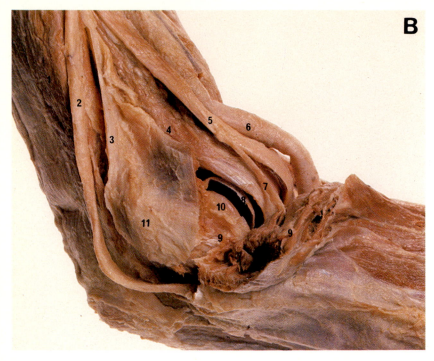

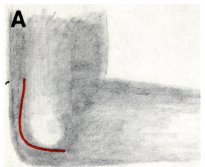

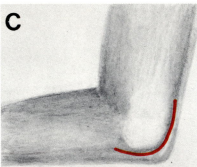

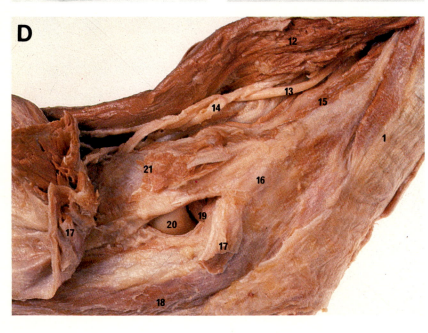

ELBOW JOINT

Background

The cavity of the elbow joint is continuous with that of the superior radio-ulnar joint. The structures of the cubital fossa lie in front of the elbow: brachialis and the tendon of biceps in the floor, with pronator teres and the common flexor origin medially and brachioradialis and the radial extensors laterally. The brachial artery and its venae commitantes are medial to the biceps tendon, with the median nerve on the medial side of the artery; the radial nerve is under cover of brachioradialis. The medial epicondyle provides a common origin for flexor muscles with the ulnar nerve behind it. In the middle at the back the tendon of triceps reaches the olecranon of the ulna, and the lateral epicondyle provides the common extensor origin with the small triangular anconeus passing to the upper part of the posterior border of the ulna.

The medial and lateral epicondyles of the humerus and the olecranon and posterior border of the ulna are subcutaneous and so easily palpable. The head of the radius and the capitulum of the humerus can also be felt at the back, below and medial to the lateral epicondyle.

The joint is commonly approached from the side (e.g. from the lateral side for exploring a damaged head of radius or medially for inspecting the trochlear surface of the humerus), or in the midline at the back above the olecranon. An anterior approach is uncommon. On the medial side the route is by detaching the common flexor origin, and laterally the approach is by opening up the interval between anconeus and extensor carpi ulnaris. At the back the lower part of triceps can be incised, and at the front brachialis is divided vertically at the lateral border of the biceps tendon so that the capsule can be visualized.

Medial Approach

With the elbow flexed to a right angle, a skin incision (A) is made behind the joint over the medial epicondyle.

The ulnar nerve is dissected free and displaced backwards (B). Above the epicondyle brachialis is stripped forwards and triceps backwards.

The common flexor origin is detached from the epicondyle and the joint capsule opened by a vertical incision in front of the epicondyle (B).

Hazards and Safeguards

The ulnar nerve is easily found behind the medial epicondyle and displaced out of danger.

The brachial artery and median nerve are in front of brachialis and protected by it as the muscle is displaced forwards.

Lateral Approach

With the elbow flexed to a right angle, a skin incision (C) is made behind the lateral epicondyle along the line of the supracondylar line of the humerus and continued down to the level of the head of the radius.

The common extensor origin is detached from the epicondyle and the joint capsule incised lateral to anconeus (D).

Alternatively the intermuscular plane between extensor carpi ulnaris anteriorly and anconeus posteriorly can be opened up to expose the capsule which is incised longitudinally.

These exposures display the capitulum of the humerus and the head and neck of the radius; for wider exposure brachioradialis and extensor carpi radialis longus can be detached from the lateral supracondylar line.

Hazards and Safeguards

The capsule incision must not extend lower than the neck of the radius to avoid damaging the posterior interosseous nerve as it winds round the upper part of the shaft from front to back within the substance of the supinator.

The radial nerve lies between brachioradialis and extensor carpi radialis longus and is protected by being sandwiched between them.

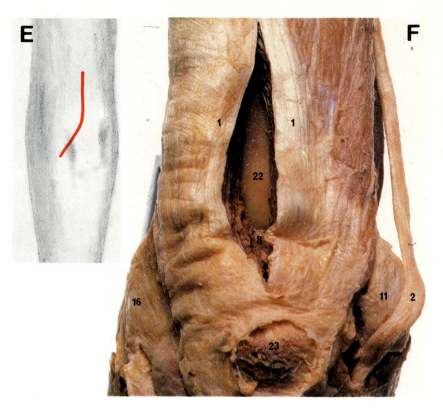

A

Incision line on the medial side.

B

Left elbow, from the medial side. The ulnar nerve is displaced backwards, the common flexor origin detached from the medial epicondyle and brachialis displaced forwards so that the capsule can be opened vertically in front of the epicondyle.

C

Incision line on the lateral side.

D

Left elbow, from the lateral side. The common extensor origin is detached from the lateral epicondyle so that the capsule can be opened, showing the head of the radius and capitulum of the humerus. Brachioradialis is displaced forwards to show the radial nerve; its posterior interosseous branch is seen entering supinator. The capsule must not be incised below the level of the head of the radius to avoid possible damage to this nerve.

E

Incision line for posterior approach.

F

Left elbow, from behind. Triceps is split vertically above the olecranon down to the posterior surface of the humerus so that the capsule can be incised at the olecranon fossa. The ulnar nerve is displaced medially to keep it as far as possible from the operation site.

1	Triceps	**13**	Radial nerve
2	Ulnar nerve	**14**	Radial recurrent artery
3	Medial intermuscular septum	**15**	Extensor carpi radialis longus
4	Brachialis	**16**	Lateral epicondyle
5	Median nerve	**17**	Common extensor origin
6	Brachial artery	**18**	Anconeus
7	Nerve to pronator teres	**19**	Capitulum
8	Capsule	**20**	Head of radius
9	Common flexor origin	**21**	Supinator
10	Medial edge of trochlea	**22**	Posterior surface of humerus
11	Medial epicondyle	**23**	Olecranon bursa
12	Brachioradialis		

Posterior Approach

With the elbow flexed to a right angle, a vertical skin incision (E) is made in the midline above the joint down to the tip of the olecranon and then laterally over the head of the radius.

Triceps is incised vertically to expose the humerus and the incision continued down to the olecranon to display the upper part of the joint capsule (F).

Hazards and Safeguards

The ulnar nerve behind the medial epicondyle should not be at risk but as a precaution it can be visualised and drawn medially.

Anterior Approach

A skin incision (A) is made along the lateral border of the tendon of biceps.

Brachialis is split vertically lateral to the biceps tendon and in the line of the skin incision to reach the front of the joint capsule (B, C and D).

Hazards and Safeguards

The brachial artery and median nerve lie medial to the biceps tendon.

The radial nerve dividing into its superficial (cutaneous) and deep (posterior interosseous) branches lies between brachialis and brachioradialis lateral to the incision line.

A

Incision line.

B

Left elbow, from the front. The capsule is incised after splitting brachialis on the lateral side of the tendon of biceps.

C

Cross section of the left elbow joint.

D

The same section as in C, showing the anterior approach to the joint by incision on the lateral side of the tendon of biceps and splitting brachialis. By keeping on the lateral side of the biceps tendon the brachial artery and median nerve are protected. The lateral cutaneous nerve of forearm and brachioradialis are displaced laterally to show the radial nerve between brachioradialis and brachialis.

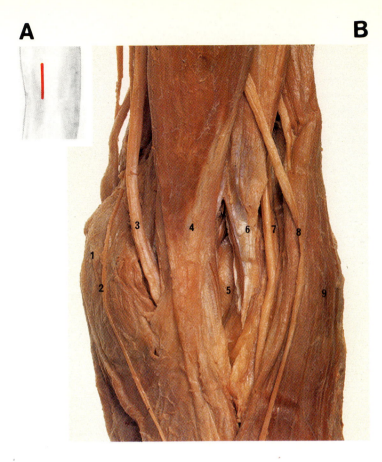

A

B

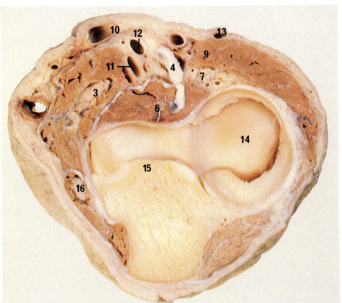

C

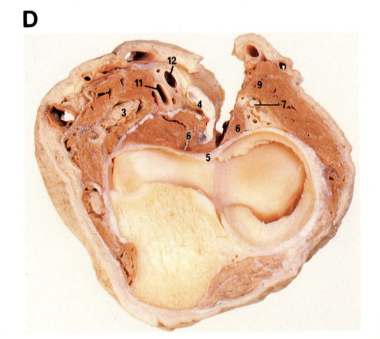

D

Puncture of the Elbow Joint

If the joint is greatly distended with fluid a needle can be inserted at the back on either side of the olecranon (E and F), with the elbow flexed to 135°.

For injection the usual site is on the posterolateral side immediately above the head of the radius, which is palpable below and medial to the lateral epicondyle of the humerus (E). The needle is inserted with the elbow flexed to a right angle.

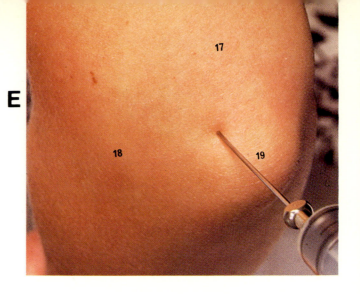

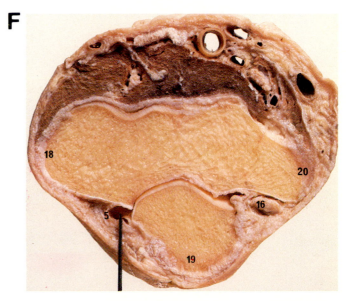

E

Puncture of the left elbow joint, from behind. The needle enters the joint cavity at the upper lateral margin of the olecranon.

F

Cross section of the left elbow joint, from below, showing the puncture at the lateral border of the olecranon.

G

Puncture of the left elbow joint, from the lateral side. The needle enters the joint just above the head of the radius.

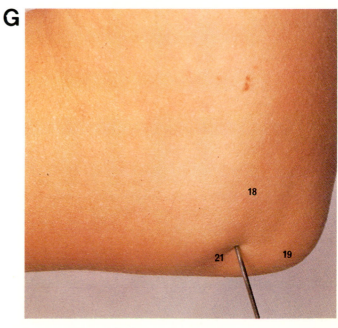

1	Common flexor origin	13	Cephalic vein
2	Medial cutaneous nerve of forearm	14	Capitulum of humerus
3	Median nerve	15	Coronoid process of ulna
4	Biceps	16	Ulnar nerve
5	Capsule	17	Triceps
6	Brachialis	18	Lateral epicondyle
7	Radial nerve	19	Olecranon
8	Lateral cutaneous nerve of forearm	20	Medial epicondyle
9	Brachioradialis	21	Head of radius
10	Median basilic vein		
11	Ulnar artry		
12	Radial artery		

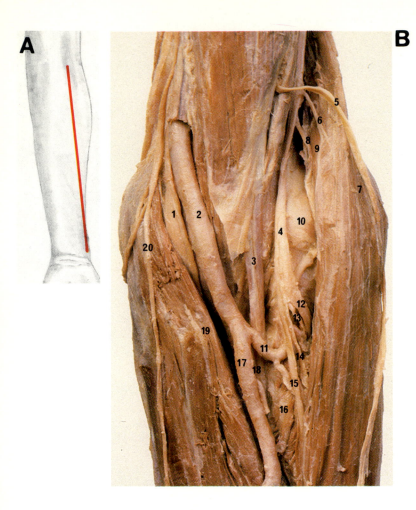

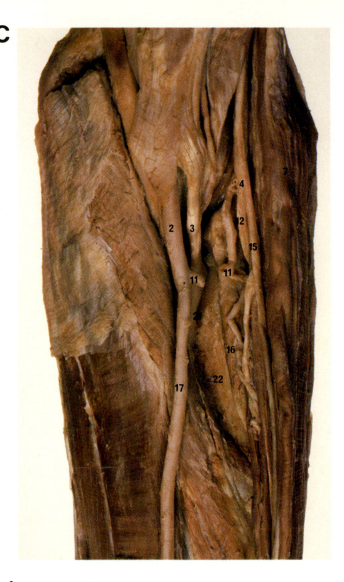

RADIUS

Background

Below the head of the radius the upper part of the bone is embraced by supinator, and the tendon of biceps is inserted into the posterior part of the radial tuberosity. Flexor pollicis longus and flexor digitorum superficialis have attachments lower down the anterior surface and anterior border respectively, and pronator teres occupies the lower anterior quarter of the shaft. The posterior surface below the oblique line gives origin to abductor pollicis longus and extensor pollicis brevis.

The usual approach to the radius is from the front, though the head is exposed through the lateral approach to the elbow joint (page 60). For exposure of the upper end below the head, brachioradialis and the two radial extensors of the wrist are displaced laterally and supinator is scraped off the bone, taking great care not to damage the posterior interosseous nerve which partly runs within the substance of that muscle. As the motor nerve to most of the extensor muscles it must not be injured. At the lower end, pronator quadratus can be removed from the front of the shaft by a route between the radial artery and the tendon of flexor carpi radialis.

Approach

With forearm supine, a skin incision (A) is made from the lateral side of the biceps tendon in the cubital fossa to the styloid process of the radius at the wrist.

The deep fascia is incised and the group of three lateral muscles at elbow level – brachioradialis and the two radial extensors – is mobilized and retracted laterally by cutting the radial recurrent artery and other muscular vessels that anchor the muscles to the radial artery (B and C).

The bursa under the biceps tendon at the radial tuberosity is opened by following the tendon down to the tuberosity, and having exposed bare bone at the bursa the supinator and the underlying periosteum are peeled off the anterior and lateral surfaces of the shaft of the radius (C, D and E).

Below the level of the supinator more of the shaft can be visualized by pulling the shaft into pronation and retracting brachioradialis and the radial extensors laterally. Lower down it can be exposed between brachioradialis laterally and flexor carpi radialis medially.

D

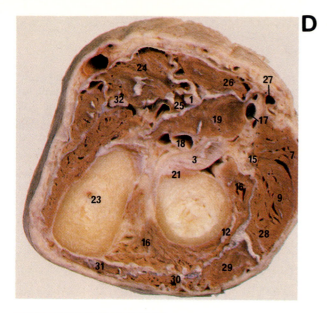

E

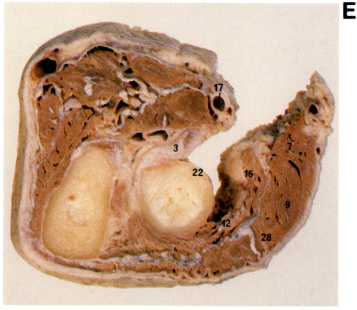

1	Median nerve	18	Ulnar artery
2	Brachial artery	19	Pronator teres
3	Tendon of biceps	20	Medial cutaneous
4	Radial nerve		nerve of forearm
5	Lateral cutaneous nerve of forearm	21	Radial tuberosity
6	Nerve to 7	22	Exposed radius
7	Brachioradialis	23	Ulna
8	Nerve to 9	24	Flexor digitorum superficialis
9	Extensor carpi radialis longus	25	Anterior interosseous nerve
10	Capsule	26	Flexor carpi radialis
11	Radial recurrent artery		and palmaris longus
12	Posterior interosseous nerve	27	Cephalic vein
13	Nerve to 16	28	Extensor carpi radialis brevis
14	Nerve to 28	29	Extensor digitorum
15	Superficial branch of 4	30	Extensor carpi ulnaris
16	Supinator	31	Anconeus
17	Radial artery	32	Ulnar nerve

For exposure of the lower end only, a skin incision (page 66, A) is made lateral to the tendon of flexor carpi radialis, beginning at the distal flexor skin crease at the wrist and extending proximally for 6 cm.

The deep fascia is incised and the tendons of flexor carpi radialis and (deeper) flexor pollicis longus are retracted medially, and the radial artery laterally.

Pronator quadratus is removed from its attachment to the anterior (lateral) margin of the radius and turned medially to expose the bone (page 66, B, C and D).

Hazards and Safeguards

The posterior interosseous nerve (deep terminal branch of the radial nerve) passes through the substance of the supinator and is not damaged if the whole thickness of the muscle is gently retracted off the bone. It is the structure at greatest risk in this exposure.

The radial nerve itself and its superficial (cutaneous) continuation lie between brachioradialis and extensor carpi radialis longus and are protected between this sandwich of muscle when the group is retracted laterally.

The radial artery begins (as a terminal branch of the brachial artery) at the medial side of the biceps tendon; it must not be damaged when incising the deep fascia.

Above the wrist, the radial artery lies to the lateral side of the tendon of flexor carpi radialis, with the median nerve on the medial side of the tendon (page 66, B and C).

A

Incision line.

B

Left cubital fossa and upper forearm. Brachioradialis and the lateral cutaneous nerve of forearm are retracted laterally and the radial artery medially to show the radial nerve and its branches and the radial recurrent artery lying in front of supinator.

C

As in B, after following the lateral side of the biceps tendon down to the radial tuberosity and opening up the bursa to expose the bone. The radial recurrent artery, which here arises almost at the bifurcation of the brachial into radial and ulnar arteries, is cut to allow lateral retraction of brachioradialis and extensor carpi radialis longus and brevis. Supinator is incised from the tuberosity downwards and with the underlying periosteum is peeled off the radius laterally. By keeping deep to the periosteum the posterior interosseous nerve which runs through the muscle is protected.

D

Cross section of the left upper forearm, from below.

E

The same section, indicating the line of approach to the upper radius along the lateral side of the biceps tendon, followed by elevating supinator from the bone and turning it laterally. The periosteum is raised with the muscle to ensure protection for the posterior interosseous nerve which is embedded in the muscle.

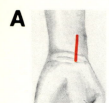

A

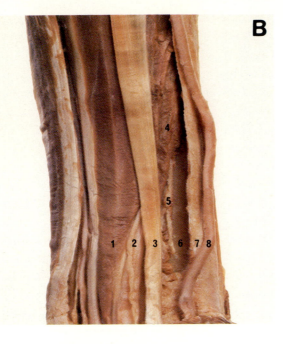

B

A
Incision line.

B
Lower left forearm, from the front. The radial artery is retracted laterally. Pronator quadratus is incised vertically lateral to flexor carpi radialis and flexor pollicis longus to expose the lower end of the radius. The median nerve lies medial to the tendon of flexor carpi radialis.

C
Cross section of the lower left forearm, from below.

D
The same section, showing the line of approach to the lower radius through the interval between the radial artery laterally and flexor carpi radialis and flexor pollicis longus medially, followed by stripping pronator quadratus off the bone in a medial direction.

1   Flexor digitorum superficialis
2   Median nerve and palmar branch
3   Flexor carpi radialis
4   Flexor pollicis longus
5   Pronator quadratus
6   Radius
7   Brachioradialis
8   Radial artery

C

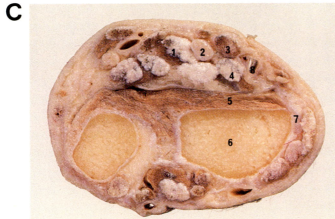

D

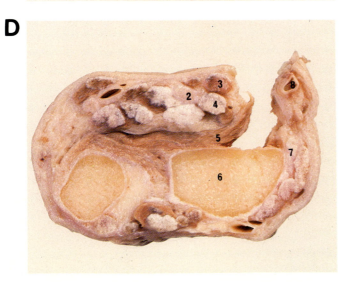

ULNA

Background

The posterior border of the ulna is subcutaneous throughout its length and easily palpable right down to the head and styloid process at the lower end. (Note that the head of the ulna is at the lower end; the head of the radius is at its upper end.) This border gives an aponeurotic origin to extensor carpi ulnaris, flexor carpi ulnaris and flexor digitorum profundus, with anconeus attached to the adjacent posterior surface at the upper end. Much of the front and side of the ulna is embraced by flexor digitorum profundus. Brachialis is attached to the coronoid process, while abductor pollicis longus, extensor pollicis longus and extensor indicis have origins from the posterior surface in that order from above downwards.

Since the posterior border of the ulna is subcutaneous, the bone is easily approached from the back.

Approach

A skin incision (E) is made along the line of the posterior border.

The periosteum is elevated and the aponeurotic origins of flexor carpi ulnaris and flexor digitorum profundus scraped off the bone and retracted medially; similarly for extensor carpi ulnaris which is retracted laterally (F and G).

Hazards and Safeguards

No major nerves or vessels are encountered near the posterior border. At the upper end the ulnar nerve passes deep to flexor carpi ulnaris.

E
Incision line.

F
Left forearm, from behind. The ulna is exposed by incising along the subcutaneous posterior border and raising the aponeurotic attachments of extensor carpi ulnaris, flexor carpi ulnaris and flexor digitorum profundus. At the top anconeus and its overlying fascia are lateral to the posterior border. The rest of the posterior border and the adjacent shaft are exposed by pushing extensor carpi ulnaris laterally, while on the medial side the fibrous attachments of flexor carpi ulnaris and flexor digitorum profundus (together with muscle fibres of the latter) are scraped off the bone.

G
Cross section of the upper third of the left forearm, orientated for comparison with F. The arrow indicates the incision line on the posterior border of the ulna.

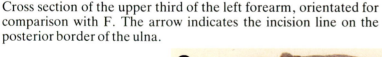

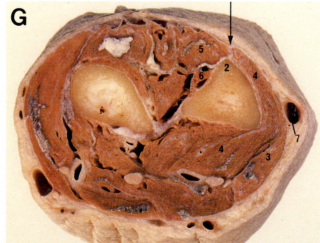

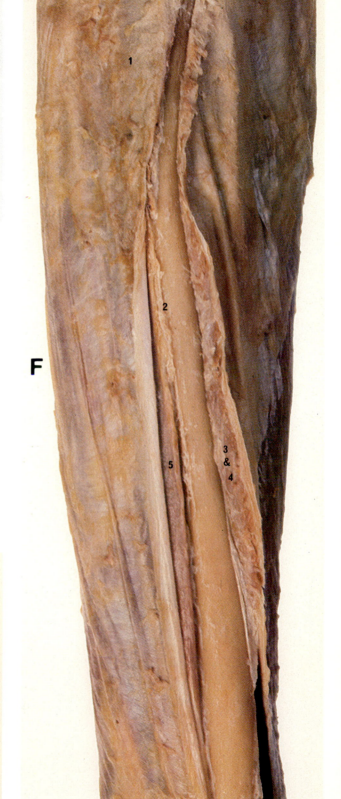

1 Fascia over anconeus
2 Posterior border of ulna
3 Flexor carpi ulnaris
4 Flexor digitorum profundus
5 Extensor carpi ulnaris
6 Extensor pollicis longus
7 Basilic vein

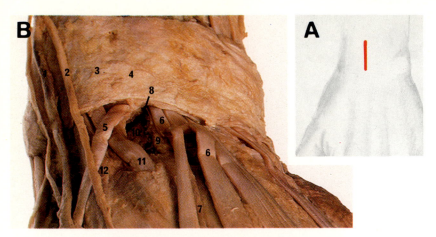

WRIST JOINT

Background

Numerous tendons, vessels and nerves cross the wrist joint, the level of which is indicated by a line drawn between the radial and ulnar styloid processes, both of which are easily palpable. On the flexor surface the tendon of flexor carpi radialis is the most prominent subcutaneous feature. The radial artery is on the radial side of this tendon, and it is here that the artery is compressed against the lower end of the radius to feel the pulse. The median nerve is on the ulnar side of the tendon and slightly overlapped from the ulnar side by the tendon of palmaris longus (but this muscle is absent in 13% of arms). The tendons of flexor pollicis longus, flexor digitorum superficialis and flexor digitorum profundus are more deeply placed and together with flexor carpi radialis and the median nerve pass into the hand deep to the flexor retinaculum. The tendon of flexor carpi ulnaris runs to the pisiform bone with the ulnar artery and ulnar nerve on the radial side of the tendon, the nerve being placed between the tendon and the artery.

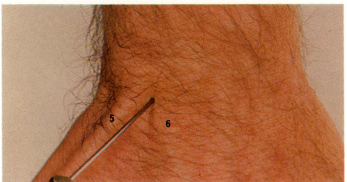

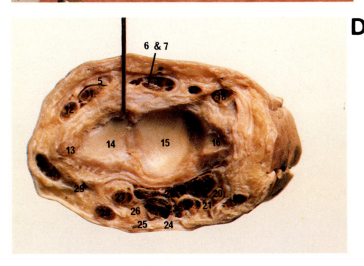

1	Cephalic vein	20	Ulnar nerve
2	Radial nerve	21	Ulnar artery
3	Extensor retinaculum	22	Flexor digitorum profundus
4	Position of dorsal tubercle	23	Flexor digitorum superficialis
5	Extensor pollicis longus	24	Flexor retinaculum
6	Extensor digitorum	25	Palmaris longus
7	Extensor indicis	26	Median nerve
8	Radius	27	Flexor pollicis longus
9	Capsule	28	Flexor carpi radialis
10	Lunate	29	Radial artery
11	Extensor carpi radialis brevis	30	Abductor pollicis longus
12	Extensor carpi radialis longus	31	Extensor pollicis brevis
13	Styloid process of radius	32	Palmar branch of 26
14	Surface for scaphoid on radius	33	Palmar branch of 20
15	Surface for lunate on radius	34	Brachioradialis
16	Surface on disc for triquetral	35	Palmar branch of 29
17	Extensor digiti minimi	36	Scaphoid
18	Extensor carpi ulnaris	37	First metacarpal
19	Flexor carpi ulnaris	38	Trapezium

A
Incision line on the dorsum.

B
Dorsum of the left wrist. The joint capsule is incised distal to the dorsal tubercle of the radius which is attached to the extensor retinaculum. The tendon of extensor pollicis longus changes direction by hooking laterally round the tubercle, and the capsule incision is made between that tendon and the tendon of extensor digitorum to the index finger. The tendon of extensor indicis is on the ulnar side of the digitorum tendon.

C
Puncture of the left wrist joint. The needle passes between the tendons of extensor pollicis longus and extensor digitorum.

D
Cross section of the left wrist joint, from below, showing the line for puncture.

On the radial side of the dorsal surface, the tendons of abductor pollicis longus and extensor pollicis brevis form the radial boundary of the anatomical snuffbox, with the tendon of extensor pollicis longus as its ulnar boundary. The tendons of extensor carpi radialis longus and brevis pass deep to extensor pollicis longus after the latter has hooked round the dorsal tubercle of the radius. Centrally the tendons of extensor digitorum and extensor indicis run on to the dorsum of the hand with the tendons of extensor digiti minimi and then extensor carpi ulnaris on the ulnar side. There are no major vessels or nerves on the dorsal surface.

The usual approach to the wrist joint is via the dorsal surface, on the ulnar side of the tendon of extensor pollicis longus. The anterior approach is hardly used except for the operative reduction of a dislocated lunate bone, but the first part of this approach forms the operation for decompression of the carpal tunnel (page 87); it involves incising the flexor retinaculum. The major hazard here is the proper identification of the median nerve from the adjacent tendons.

Posterior Approach

A longitudinal skin incision (A) is made on the back of the wrist above and below the level of the joint and medial to the dorsal tubercle of the radius.

The tendons of extensor digitorum and extensor indicis are displaced medially and the joint capsule exposed for incision on the ulnar side of the tendon of extensor pollicis longus (B).

Hazards and Safeguards

On the extensor surface of the wrist only minor vessels are involved in the incision line.

Puncture of the Wrist Joint

The joint is entered on the dorsal surface (C) between the tendon of extensor pollicis longus and the index finger tendon of extensor digitorum (a similar site to that for dorsal exposure of the joint).

The styloid process of the radius is palpated in the anatomical snuffbox as a guide to the line of the joint. The two extensor tendons are then palpated and the needle inserted between them in the line of the joint (C and D).

E
Incision line for scaphoid exposure.

F
Palmar surface of the left wrist. The scaphoid is exposed by opening the wrist joint capsule between the radial artery laterally and the tendon of flexor carpi radialis medially. The median nerve is on the ulnar side of the tendon. The palmar branch of the radial artery is here small and enters the thenar muscle mass; it may be larger and can lie superficial to the thenar muscles.

G
Incision line for trapezium exposure.

H
Left wrist, from the lateral side. The joint between the trapezium and the base of the first metacarpal is opened in the anatomical snuffbox behind the tendon of extensor pollicis brevis. The cephalic vein and radial nerve lie superficially in the snuffbox and are retracted backwards; the radial artery is in the floor.

E **F**

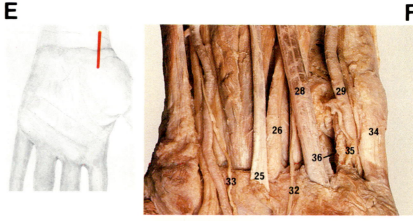

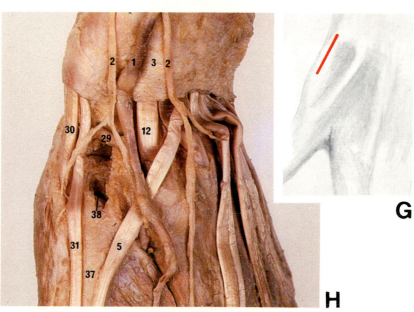

G

H

CARPAL BONES

Background
Of all the carpal bones, the scaphoid is the one most commonly fractured, while the lunate is the most liable to dislocation, but damage to any of the other carpal bones is possible. Many injuries can be successfully treated by manipulation but sometimes operation is required. As examples, approaches to the scaphoid (for the operative treatment of certain fractures) and to the trapezium (for its removal because of arthritic disease) are described here. (The lunate can be exposed through the anterior approach to the wrist joint.)

The scaphoid is approached from the front between the tendon of flexor carpi radialis and the radial artery, and the trapezium from the side through the anatomical snuffbox.

Approach to the Scaphoid
The tubercle of the scaphoid is palpated distal to the lower visible or palpable end of the flexor carpi radialis tendon, and a skin incision (page 69, E) is made upwards from the tubercle for 3 cm, between the flexor carpi radialis tendon medially and the radial artery laterally.

Retraction of these structures enables the scaphoid to be exposed by incising the capsule of the wrist joint (page 69, F).

Hazards and Safeguards
The radial artery and its palmar branch are on the radial side of the flexor carpi radialis tendon; the median nerve and its palmar branch are on the ulnar side of the tendon.

Approach to the Trapezium
With the forearm in the midprone position and the thumb uppermost, a skin incision (page 69, G) is made over the anatomical snuffbox immediately posterior to and parallel with the tendon of extensor pollicis brevis (which with abductor pollicis longus forms the radial boundary of the snuffbox).

The radial nerve and cephalic vein are retracted, and the radial artery and the base of the first metacarpal are identified so that the joint between the metacarpal and the trapezium can be opened (page 69, H).

Hazards and Safeguards
The radial nerve and cephalic vein lie superficially in the snuffbox, with the radial artery in the floor.

When manipulating the trapezium to remove it the tendon of flexor carpi radialis that lies in the groove on the bone must not be damaged.

BRACHIAL PLEXUS

Background
The brachial plexus is usually formed by the ventral rami of the fifth, sixth, seventh and eighth cervical nerves and first thoracic nerve, and can be described as having supraclavicular and infraclavicular parts.

The supraclavicular part consists of the roots and trunks of the plexus. The roots lie in the neck between scalenus anterior and scalenus medius, and the trunks are in the posterior triangle of the neck. These parts of the plexus can be explored by dissection in the posterior triangle.

The divisions of the plexus are behind the clavicle, and these give rise to the infraclavicular part which consists of the cords of the plexus and their branches. The three cords – lateral, medial and posterior – are arranged round the second part of the axillary artery according to their names.

The lateral cord gives off the lateral pectoral nerve and then divides into the musculocutaneous nerve and the lateral root of the median nerve.

The medial cord gives off the medial pectoral nerve, the medial cutaneous nerve of arm and the medial cutaneous nerve of forearm and then divides into the ulnar nerve and the medial root of the median nerve.

The posterior cord gives off the upper and lower subscapular nerves and the thoracodorsal nerve and then divides into the axillary and radial nerves.

A
Incision lines for supraclavicular (A) and infraclavicular (B) approaches.

B
Right brachial plexus in the posterior triangle. The fat in the lower part of the triangle, inferior belly of omohyoid and superficial vessels are removed and the fascial sheath of the plexus is being cut open.

C
Deeper dissection with the sheath opened. Scalenus anterior is being transected to give easier access to the lower part of the plexus. The phrenic nerve is retracted medially.

D
Infraclavicular part of the right brachial plexus. The deltopectoral groove is opened up by detaching part of pectoralis major from the clavicle (at operation it can simply be retracted medially). Pectoralis minor is divided and the axillary sheath opened to display the neural elements round the axillary artery.

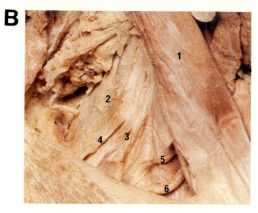

B

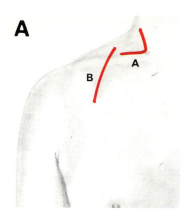

A

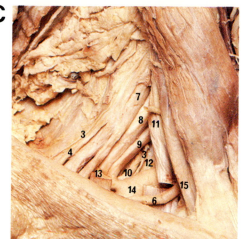

C

The cords and their branches, which include all the main nerves of the upper limb, can be displayed by opening up the axilla from below.

Approach to the Supraclavicular Part

An L-shaped skin incision (A) is made along the posterior border of sternocleidomastoid and 2 cm below the clavicle.

A triangular piece of skin (with the underlying platysma) is reflected and the external jugular vein is ligated above the clavicle.

The inferior belly of omohyoid and superficial cervical vessels are removed. Scalenus anterior is identified together with the roots of the plexus that lie between it and scalenus medius and which form the trunks of the plexus (B and C). The upper and middle trunks should be found easily; the upper trunk gives off the suprascapular nerve, a prominent branch arising from the junction of the fifth and sixth cervical ventral rami and which when followed proximally may be a useful guide to the upper trunk. To expose the lower trunk it may be necessary to transect scalenus anterior and detach part of sternocleidomastoid from the clavicle.

Hazards and Safeguards

When transecting scalenus anterior the phrenic nerve must be carefully preserved. The nerve lies deep to the prevertebral fascia and runs straight downwards, but since scalenus anterior passes not only downwards but *laterally* the nerve appears to cross the front of the muscle obliquely from lateral to medial side. The superficial cervical and suprascapular vessels lie superficial to the prevertebral fascia and cross the nerve transversely.

On the left the thoracic duct (and on the right the right lymphatic duct) also lie in front of the prevertebral fascia, crossing the phrenic nerve and running along the medial border of scalenus anterior to enter the junction of the internal jugular and subclavian veins.

Approach to the Infraclavicular Part

A skin incision (A) is made from the anterior border of trapezius above the clavicle, then down over the clavicle and along the line of the deltopectoral groove.

The deltopectoral groove is opened up to expose the pectoralis minor which is detached 1 cm from the coracoid process.

The axillary vessels and the cords of the plexus with their branches can then be dissected out from the fascial axillary sheath (D).

If a more proximal exposure is required the cephalic vein is ligated and the middle third of the clavicle stripped of attached muscles (pectoralis major and subclavius) and removed if necessary.

Hazards and Safeguards

The medial and lateral pectoral nerves are at risk when reflecting pectoralis minor. The *lateral* nerve from the lateral cord passes above the *medial* (upper) border of the muscle, while the *medial* nerve from the medial cord is related to the *lateral* (lower) border.

The axillary fascia is tough, and tributaries of the axillary vein may obscure nerves.

1	Sternocleidomastoid
2	Scalenus medius behind prevertebral fascia
3	Cut edge of sheath
4	Suprascapular nerve
5	Superficial cervical artery
6	Suprascapular artery
7	Upper trunk
8	Middle trunk
9	Eighth cervical ventral ramus
10	First thoracic ventral ramus
11	Scalenus anterior and phrenic nerve
12	Suprapleural membrane
13	Dorsal scapular artery
14	Subclavian artery
15	Internal jugular vein

16	Deltoid	26	Medial cutaneous nerve of arm
17	Cephalic vein	27	Medial cutaneous nerve of forearm
18	Clavipectoral fascia	28	Ulnar nerve
19	Lateral pectoral nerve	29	Median nerve
20	Pectoralis major	30	Axillary artery
21	Thoraco-acromial artery	31	Coracobrachialis and short head of biceps
22	Axillary vein	32	Musculocutaneous nerve
23	Lateral thoracic artery	33	Lateral cord
24	Pectoralis minor		
25	Medial pectoral nerve		

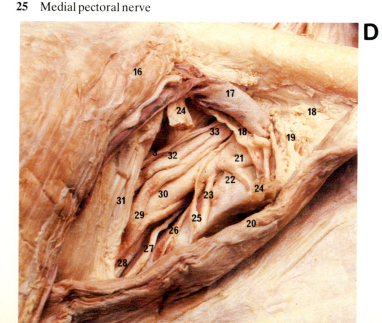

D

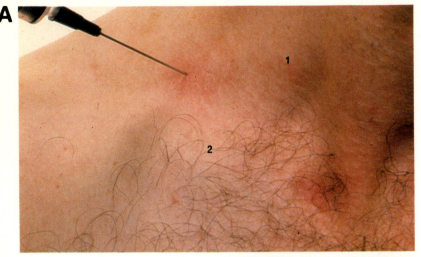

A

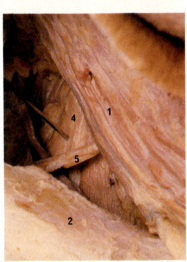

B

1 Sternocleidomastoid
2 Clavicle
3 Superficial cervical vessels
4 Sheath over brachial plexus
5 Omohyoid
6 Pectoralis major
7 Coracobrachialis
8 Biceps
9 Cut edge of axillary sheath
10 Median nerve

A
Supraclavicular brachial plexus block. The needle is passed for 2.5 cm from above the midpoint of the clavicle in the direction of the third thoracic spine.

B
Companion dissection for A. Fat in the posterior triangle is removed to show the needle just entering the sheath of the plexus (prevertebral fascia).

C
Axillary brachial plexus block. The axillary artery is palpated and the needle inserted just anterior to it.

D
Companion dissection for C. The front of the axillary sheath is being opened and the needle tip is adjacent to the median nerve which obscures the axillary artery. For a deeper dissection see page 74, D.

Brachial Plexus Block

The component parts of the brachial plexus and the subclavian and axillary vessels are enclosed in a connective tissue sheath (perivascular sheath) derived from the prevertebral fascia. Successful local anaesthesia can be obtained when the inside of the sheath is infiltrated with anaesthetic solution. In the supraclavicular approach the roots and trunks of the plexus are anaesthetized in the posterior triangle as they emerge between scalenus anterior and scalenus medius and pass towards the first rib. The axillary approach affects the cords of the plexus and the origins of individual nerves.

Supraclavicular Block

The needle is inserted 2 cm above the midpoint of the clavicle (A and B) and is directed downwards, medially and backwards in a line towards the third thoracic vertebral spine.

The tip of the needle reaches the first rib about 2.5 cm from the skin surface. The needle is withdrawn slightly and after aspiration to ensure it is not in a vessel the injection is made.

Alternative methods involve palpating the subclavian artery low in the posterior triangle and inserting the needle into the perivascular sheath there, or inserting it into the sheath higher up between scalenus anterior and scalenus medius, using the posterior border of sternocleidomastoid as the guide to the interscalene groove.

Hazards and Safeguards

The greatest danger in the first approach is pneumothorax caused by penetration of the needle into the pleural cavity through the suprapleural membrane above the first rib. The syringe must not be removed from the needle.

The subclavian vessels or their branches must not be damaged causing local haemorrhage or even haemothorax if the pleural cavity has also been entered.

Diffusion of the anaesthetic solution may rarely cause a block of the cervicothoracic (stellate) ganglion giving rise to Horner's syndrome (page 19), a block of the phrenic nerve or a block of the recurrent laryngeal nerve (but only on the right side, where this nerve loops round the subclavian artery; on the left it loops round the arch of the aorta).

Anaesthesia in the distribution of the ulnar nerve may not be satisfactory; the nerve receives its fibres from the lower three roots of the plexus (C7, 8 and T1) and diffusion of the solution may not reach the lowest levels.

Axillary Block

With the subject lying down, the arm is abducted to 90°.

The axillary artery is palpated and the needle inserted just anterior to it (C and D). Pulsation transmitted to the needle suggests that it is correctly placed within the sheath and after aspiration to ensure that the needle is not in a vessel the injection is made.

Finger pressure distal to the injection site (or a tourniquet on the upper arm close to the axilla) prevents the solution from diffusing down the arm.

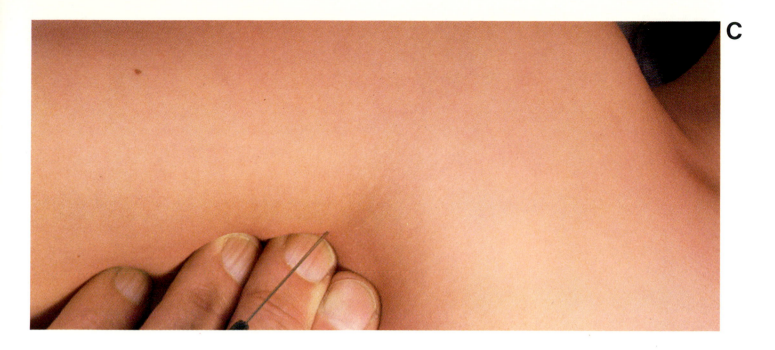

C

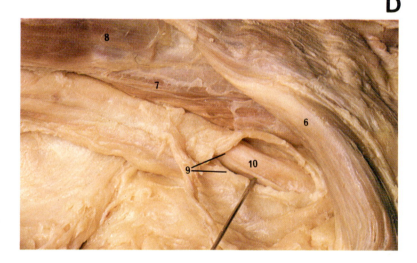

D

SUBCLAVIAN AND AXILLARY ARTERIES

Background

The left subclavian artery is a direct branch from the aortic arch but the right arises from the brachiocephalic artery. Each grooves the cervical pleura and the apex of the lung and crosses the first rib behind the attachment of scalenus anterior, which separates the artery from its companion vein lying in front of the muscle at a lower level. The muscle traditionally divides the artery into first, second and third parts – proximal to, behind and distal to the muscle respectively. At the outer border of the first rib the vessel becomes the axillary artery. The subclavian artery can be palpated in the root of the neck by pressing it against the first rib; with the shoulder depressed, the index and middle fingers are hooked over the clavicle downwards, backwards and medially in the angle between sternocleidomastoid and the clavicle.

The subclavian artery can be exposed in the root of the neck by detaching scalenus anterior from the first rib (but to display the origin on the left a thoracotomy is required).

The axillary artery is the continuation of the subclavian distal to the first rib, and the three parts lie in the axilla proximal to, behind and distal to pectoralis minor respectively. The lower part can be palpated in the axilla by pressing laterally against the humerus. The vessel (or its continuation the brachial artery) is a possible alternative to the femoral artery for arteriography (page 196). A catheter in the left axillary artery can be pushed into the aortic arch and often into the thoracic aorta (unless the origin of the subclavian is too acute).

The first part of the axillary artery can be exposed from the front by splitting the clavicular head of pectoralis major and going through the clavipectoral fascia. The second and third parts are approached from below through the axilla.

Hazards and Safeguards

The plexus in the axilla is perhaps more superficial than expected and the injection must not be too deep.

The tough axillary fascia envelops the nerves and vessels and can inhibit the diffusion of anaesthetic solution if the needle point is not entirely within the sheath, but with a needle inserted correctly the sheath ensures proper diffusion round the nerves. As much as 40 ml of solution may be required.

The axillary vessels may be pierced; aspiration before injection is essential to check that the needle is not in a vessel.

The axillary approach avoids the possibility of pneumothorax and other complications associated with supraclavicular approach, but the high origin of the musculocutaneous nerve (from the lateral cord) may mean that this nerve is not effectively blocked.

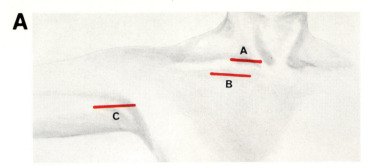

A

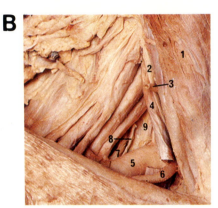

B

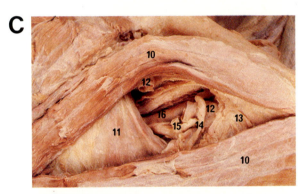

C

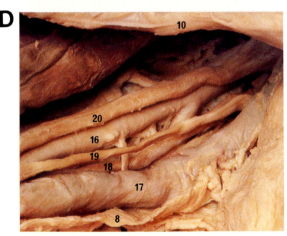

D

Approach to the Subclavian Artery

A skin incision (A) is made just above and parallel to the medial third of the clavicle, and is deepened to include platysma.

The clavicular head of sternocleidomastoid and the adjacent investing layer of deep cervical fascia are divided, and the fat in this lowest part of the posterior triangle is dissected to expose the prevertebral fascia overlying the phrenic nerve and scalenus anterior. The third part of the artery is seen lateral to the muscle (B).

The phrenic nerve is freed and displaced medially before incising scalenus anterior transversely above its rib attachment to reveal the second part of the artery behind it.

A more extensive exposure to show the continuity with the axillary artery can be obtained by removing part of the clavicle.

Hazards and Safeguards

The division of scalenus anterior must avoid damage to the underlying artery and other vessels. The suprascapular and superficial cervical arteries (from the thyrocervical trunk) and their accompanying veins cross scalenus anterior and the phrenic nerve superficial to the prevertebral fascia.

The internal jugular vein and (on the left) the thoracic duct are at the medial edge of scalenus anterior, and the phrenic nerve must be very carefully retracted.

The lower trunk of the brachial plexus is posterolateral to the artery, with the contribution from the first thoracic nerve crossing the first rib behind the artery.

Accidental damage to the lung and pleura must be avoided.

Approach to the First Part of the Axillary Artery

With the arm abducted to a right angle, a skin incision (A) is made just below and parallel to the medial half of the clavicle.

The clavicular head of pectoralis major is split in half in the line of its fibres and the edges separated to expose the clavipectoral fascia.

The axillary artery is palpated and the clavipectoral fascia and axillary sheath incised over the vessel (C).

Hazards and Safeguards

The axillary vein lies below and medial to the artery within the sheath, with the medial cord of the brachial plexus behind the artery and the posterior and lateral cords above it. To clear the artery the vein is displaced downwards and the parts of the plexus retracted upwards.

Branches of the thoraco-acromial vessels that cross the incision line may have to be ligated but the lateral pectoral nerve which pierces the clavipectoral fascia to enter pectoralis major should be preserved.

Approach to the Second and Third Parts

With the arm abducted to right angle, the artery is palpated above the posterior fold of the axilla and a skin incision (A) made over it. If there are no pulsations in the artery the incision line is the groove between coracobrachialis and the long head of triceps.

Pectoralis major and minor are retracted upwards and medially (and divided if necessary) to expose the axillary sheath.

The sheath is opened and the artery exposed on the lateral side of the axillary vein (D).

Hazards and Safeguards

The three cords of the brachial plexus (medial, lateral and posterior) are arranged round the second part of the artery according to their names, and are vitally important hazards when dissecting the axillary sheath which is a dense structure.

The subscapular artery may be followed upwards as a guide to the axillary artery.

MUSCULOCUTANEOUS NERVE

Background

The musculocutaneous nerve arises from the lateral cord of the brachial plexus and passes through coracobrachialis – a feature that confirms the proper identification of the nerve. After supplying that muscle, biceps and brachialis, it becomes superficial above the elbow at the medial border of biceps at the point where the muscular fibres become tendinous, and changes its name to the lateral cutaneous nerve of the forearm.

Damage to this nerve and the need to explore it are unusual, but it may need to be examined at its origin.

Approach

A skin incision (E) is made along the line of the deltopectoral groove, which is opened up to expose pectoralis minor.

Deep to pectoralis minor the lateral cord of the brachial plexus is identified and the musculocutaneous nerve dissected out (F).

Hazards and Safeguards

The lateral cord of the plexus lies on the lateral side of the second part of the axillary artery, deep to pectoralis minor. The musculocutaneous nerve is the large *lateral* branch of the cord; the large *medial* branch of the cord is the lateral root of the median nerve which passes medially on the surface of the artery. Occasionally a supernumerary root of the median nerve may branch off the musculocutaneous nerve at a lower level. The musculocutaneous nerve is identified by the fact that it enters the substance of coracobrachialis.

A

Incision lines for subclavian artery (A), first part of axillary artery (B) and second and third parts of axillary artery (C).

B

Right posterior triangle. Scalenus anterior is being transected to display the subclavian artery. The phrenic nerve is retracted medially.

C

Right infraclavicular region, with pectoralis major split and the clavipectoral fascia divided to show the first part of the axillary artery.

D

Right axilla, with the axillary sheath opened to show the artery and adjacent nerves.

E

Incision line for the musculocutaneous nerve.

F

Right infraclavicular region. The deltopectoral groove is opened up and the musculocutaneous nerve displayed below pectoralis minor and entering coracobrachialis.

1   Sternocleidomastoid
2   Phrenic nerve
3   Superficial cervical artery
4   Scalenus anterior
5   Subclavian artery
6   Suprascapular artery
7   First thoracic ventral ramus
8   Cut edge of sheath
9   Suprapleural membrane
10 Pectoralis major
11 Pectoralis minor
12 Cephalic vein
13 Clavipectoral fascia
14 Lateral pectoral nerve
15 Thoraco-acromial artery
16 Axillary artery
17 Axillary vein
18 Ulnar nerve
19 Medial cutaneous nerve of forearm
20 Median nerve
21 Musculocutaneous nerve
22 Lateral root of 20
23 Coracobrachialis

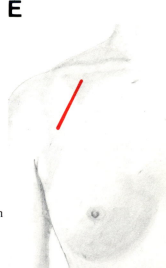

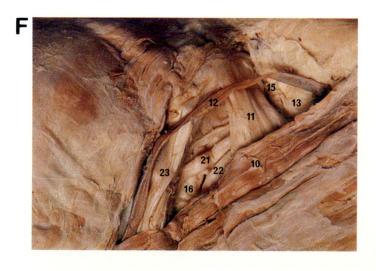

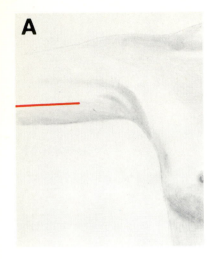

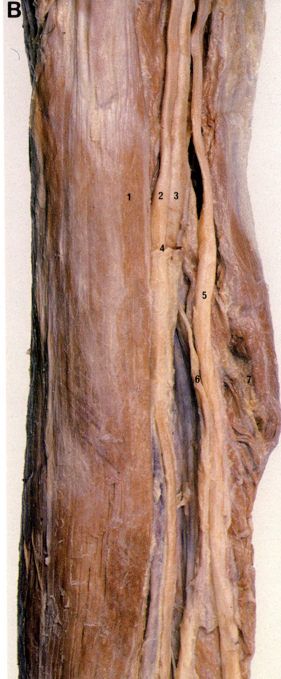

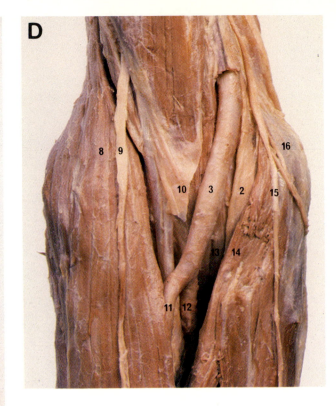

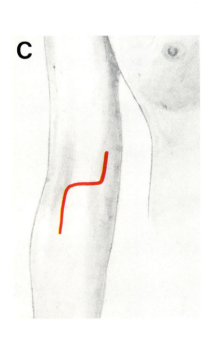

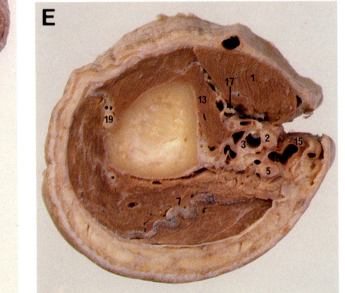

BRACHIAL ARTERY, MEDIAN NERVE AND ULNAR NERVE IN THE ARM

Background

The brachial artery is the continuation of the axillary artery and lies on the medial side of the arm under cover of the medial border of biceps. It is closely accompanied throughout its length by the median nerve which at the cubital fossa is on the medial side of the artery (which in turn is medial to the biceps tendon). The artery is normally palpable, but in the upper part of the arm pressure should be exerted in a *lateral* direction, not backwards, since the artery is medial to the humerus here. Lower down and especially in the cubital fossa, which is the usual site for palpating it, the vessel is in front of the humerus (brachialis intervening), and here backward pressure is satisfactory. The artery is the one used for taking the blood pressure. The cuff of the sphygmomanometer is inflated to stop arterial flow, and when listening for the appropriate sounds after slowly releasing the pressure in the cuff to allow flow to return, the stethoscope is placed over the artery in the fossa, the correct position being defined by palpation. The artery may also be punctured here as a possible site for catheterization for arteriography, passing the catheter through into the aortic arch, but the femoral artery is often the preferred site (page 196) since the incidence of thrombotic complications is greater in arm vessels which are usually smaller in diameter than those in the leg.

The ulnar nerve is on the medial side of the brachial artery in the upper part of the arm but lower down it enters the posterior compartment to become subcutaneous behind the medial epicondyle.

The median nerve slowly crosses in front of the brachial artery from lateral to medial side in its course down the arm and there are venae commitantes accompanying it. The basilic vein perforates the deep fascia from superficial to deep near the middle of the arm.

Approach in the Arm

With the arm abducted and the elbow extended, a skin incision (A) is made along the groove at the medial border of biceps, between biceps and triceps.

The deep fascia is divided and the groove opened up to display the neurovascular bundle embedded in connective tissue that is the continuation of the axillary sheath (B and E).

Hazards and Safeguards

After incising the deep fascia the vessels and nerves require careful dissection from their surrounding connective tissue: their relationships have been noted above.

Approach at the Elbow

For exposing the brachial artery and the median nerve, a skin incision (C) is made over the lower part of the brachial artery in the arm, continued laterally across a skin crease in the front of the cubital fossa and then downwards over the upper part of brachioradialis (i.e. an almost Z-shaped incision – it heals better than a longitudinal one that can lead to flexion contracture).

The superficial veins are ligated as necessary and the bicipital aponeurosis is divided to expose the artery (and its bifurcation into radial and ulnar vessels) at the medial side of the biceps tendon, with the median nerve on the medial side of the artery (D).

At the elbow the ulnar nerve is subcutaneous behind the medial epicondyle where it is easily exposed by an overlying incision.

Hazards and Safeguards

The pattern of superficial veins in the cubital fossa is variable (page 93) and they can be avoided or ligated as necessary.

The medial and lateral cutaneous nerves of the forearm lie deep to the superficial veins, although part of the medial cutaneous nerve above the elbow usually lies superficial to the basilic vein.

The most important structure adjacent to the artery at the elbow is the median nerve which is on the medial side of the artery; the biceps tendon is lateral to the artery (D).

Muscular branches of the nerve are not usually given off above the level of the elbow joint, but occasionally the nerve to pronator teres arises several centimetres above this level (as in B on page 60).

A

Incision line in the arm.

B

Right arm, from the front, with deep fascia, superficial nerves and veins removed. The upper part of the fascial sheath is removed but remains round the brachial vessels and median nerve lower down. The ulnar nerve passes behind the medial intermuscular septum to enter the posterior compartment.

C

Incision line at the elbow.

D

Right cubital fossa, with deep fascia and superficial veins removed. The bicipital aponeurosis is removed as part of the deep fascia to show the brachial artery medial to the biceps tendon, and the median nerve medial to the artery.

E

Cross section of the middle of the right arm, from below, with the incision line for exploring the neurovascular bundle.

1	Biceps	**11**	Radial artery
2	Median nerve	**12**	Ulnar artery
3	Brachial artery	**13**	Brachialis
4	Cut edge of sheath	**14**	Pronator teres
5	Ulnar nerve	**15**	Medial cutaneous nerve of forearm
6	Medial intermuscular septum		
7	Triceps	**16**	Medial epicondyle
8	Brachioradialis	**17**	Musculocutaneous nerve
9	Lateral cutaneous nerve of forearm	**18**	Basilic vein
		19	Radial nerve
10	Cut edge of bicipital aponeurosis		

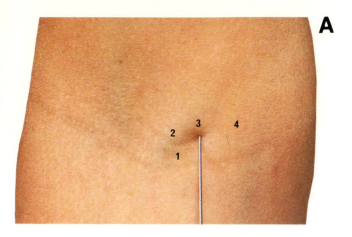

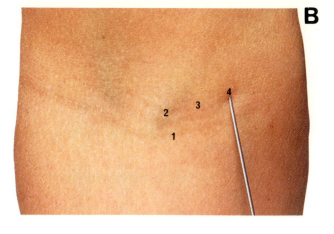

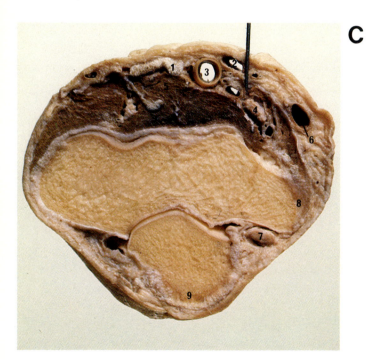

Puncture of the Brachial Artery

The artery is identified by palpation in the cubital fossa, on the medial side of the biceps tendon, and the needle is inserted on a line level with the medial and lateral epicondyles, avoiding any obvious superficial veins and also the median nerve which is on the medial side of the artery (A). The artery and nerve are both deep to the deep fascia.

Median Nerve Block at the Elbow

With the elbow extended the brachial artery is palpated in the upper part of the cubital fossa, medial to the biceps tendon.

The median nerve lies medial to the artery and the injection is made level with a line drawn between the medial and lateral epicondyles (B and C).

Hazards and Safeguards

Injection into vessels, particularly superficial veins, must be avoided. The median nerve is deep to the deep fascia.

Ulnar Nerve Block at the Elbow

With the elbow flexed to a right angle, the ulnar nerve is palpated as it lies behind the medial epicondyle, and the injection is made here into the surrounding tissue (D and E).

Hazards and Safeguards

With such a superficial nerve near bone, it is important not to transfix the nerve to the bone with the needle; as with other nerve blocks the object is to infiltrate the *surrounding* tissue.

A

Puncture of the right brachial artery. Pulsation in the artery is identified in the cubital fossa medial to the tendon of biceps (see page 76, C) and the needle is inserted here, avoiding superficial veins. In this arm there is a prominent median cubital vein.

B

Right median nerve block at the elbow. The brachial artery is identified by palpation medial to the tendon of biceps; the nerve lies medial to the artery.

C

Cross section of the right elbow, showing the site for median nerve block, medial to the brachial artery.

D

Right ulnar nerve block at the elbow. The nerve is palpable behind the medial epicondyle and the injection is made here, with the elbow flexed to a right angle.

E

Cross section of the right elbow, showing the site for ulnar nerve block behind the medial epicondyle.

1 Tendon of biceps
2 Median cubital vein
3 Brachial artery
4 Median nerve
5 Brachialis
6 Basilic vein
7 Ulnar nerve
8 Medial epicondyle
9 Olecranon

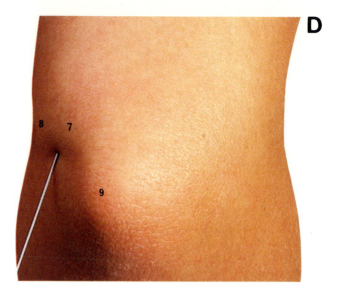

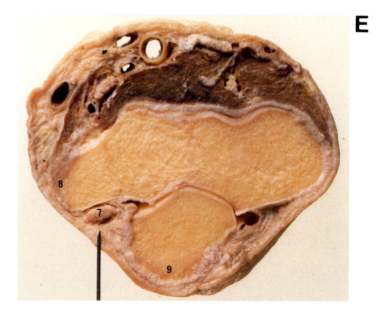

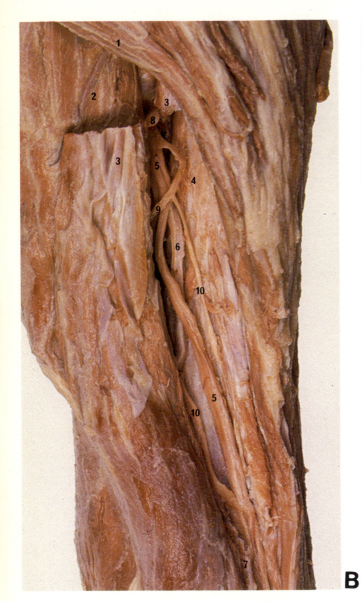

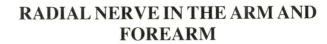

RADIAL NERVE IN THE ARM AND FOREARM

Background

The radial nerve, the largest branch of the brachial plexus, is the continuation of the posterior cord, and after leaving the axilla by crossing the tendon of latissimus dorsi and teres major it passes behind the humerus between the long and medial heads of triceps and under cover of the lateral head, crossing the upper end of the medial head obliquely from the medial to the lateral side to come into contact with the radial groove of the humerus. It is most commonly injured here by fractures of the bone. The nerve can be exposed from behind by separating the long and medial heads of triceps.

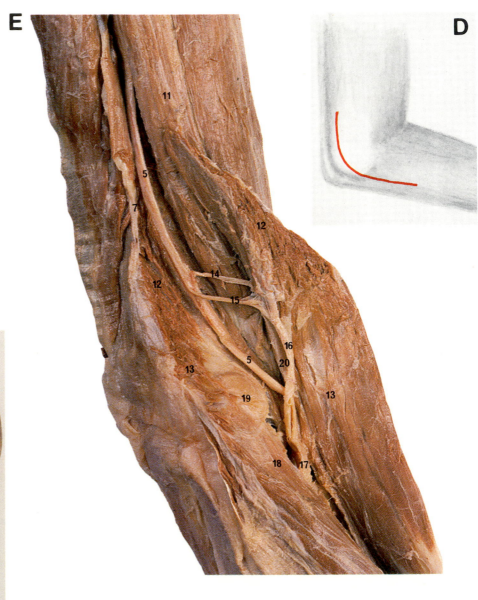

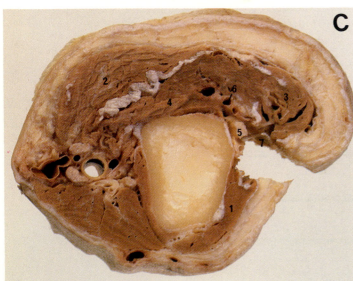

In the lower part of the arm it enters the anterior compartment by piercing the lateral intermuscular septum and comes to lie between brachialis and brachioradialis. Here it can be exposed from the front by opening up the groove between those two muscles, while from the back exposure can be obtained by detaching brachioradialis and extensor carpi radialis longus from the lateral supracondylar line of the humerus.

At the level of the lateral epicondyle of the humerus as it lies between brachialis and brachioradialis the radial nerve divides into its two terminal branches – the superficial branch which is only cutaneous in distribution, and the deep or posterior interosseous branch which is of great importance as the motor nerve to extensor muscles of the forearm and hand. The posterior interosseous nerve spirals backwards through the supinator muscle, and it can be exposed from behind by following down from the lower end of the radial nerve.

Approach to the Radial Nerve in the Arm

A skin incision (A) is made along the lower part of the posterior border of deltoid and continued down the lateral side of the arm.

The lateral head of triceps is reflected off the humerus to expose the radial nerve as it crosses the uppermost part of the medial head of triceps and comes to lie on the radial groove of the humerus (B and C).

The lower part of the nerve can be visualized by following the anterior border of brachioradialis; the nerve lies under cover of the muscle.

Hazards and Safeguards

As the radial nerve enters the arm from the axilla it is accompanied by the profunda brachii vessels.

The four branches of the radial nerve to triceps – to the long, medial, lateral and medial heads in that order from above downwards – are all given off before or as the nerve enters the radial groove of the humerus.

Approach to the Radial and Posterior Interosseous Nerves at the Elbow

A skin incision (D) is made over the lateral supracondylar line of the humerus and then from the lateral epicondyle for 10 cm along the posterior border of the extensor carpi muscles.

The origins of brachioradialis and extensor carpi radialis longus are detached from the humerus and turned forward to expose the radial nerve (E). Its posterior interosseous branch can be traced

downwards into supinator, whose superficial part can be incised if further exposure of the nerve is necessary.

Hazards and Safeguards

The radial recurrent artery passes upwards on the surface of supinator and gives off a number of muscular branches.

The radial nerve itself gives off branches to brachioradialis and extensor carpi radialis longus before the origin of the posterior interosseous branch (E).

A
Incision line for the radial nerve in the arm.

B
Right arm, from behind. The lateral head of triceps is transected and retracted medially to reveal the radial nerve crossing the uppermost part of the medial head, running in the radial groove of the humerus and then piercing the lateral intermuscular septum to enter the anterior compartment.

C
Cross section above the middle of the right arm, orientated for comparison with B. The radial nerve is deep to the gap opened up between deltoid and the lateral head of triceps and is still in the posterior compartment behind the lateral intermuscular septum.

D
Incision line for the radial nerve at the elbow.

E
Right elbow, from the lateral side. Brachioradialis and extensor carpi radialis longus are detached from the lateral supracondylar line of the humerus and turned forwards, showing the posterior interosseous nerve entering supinator.

1	Deltoid	11	Brachialis
2	Long head of triceps	12	Brachioradialis
3	Lateral head of triceps	13	Extensor carpi radialis longus
4	Medial head of triceps	14	Nerve to 12
5	Radial nerve	15	Nerve to 13
6	Profunda brachii artery	16	Radial recurrent artery
7	Lateral intermuscular septum	17	Posterior interosseous nerve
8	Nerve to 2	18	Supinator
9	Nerve to 3	19	Lateral epicondyle
10	Nerve to 4	20	Tendon of biceps

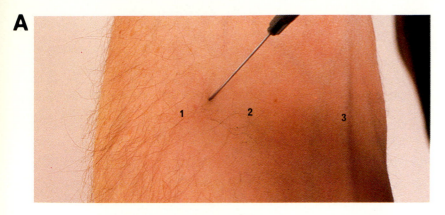

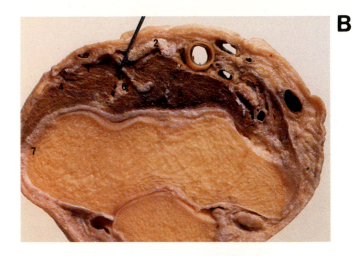

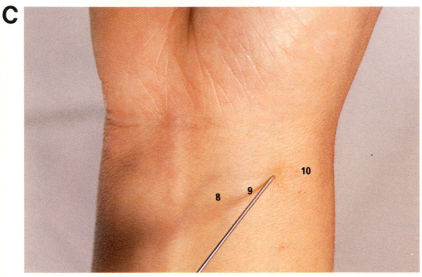

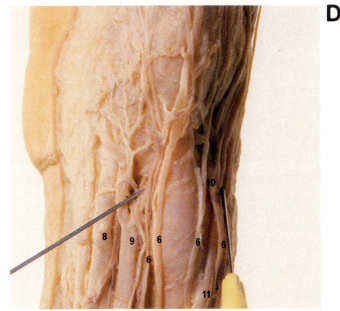

Radial Nerve Block at the Elbow

With the elbow extended the tendon of biceps is palpated in the upper part of the cubital fossa.

The needle is inserted between the biceps tendon and brachioradialis (which lies laterally) in the direction of the lateral epicondyle (A). The radial nerve is under cover of brachioradialis (B), and after the needle point has contacted bone it is withdrawn slightly and the injection made as withdrawal continues.

Hazards and Safeguards

The radial nerve is situated between brachialis and brachioradialis; the needle point should ideally find the plane between these two muscles (B).

Radial Nerve Block at the Wrist

Several subcutaneous injections are made at the level of the styloid process of the radius, beginning lateral to the tendon of flexor carpi radialis (C) and continuing on to the radial side of the dorsum.

Hazards and Safeguards

Multiple injections are necessary as the nerve at this level is not a single trunk but has divided into a sheaf of branches (D).

A
Right radial nerve block at the elbow. The needle is inserted lateral to the biceps tendon and in a lateral direction to infiltrate the nerve as it lies between brachialis and brachioradialis.

B
Cross section of the right elbow, showing the line of approach for radial nerve block.

C
Right radial nerve block at the wrist. Subcutaneous injections are made at the level of the radial styloid, beginning lateral to the tendon of flexor carpi radialis.

D
Right wrist, seen obliquely from the lateral side, showing numerous branches of the radial nerve which explain the necessity for multiple injections.

D

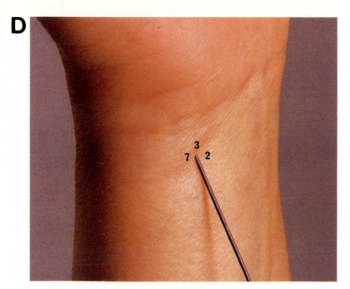

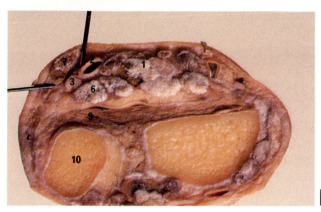

F

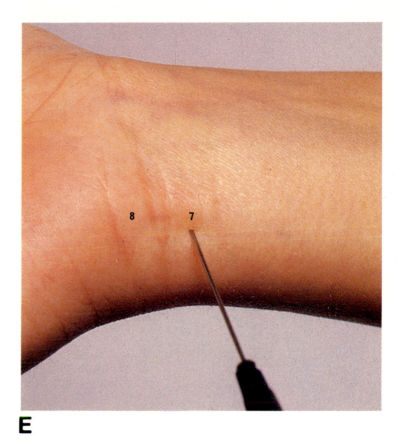

E

between the artery and the tendon (D and F).

An alternative approach is from the ulnar side of the wrist, introducing the needle *behind* the tendon (E and F).

Hazards and Safeguards

Aspiration must ensure that the needle is not in the artery or any other vessel.

A

Incision line.

B

Lower right forearm, from the front and ulnar side. Flexor carpi ulnaris is partly detached from the pisiform bone and retracted medially (at operation it is simply retracted) to show the ulnar artery and nerve, with the origins of the nerve's dorsal and palmar branches. These must be remembered when following the nerve upwards. The nerve is on the ulnar side of the artery.

C

Puncture of the right ulnar artery. The artery is entered on the radial side of the tendon of flexor carpi ulnaris.

D

Right ulnar nerve block at the wrist. The artery is palpated on the radial side of the pisiform and the flexor carpi ulnaris tendon, and the injection made between the artery and the tendon, the nerve being on the ulnar side of the artery.

E

Right ulnar nerve block at the wrist. An alternative approach to the nerve, passing *behind* the tendon of flexor carpi ulnaris from the ulnar side.

F

Cross section above the right wrist, showing the two approaches for ulnar nerve block.

1 Flexor digitorum superficialis
2 Ulnar artery
3 Ulnar nerve
4 Dorsal branch
5 Palmar branch
6 Flexor digitorum profundus
7 Flexor carpi ulnaris
8 Pisiform
9 Pronator quadratus
10 Ulna

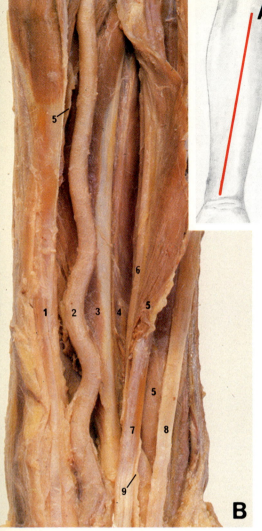

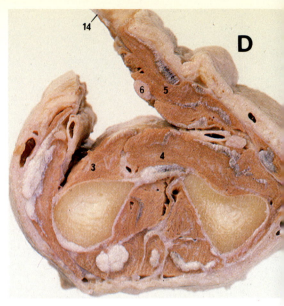

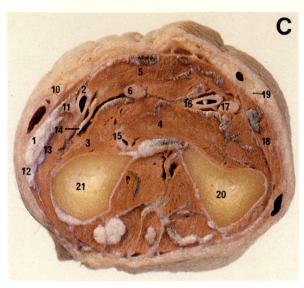

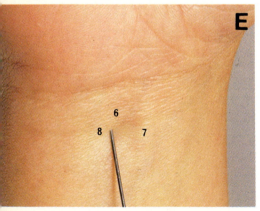

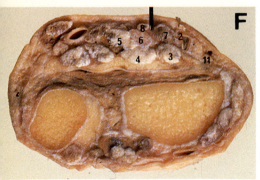

MEDIAN NERVE IN THE FOREARM AND HAND

A
Incision line for approach in the forearm.

B
Right forearm, from the front. The radial head of flexor digitorum superficialis is detached from the radius and turned over medially to show the median nerve adhering to the under surface of the muscle.

C
Cross section of the middle to the right forearm, from below.

D
The same section, with detachment of the radial head of flexor digitorum superficialis and showing the median nerve adhering to it.

E
Right median nerve block at the wrist. The injection is made on the ulnar side of the tendon of flexor carpi radialis.

F
Cross section of the right forearm above the wrist, from below, showing the injection site for median nerve block.

Background
After leaving the cubital fossa by passing deeply between the two heads of pronator teres, the median nerve runs down the forearm adhering by connective tissue to the deep surface of flexor digitorum superficialis. Above the wrist it becomes superficial by curving round the lateral border of that muscle. Before passing into the hand under the flexor retinaculum (through the carpal tunnel) it is overlapped from the ulnar side by the tendon of palmaris longus (if present), with the tendon of flexor carpi radialis on its radial side. Exposure or block of the nerve here is easy but it must be distinguished from the adjacent tendons. At a higher level the nerve can be visualized by detaching the radial head of flexor digitorum superficialis from the radius and turning the muscle over to see the nerve adhering to it. In the carpal tunnel the nerve may be subject to compression, usually because of swelling of the synovial sheaths of the flexor tendons that also lie beneath the retinaculum. Immediately distal to the retinaculum the nerve gives off the important muscular (recurrent or thenar) branch which usually supplies abductor pollicis brevis, flexor pollicis brevis and opponens pollicis, and then divides into various digital branches for the cutaneous supply of the radial three-and-a-half digits. Pressure on the nerve in the tunnel can be released by incising the retinaculum.

Approach in the Forearm
A skin incision (A) is made from the medial side of the biceps tendon in the cubital fossa and down the forearm along the line of the radius.

To expose the nerve in the middle of the forearm, the deep fascia is incised and the radial head of flexor digitorum superficialis is detached from the bone and turned over medially to show the nerve adhering to the under surface of the muscle (B, C and D).

Above the wrist the nerve is identified at the lateral border of the superficialis muscle, overlapped by the palmaris longus tendon (if present) and with the tendon of flexor carpi radialis on the radial side of the nerve.

Hazards and Safeguards

The distinction between the median nerve and the flexor tendons at the wrist has already been mentioned on page 68 but is so important that it is repeated below (under the Carpal Tunnel heading).

Median Nerve Block at the Wrist

With the wrist in extension, the needle is inserted at the level of the proximal skin crease at the wrist (level with the styloid process of the ulna), between the tendons of flexor carpi radialis lateral to the nerve and palmaris longus which if present partially overlaps the nerve from the ulnar side (E and F).

Hazards and Safeguards

After curving round the lateral border of flexor digitorum superficialis, the median nerve lies very close to the surface and must not be transfixed by the needle.

Approach in the Carpal Tunnel

A skin incision (G) is made in the palm along the proximal part of the curved skin crease at the base of the thenar eminence and continuing proximally as far as the distal skin crease of the wrist.

The palmar aponeurosis and the distal end of the flexor retinaculum are identified and incised longitudinally to expose the median nerve (H and J). A guide is passed proximally under the retinaculum so that the incision in it can be continued proximally. The incision line must be kept to the ulnar side of the median nerve and the palmaris longus tendon (if present) to avoid damaging the muscular branch of the nerve.

Alternatively the retinaculum can be incised from its proximal edge after carefully identifying the median nerve and keeping to its ulnar side.

Hazards and Safeguards

Above the wrist it is vitally important to distinguish the median nerve from the flexor tendons. The nerve at this level may resemble a tendon because it is flattened rather than round, but in the living body the nerve is normally whiter and has fine vessels on its surface. The tendon of flexor carpi radialis is on the radial side of the nerve and the tendon of palmaris longus slightly overlaps the nerve from the ulnar side. It must be remembered that palmaris longus is absent in 13% of arms.

The incision in the retinaculum is made on the *ulnar* side of the median nerve to avoid damage to the muscular (recurrent or thenar) branch which arises from the radial side of the nerve immediately distal to the retinaculum (H).

The palmar branches of the median and ulnar nerves both arise from their parent trunks about 5 cm proximal to the retinaculum, and both pass into the palm superficial to the retinaculum (H). An incision on the ulnar side of the median nerve should avoid both of them.

The superficial palmar arch is near the distal end of the incision (H).

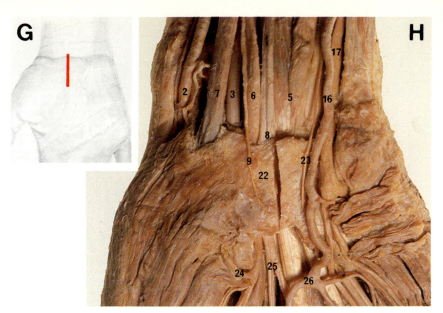

G
Incision line for approach in the carpal tunnel.

H
Right flexor retinaculum, incised along the ulnar side of the median nerve to avoid damage to the muscular branch to the thenar muscles which arises from the radial side of the nerve.

J
Cross section of the right wrist through the flexor retinaculum, from below.

1	Brachioradialis	17	Ulnar nerve
2	Radial artery	18	Flexor carpi ulnaris
3	Flexor pollicis longus	19	Medial cutaneous nerve of forearm
4	Flexor digitorum profundus		
5	Flexor digitorum superficialis	20	Ulna
6	Median nerve	21	Radius
7	Flexor carpi radialis	22	Flexor retinaculum
8	Palmaris longus	23	Palmar branch of 17
9	Palmar branch of 6	24	Muscular branch of 6
10	Lateral cutaneous nerve of forearm	25	Palmar digital branches of 6
11	Radial nerve	26	Superficial palmar arch
12	Extensor carpi radialis longus	27	Pisiform
13	Extensor carpi radialis brevis	28	Triquetral
14	Radial origin of 5	29	Surface for capitate on lunate
15	Anterior interosseous nerve and vessels	30	Scaphoid with surface for capitate
16	Ulnar artery		

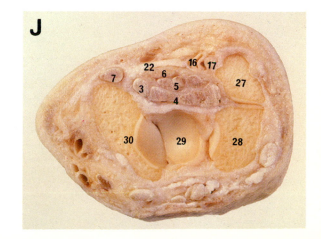

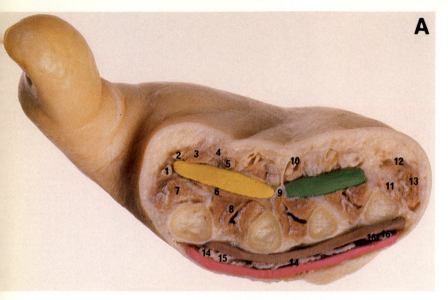

A

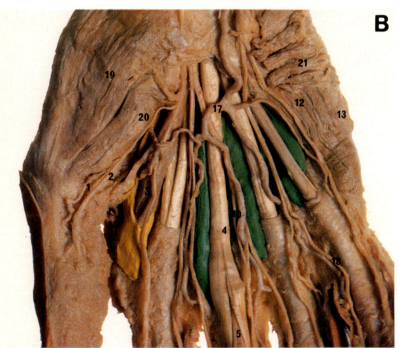

B

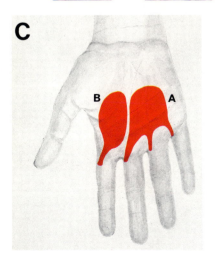

C

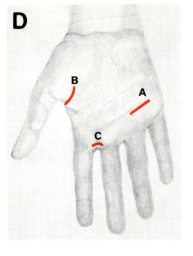

D

HAND SPACES, SYNOVIAL SHEATHS AND DIGITAL NERVES

Background

Antibiotic therapy has greatly reduced the incidence of severe hand infections, but when they do occur it may be necessary to make incisions to release accumulations of pus. The sites where pus collects are determined by the anatomy of the various fascial planes and tendon sheaths, and a number of 'spaces' are described; in the normal hand they are really planes rather than true spaces or gaps, and they only become defined with circumscribed boundaries when collections of pus develop. The synovial sheaths on the dorsum of the wrist (page 91, F) are not normally subject to infection.

Dorsal Subcutaneous and Subaponeurotic Spaces

The dorsal subcutaneous space (A) lies between the skin of the dorsum of the hand and the underlying flat extensor tendons. The subcutaneous tissue of the dorsum is very loose and readily becomes oedematous even from infections in the palm. The dorsal subaponeurotic space (A) is between the extensor tendons and the underlying metacarpals and interossei.

A

Cross section of the right hand, with coloured representations of some tissue spaces. Yellow: thenar space. Green: midpalmar space. Brown: dorsal subaponeurotic space. Red: dorsal subcutaneous space.

B

Palm of the right hand, with coloured representations of the thenar space (yellow) and the midpalmar space (green). Infections in the thenar space, largely hidden by the flexor tendons to the index finger and the first lumbrical, may invade the sheath of the first lumbrical, as indicated here by partial engulfment of the muscle. Infections in the midpalmar space may invade the other lumbrical canals.

C

Diagram of the midpalmar (A) and thenar (B) spaces.

D

Incision lines for draining the midpalmar space (A), the thenar space (B) and a web space (C).

1	Radialis indicis artery	11	Opponens digiti minimi
2	Palmar digital nerve	12	Flexor digiti minimi brevis
3	First lumbrical	13	Abductor digiti minimi
4	Flexor digitorum superficialis	14	Extensor digitorum
5	Flexor digitorum profundus	15	Extensor indicis
6	Adductor pollicis	16	Extensor digiti minimi
7	First dorsal interosseous	17	Superficial palmar arch
8	Other interossei	18	Palmar digital artery and nerve
9	Septum	19	Abductor pollicis brevis
10	Common palmar digital artery and nerve	20	Flexor pollicis brevis
		21	Palmaris brevis

Approach

Abscesses in the dorsal subcutaneous or subaponeurotic spaces are incised longitudinally over the area of pointing or maximal fluctuation.

Hazards and Safeguards

Apart from the dorsal venous arch and its tributaries there are no major vessels or nerves on the dorsum.

Damage to extensor tendons must be avoided.

Palmar Subaponeurotic Space

The palmar subaponeurotic space lies between the palmar aponeurosis and the long flexor tendons of the fingers. It contains the superficial palmar (arterial) arch and the various palmar digital vessels and nerves. There is no palmar *subcutaneous* space since in the centre of the palm the skin and aponeurosis are firmly adherent to one another but the skin can become infected via an entry wound to the subaponeurotic space.

Approach

An abscess in the palmar subaponeurotic space is drained by an incision in whichever skin crease lies over the site.

Hazards and Safeguards

Flexor tendons, the superficial palmar arch and the various palmar digital vessels and nerves are all at risk. In the more proximal part of the palm the vessels lie superficial to the nerves.

Midpalmar Space

The midpalmar space (A, B and C) lies deeply in the *medial* part of the palm, between the flexor tendons (within their synovial sheath) of the middle, ring and little fingers in front, and the third, fourth and fifth metacarpals and intervening interossei behind. Infection in the midpalmar space readily breaks through into the connective tissue sheaths of the adjacent lumbrical muscles (lumbrical canals), so that the space is usually considered to be continuous distally with the second, third and fourth lumbrical canals. The space is limited medially by the hypothenar muscle mass and laterally by a septum attached to the third metacarpal (see Thenar Space, below).

Approach

A transverse incision is made in the distal palmar skin crease from the third to the fifth metacarpal (D), and the midpalmar space can be entered on either side of the tendons to the ring finger.

An alternative approach is an extension of that used for the ulnar bursa (see below), or the web space between the middle and ring fingers can be incised longitudinally to enter the lumbrical canal of the ring finger.

Hazards and Safeguards

At about the level of the distal palmar skin crease the palmar digital vessels and nerves are beginning to change places, the nerves coming to lie superficial to the vessels.

The ring finger tendons are used as the guide to the space which can be entered on either side of the tendons.

Thenar Space

The thenar space (A, B and C) lies deeply in the *lateral* part of the palm, between the flexor tendons of the index finger and the first and second lumbricals in front, and the adductor pollicis behind. The space is continued distally in the connective tissue sheath of the first lumbrical (and occasionally in that of the second lumbrical as well). It is limited laterally by the thenar muscle mass and medially by a connective tissue septum that passes from the under surface of the palmar aponeurosis round the radial side of the mass of flexor tendons to the fingers to reach the front of the shaft of the third metacarpal. This septum separates the thenar and midpalmar spaces.

Approach

A curved incision is made parallel and medial to the distal end of the metacarpophalangeal thumb crease, extending distally to the thumb web (D). The space is entered in front of the distal border of adductor hallucis.

An alternative approach is by a short longitudinal or transverse incision on the *dorsal* surface of the thumb web, entering the space over the distal border of adductor hallucis.

Hazards and Safeguards

The palmar digital branch of the median nerve to the thumb is at risk in the curved incision. The incision must be kept well clear of the curved palmar thumb crease to avoid damage to the muscular (recurrent) branch to the thenar muscles.

Web Spaces

The three interdigital web spaces are between the bases of the fingers and therefore between the digital slips of the palmar aponeurosis. They contain the superficial and deep transverse metacarpal ligaments, a lumbrical muscle, and palmar digital vessels and nerves embedded in loose fatty tissue. Although the web spaces contain a lumbrical muscle, web infections do not usually break through into a lumbrical canal to involve the midpalmar space.

Approach

Infections of the web spaces are drained by a short transverse incision made parallel and just proximal to the edge of the web (D).

Hazards and Safeguards

Digital vessels and nerves may be at risk. At this level in the hand the nerves lie superficial to the vessels.

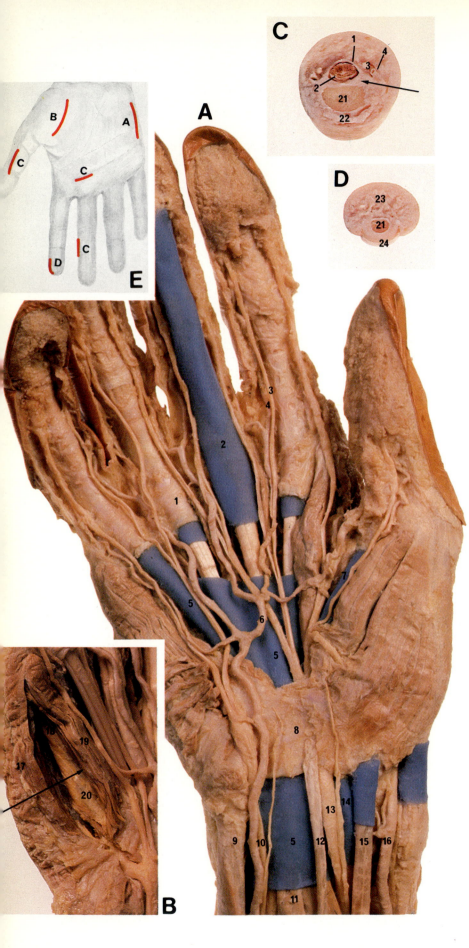

A

Wrist and palm of the right hand, with synovial sheaths (blue). The fibrous flexor sheath of the middle finger is removed to show the whole length of the synovial sheath. The synovial sheath of flexor pollicis longus continues proximally as the radial bursa and that of the little finger as the ulnar bursa, which also incorporates the other finger tendons in the *palm* but not in the index, middle or ring *fingers* where the sheaths usually remain separate.

B

Ulnar side of the right hand, showing the approach line (arrow) to the ulnar bursa between flexor and abductor digiti minimi with detachment of opponens from the fifth metacarpal.

C

Cross section of the proximal phalanx of the right index finger. The main digital arteries and nerves lie alongside the fibrous flexor sheath; the nerve is anterior to the artery. The arrow indicates the line of incision for entering the synovial sheath, dorsal to the nerve and vessels.

D

Cross section of the distal phalanx of the index finger, showing the pulp.

E

Incision lines for draining the ulnar bursa (A), radial bursa (B), a digital synovial sheath (C) and a pulp space (D).

F

Wrist and dorsum of the right hand, with synovial sheaths (blue). The sheaths envelop the tendons as they pass beneath the extensor retinaculum but they do not extend far distally.

1	Fibrous sheath	19	Flexor digiti minimi brevis
2	Synovial sheath	20	Fifth metacarpal
3	Palmar digital nerve	21	Phalanx
4	Palmar digital artery	22	Extensor expansion
5	Ulnar bursa	23	Pulp
6	Superficial palmar arch	24	Nail
7	Radial bursa	25	Abductor pollicis longus
8	Flexor retinaculum	26	Extensor pollicis brevis
9	Flexor carpi ulnaris	27	Cephalic vein
10	Ulnar artery and nerve	28	Radial nerve
11	Flexor digitorum superficialis	29	Sheath for extensor carpi radialis longus and brevis
12	Palmaris longus		
13	Median nerve	30	Extensor retinaculum
14	Flexor pollicis longus and 7	31	Extensor pollicis longus
15	Flexor carpi radialis	32	Extensor digitorum
16	Radial artery	33	Extensor indicis
17	Abductor digiti minimi	34	Extensor digiti minimi
18	Opponens digiti minimi	35	Extensor carpi ulnaris

Ulnar Bursa

The ulnar bursa (A) is the name given to the combined synovial sheath for all the finger tendons in the palm. It extends proximally under the flexor retinaculum, and distally it is continuous with the synovial sheath of the flexor tendons of the little finger (see below).

Approach

A skin incision (E) is made on the anterolateral side of the fifth metacarpal.

Abductor and flexor digiti minimi are separated to expose opponens digiti minimi which is detached from the fifth metacarpal (B). The bursa can now be entered in front of the metacarpal.

Since the bursa is continuous with the synovial sheath of the little finger, an additional incision is made on the radial side of the little finger (see below) to ensure through-and-through drainage.

Hazards and Safeguards

This approach from the side but in front of the fifth metacarpal enables the infected bursa to be entered without the risk of damaging the palmar vessels and nerves. The bursa will have been opened before the tendons of the little finger are reached but the approach can be extended deep to these tendons to enter the mid-palmar space if necessary.

Radial Bursa

The radial bursa (A) is the name given to the proximal part of the synovial sheath of the flexor pollicis longus tendon. Like the ulnar bursa it extends proximally under the flexor retinaculum and in about 10% of hands it communicates here with the ulnar bursa.

Approach

A skin incision (E) is made on the thenar eminence about 2 cm on the radial side of the curved skin crease at the base of the eminence, and the bursa entered.

Since the bursa is continuous with the synovial sheath of the thumb an additional incision is made on the thumb (see below).

Hazards and Safeguards

The incision must not extend proximally to less than 2 cm beyond the flexor retinaculum, to avoid damage to the muscular (recurrent) branch of the median nerve. This branch arises immediately the parent trunk emerges beneath the distal edge of the retinaculum and curves laterally to enter the thenar muscle mass (page 87, H).

Digital Synovial Sheaths

The synovial sheaths of the flexor tendons of the fingers and thumb lie inside the relatively much tougher fibrous flexor sheaths (A and C). The fibrous sheaths are thinnest or even deficient over the finger flexion creases; these are therefore the likeliest sites for a pinprick to set up a synovial sheath infection. On the index, middle and ring fingers the synovial sheaths extend for a few millimetres proximal to the ends of the fibrous sheaths (level with the heads of the metacarpals). This is the weakest part of the sheath and if distended with pus it may burst here, so infecting the lumbrical canals and through them the midpalmar and thenar spaces. The synovial sheath of the thumb is continuous with the radial bursa. The synovial sheath of the flexor tendons of the little finger is continuous with the ulnar bursa; the sheaths of the ring, middle and index fingers usually remain separate but occasionally any one or even all of them may communicate with the ulnar bursa.

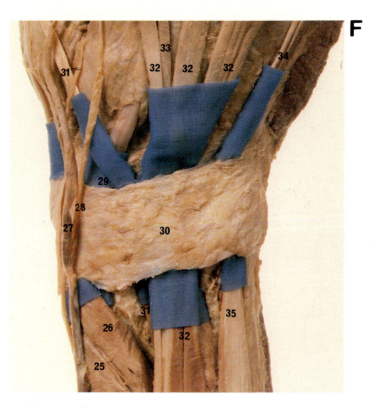

F

Approach

For opening an infected synovial sheath of a finger, two incisions (E) are required so that the sheath can be opened at each end; a single opening will not provide sufficient drainage for this tubular structure.

The distal skin incision is made on the radial side of the middle phalanx (C and E), on a line level with the dorsal ends of interphalangeal joint skin creases. (Alternatively a transverse incision can be made along the distal crease.) The tough fibrous sheath is incised in the same line to expose the bulging synovial sheath which can then be opened.

The proximal skin incision is made transversely opposite the base of the finger in the distal palmar crease (or in the equivalent position in the case of the index finger, to which the distal crease does not extend). The bulging proximal end of the synovial sheath is then opened.

For entering the synovial sheath of the thumb, the skin and sheath incisions are made on the lateral side of the proximal phalanx, in a corresponding position to those made on the fingers.

Hazards and Safeguards

At the side of the finger the incision line lies dorsal to the palmar digital nerve and vessels, which should thus be avoided (C).

In the palm similar vessels and nerves will also be at risk, but the bulging of the infected synovial sheath which extends proximal to the end of the fibrous sheath will indicate where it should be incised.

As the little finger and thumb synovial sheaths are continuous with the ulnar and radial bursae respectively, either of these may have to be opened up as well (see above).

Pulp Spaces

The pulp spaces (page 90 D) are on the palmar side of the tips of the fingers and thumb. They contain fatty tissue that is divided into numerous compartments by fibrous septa that pass between the terminal phalanx and the skin. Terminal branches of the palmar digital vessels course distally through the space and some of them supply most of the terminal phalanx; infection and death of the bone may follow their occlusion. The pulp space is limited proximally by the firm adherence of the skin of the distal flexion crease to the underlying tissue, so that pulp infection does not spread proximally along the finger.

Approach

An incision is made on the radial side of the finger tip and may be curved in a hockey-stick fashion on to the tip but avoiding extension on to the normal tactile area of the finger pad (page 90 E).

The knife is then passed transversely through the pulp to break through the numerous septa that connect the phalanx with the skin.

Hazards and Safeguards

The division of the pulp into small compartments by connective tissue septa means that when infection is present care must be taken to ensure that *all* the affected pockets are opened up.

Subungual Spaces

The subungual space lies deep to the base of the nail, and is continuous with the tissue of the nail fold at the sides and base of the nail. Infection in the nail fold (paronychia) can thus spread beneath the nail to form a subungual abscess, and this can only be drained by removing the proximal part of the nail.

Approach

For a paronychial abscess a longitudinal incision is carried proximally in the line of the lateral nail fold.

For a subungual abscess the proximal part of the nail is removed.

Hazards and Safeguards

When the proximal part of a nail requires to be removed, the distal part should be left in situ to keep covered as much as possible of the sensitive nail bed.

Digital Nerves

Although the nerves of each digit – dorsal and palmar on each side – can be blocked by a 'ring infiltration' that completely encircles the base of the digit, this method is not usually recommended because of the danger of inducing spasm in the arteries and causing ischaemic damage.

The preferred technique is to infiltrate the tissues in the distal part of the palm where the common palmar digital nerve divides into the proper palmar digital nerves, or to use a dorsal approach at the finger base.

Digital Nerve Block

For the palmar approach, the needle is inserted proximal to the web space level with the distal palmar crease (A) to infiltrate the tissues before the palmar digital nerve reaches the finger (B).

For the dorsal approach, the needle is inserted at the side of the digit immediately proximal to the web margin (C), and the tissue over the extensor expansion is infiltrated to anaesthetize the dorsal digital nerve. The needle tip is then directed towards the palm just distal to the web margin, to block the palmar digital nerve. The procedure is repeated on the opposite side of the digit.

Hazards and Safeguards

A completely circumferential infiltration of the base of the digit is avoided by the above methods, but the injection of too much solution may still cause the arterial constriction that the methods were designed to avoid.

A
Digital nerve block of the right index finger, showing the injection site for infiltration of the palmar digital nerve of the ulnar side of the finger.

B
Distal part of the right palm. The infiltration affects the palmar digital nerve *before* it reaches the finger.

C
Digital nerve block of the right index finger from the dorsal surface.

1	Palmar digital nerve	4	Flexor digitorum superficialis
2	Palmar digital artery	5	Flexor digitorum profundus
3	First lumbrical		

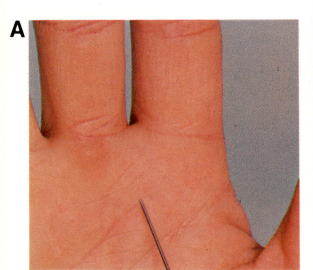

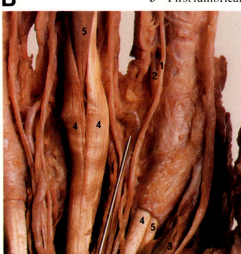

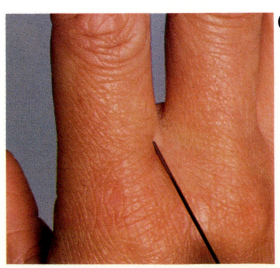

SUPERFICIAL VEINS OF THE UPPER LIMB

Background

From a dorsal venous network on the back of the hand (D), the cephalic and basilic veins emerge to run superficial to the deep fascia on the radial and ulnar sides respectively of the front of the forearm. They are commonly joined in the front of the cubital fossa by a median cubital vein to give an approximately H-shaped pattern of major vessels. A common variation is seen when there is a median forearm vein which bifurcates in front of the cubital fossa giving median cephalic and median basilic vessels that join the cephalic and basilic veins respectively, so forming an M-shaped pattern, but there can be many other variations (E). The lateral cutaneous nerve of the forearm and its branches are usually deep to the neighbouring veins but branches of the medial cutaneous nerve of the forearm are often superficial to veins. The cephalic vein continues up the arm to the deltopectoral groove and then pierces the clavipectoral fascia just below the clavicle to enter the axillary vein. The basilic vein perforates the deep fascia near the middle of the upper arm and runs upwards medial to the brachial artery, being joined by its venae commitantes and becoming the axillary vein at the lower border of the axilla.

1   Cephalic vein
2   Radial nerve
3   Dorsal venous network
4   Basilic vein
5   Lateral cutaneous nerve of forearm

D
Superficial veins of the right wrist and dorsum of the hand. On the radial side, the cephalic vein begins in the anatomical snuffbox as a continuation of the dorsal venous network.

E
Superficial veins of the front of the right elbow. Here the cephalic and basilic veins are joined by a median cubital vein into which a median forearm vein drains.

6   Tendon of biceps
7   Brachial artery under fascia
8   Median cubital vein
9   Median forearm vein
10   Medial cutaneous nerve of forearm
11   Medial epicondyle

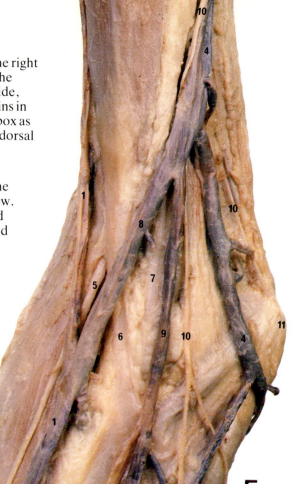

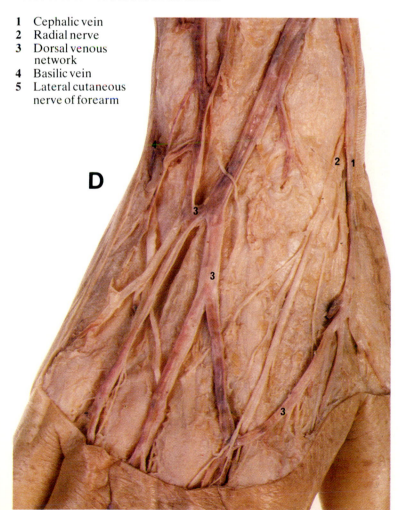

Approach

For venepuncture (taking specimens of blood, giving transfusions or injecting drugs such as anaesthetic solutions), any of the above hand or forearm veins can be used as convenient; those on the dorsum of the hand or in the region of the cubital fossa are most commonly used. Being subcutaneous they can usually be entered easily when distended by a temporary tourniquet, unless they are unusually small or obscured by fat. For prolonged use (e.g. many hours of transfusion), insertion of the needle at sites where the veins cross elbow flexion creases should be avoided if at all possible, otherwise the limb will have to be immobilised in extension which is uncomfortable for prolonged periods.

Hazards and Safeguards

The needle point should not be allowed to perforate the oppostie side of the vein and produce a possibly painful haematoma, and it must not perforate the deep fascia.

The brachial artery at the level of the cubital fossa is protected by being deep to the bicipital aponeurosis which separates the artery from the overlying median cubital vein or similar vessel, but a high division of the brachial artery may give rise to a subcutaneous radial or ulnar artery in the cubital fossa that must be distinguished from veins by its pulsation. The normal brachial artery is medial to the tendon of biceps, with the median nerve medial to the artery.

THORAX

THORACIC WALL

Background

The heart within the pericardial sac, the lungs within their pleural sacs, the great vessels, oesophagus, thymus and the sympathetic trunks are structures that may require surgical attention within the thorax. Access can be obtained through intercostal spaces or by stripping the periosteum from a rib and going through the bed of the rib (anterolateral and posterolateral thoracotomy depending on the extent of the incision), or through an anterior midline approach by splitting the whole sternum vertically (anterior thoracotomy, median sternotomy). With suitable retraction of ribs or the cut edges of the sternum surprisingly wide access to thoracic contents can be obtained, and the anatomy of these approaches is described below, together with some examples of dealing with specific structures within the thorax. The relatively simpler procedures of removing fluid from the pleural and pericardial cavities are also considered, as is the important topic of cardiac massage.

Intercostal Drainage

Through a wheal of local anaesthesia that includes the whole thickness of the chest wall including the pleura, a suitable needle (or trocar and cannula) is inserted into the posterolateral chest wall (A and B) in the posterior axillary line in an appropriate interspace (frequently the eighth or ninth), depending on the level of fluid as revealed radiologically.

For more permanent drainage through an in-dwelling tube, a short portion of rib is removed after elevating it from its periosteal sleeve, and the tube is inserted through the bed of the rib.

Hazards and Safeguards

The posterior intercostal vessels and intercostal nerve lie in the costal groove along the lower border of the rib at the *upper boundary* of the intercostal space (A). They will be avoided if the needle or trocar is inserted close to the rib at the *lower boundary* of the space (B), but the instrument must not be too far back near erector spinae because here the vessels are in the *middle* of the space and only reach the costal groove farther laterally.

Median Sternotomy

A skin incision is made from the jugular notch of the manubrium to just below the xiphoid process, and is deepened to include the periosteum of the sternum.

The attachment of the diaphragm to the xiphoid process is divided, and the tissues on the deep surface of the sternum are freed from it by blunt dissection from above and below, using a finger introduced from above the jugular notch and below the xiphoid process.

The sternum is split vertically in the midline with a sternal saw, and the cut edges are retracted laterally (see D on page 67) and held apart by an appropriate type of retractor.

Hazards and Safeguards

The edges of the pleural sacs, which are adjacent from second to fourth costal cartilage levels, should be defined. The right pleural sac may extend across the midline (as in D, page 97) and may be entered when separating tissues from the back of the sternum. The so-called sternopericardial ligaments that attach the fibrous pericardium to the sternum vary greatly in density.

Bleeding from the cut edges of the sternum is controlled by bone wax.

Anterolateral and Posterolateral Thoracotomy

The lateral approach to structures within the thorax often involves a combination of anterolateral and posterolateral incisions depending on the amount of access required, and one is easily extended into the other.

For anterolateral thoracotomy the patient lies on the back but tilted obliquely with supports under the appropriate shoulder and hip.

A skin incision (C) is made in the line of the chosen rib, usually the fifth or sixth, from the midline to the midaxillary line but curving below the breast in the female. Pectoralis major is divided in the line of the skin incision together with part of rectus abdominis and serratus anterior.

For posterolateral thoracotomy the patient lies on the opposite side and with the arm of the affected side abducted.

The skin is incised in a curved line following the required rib from near the midline posteriorly to beyond the midaxillary line (C). Trapezius and latissimus dorsi are incised in the line of the skin incision, exposing rhomboid major and serratus anterior which are in turn divided.

The periosteum of the chosen rib is incised longitudinally along the middle of the rib and then stripped off the upper half of its front and back (A). The periosteal bed is then incised through to the pleural cavity and a rib spreader inserted.

Hazards and Safeguards

The required rib must be properly identified by counting down from the second at the level of the manubriosternal joint.

Traction to spread ribs may stretch the intercostal nerve and vessels of the space entered. The vessels can be ligated and the nerve deliberately cut to avoid a traction injury but this may not be considered necessary. Stripping the periosteum immediately *above* a rib rather than below it reduces the risk of injury to the main intercostal nerve; the collateral branch that runs along the upper border of a rib is very small and can be ignored.

An incision in serratus anterior may involve the long thoracic nerve which supplies the muscle but it may have to be sacrificed to give adequate exposure.

A
Right intercostal muscles, vessels and nerves, in a stepped dissection. The vessels and nerves are between the second and third layers of muscles. The periosteum is being stripped off the upper part of the seventh rib.

Thoraco-abdominal Incision

Used on the appropriate side for providing wide upper abdominal exposure, e.g. to the kidney, spleen, liver and cardio-oesophageal junction.

With the patient slightly tilted towards the opposite side and with the arm flexed, a skin incision (C) is made in the line of the ninth intercostal space from the midaxillary line to the lateral border of the rectus sheath level with the umbilicus.

The anterior edge of latissimus dorsi, serratus anterior and external oblique are incised, followed by incision of the intercostal muscles above the ninth rib (or incision through the bed of the rib). The pleura is incised to enter the pleural space and reveal the diaphragm (D).

A short length of the ninth costal cartilage at the costal margin is removed.

The diaphragm is incised and the incision continued into the anterior abdominal wall and peritoneum, and the wound edges are widely retracted.

Hazards and Safeguards

For approaching the cardio-oesophageal junction on the left, the diaphragm is incised radially in the direction of the oesophageal hiatus; otherwise the diaphragm should be incised near its peripheral attachment to ribs and costal cartilages. Radial or peripheral incisions are the least likely to damage the motor innervation from the branches of the phrenic nerves which fan out from their points of entry at the oesophageal and vena caval openings.

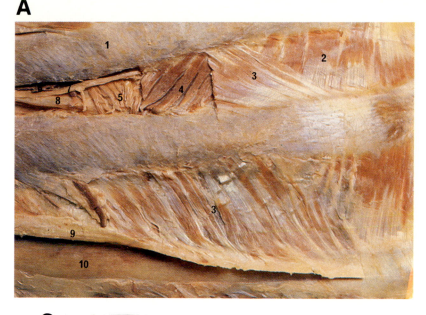

A

1 Fifth rib
2 Anterior intercostal membrane over 4
3 External intercostal
4 Internal intercostal
5 Innermost intercostal
6 Intercostal vessels
7 Intercostal nerve
8 Pleura
9 Periosteum
10 Seventh rib

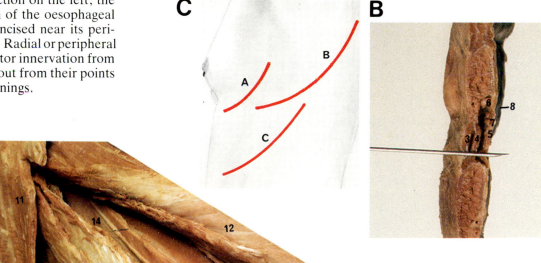

B

Cross section of ribs and intercostal muscles, showing the route for draining the pleural sac with the needle *above* a rib, so avoiding the vessels and nerves that run along the upper border of an intercostal space.

C

Incision line for anterolateral thoracotomy (A), posterolateral thoracotomy (B) and thoraco-abdominal incison (C).

D

Right thoraco-abdominal incision in the eighth intercostal space. The pleural cavity is entered and then the diaphragm incised to enter the peritoneal cavity.

11 Latissimus dorsi
12 External oblique
13 Intercostal muscles
14 Diaphragmatic pleura
15 Diaphragm
16 Peritoneum
17 Liver
18 Ninth costal cartilage

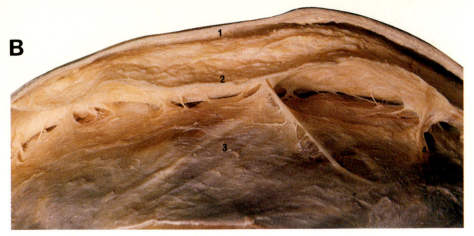

B

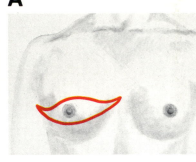

A

1 Skin
2 Mammary gland
3 Fascia over
  pectoralis major
4 Mammary branch
  of intercostal vessel

BREAST

Background

The female breast (mammary gland) extends from the second to fourth ribs and from the midline to the midaxillary line, two thirds of it overlying pectoralis major and one third over serratus anterior, with the lower margin contacting the upper end of the rectus sheath and external oblique. It lies in the superficial fascia (being a modified sweat gland) but the axillary tail penetrates below it to lie adjacent to the anterior and central groups of axillary lymph nodes. About 15-20 lactiferous ducts from the lobules of breast tissue converge on the nipple, which is surrounded by the areola. The shape and bulk of the non-lactating breast depend on the amount of adipose tissue, not on variations in the number of potential secretory elements, though these proliferate in pregnancy, when the areola also enlarges and becomes more deeply pigmented. The pigment fades after childbirth but the enlarged areola remains as a sign of a previous pregnancy. The blood supply of the breast comes from penetrating branches of the upper four anterior intercostal arteries, with others from the lateral thoracic and thoraco-acromial vessels. The lymphatic drainage is of the greatest importance in view of the high incidence of carcinoma of the breast, and the essentials are simple: the lateral parts tend to drain to axillary nodes and the medial parts drain through the upper intercostal spaces to internal thoracic nodes. Complications arise because normal channels may become blocked by disease or treatment and more extensive spread may result: to the opposite breast, to cervical nodes, into the peritoneum through the rectus sheath, or even to inguinal nodes through the subcutaneous tissues of the abdominal wall.

The rudimentary male breast consists of little more than the nipple and areola, but it must be remembered that 1% of breast cancers occur in males, in whom lymphatic spread is early and extensive.

Cysts or other benign breast lesions can be removed by local excision, but for carcinoma a variety of procedures can be used depending on the extent of the disease. Simple mastectomy implies removal of all breast tissue and may be extended to include removal of axillary fat and lymph nodes, while in radical mastectomy the nodes and fat are removed with pectoralis minor and perhaps pectoralis major as well, although the extent of muscle removal is a controversial issue. However much tissue is removed, the object is to remove it all as a single mass in order to eliminate as far as possible any contamination of the operation site by cancer cells that might escape from cut lymphatic channels or diseased tissue.

Approach

For most mastectomies, elliptical skin incisions (A) are made transversely or slightly obliquely towards the axilla, above and below the nipple and from near the midline to the anterior fold of the axilla.

For simple mastectomy, upper and lower skin flaps are raised off the breast tissue, and then the breast tissue itself is stripped off the pectoral fascia overlying pectoralis major (B), from the level of the second costal cartilage downwards and laterally. The axillary tail and the lateral part overlying serratus anterior and latissimus dorsi are freed, together with axillary fat and nodes.

For more radical procedures, pectoralis minor can be removed to assist in clearing the axilla, or pectoralis minor and major can both be removed.

Hazards and Safeguards

Skin is closely attached to breast tissue especially in thin individuals, and care must be taken not to perforate the skin flaps.

In the axilla the intercostobrachial nerve (lateral cutaneous branch of the second intercostal nerve) will be cut when clearing fat and lymph nodes, but the long thoracic nerve (to serratus anterior) and the thoracodorsal nerve (to latissimus dorsi) must be carefully preserved (they are shown on page 109), together with all the other branches of the brachial plexus in the axilla. If both pectoral muscles are being removed there is obviously no need to keep the pectoral nerves, but if pectoralis major remains then the lateral pectoral nerve which pierces the clavipectoral fascia at the upper border of pectoralis minor must be preserved so that at least part of the muscle retains a nerve supply.

The cephalic vein is preserved if the clavipectoral fascia is removed but tributaries of the axillary vein are ligated as necessary (but not the vein itself). Major branches of the axillary artery such as the subscapular are retained.

Removal of axillary nodes interferes with the lymphatic drainage of the upper limb, and a variable amount of oedema may occur.

THYMUS

Background

The thymus lies in the superior and anterior mediastinum, behind the sternum and in front of the aorta and the three branches of its arch (the brachiocephalic, left common carotid and left subclavian arteries), with the left brachiocephalic vein between these branches and the thymus. Although it normally undergoes considerable involution after puberty, a persistent thymus in the adult may be expected to extend from the level of the fourth costal cartilage upwards to the lower poles of the thyroid gland. It lies behind the pretracheal fascia and may appear to be approximately H-shaped, but in fact it consists of two unequal-sized lobes, each of which receives a branch from the corresponding internal thoracic artery and perhaps from the inferior thyroid artery also. Thymic veins drain mainly into the left brachiocephalic vein but others may reach internal thoracic or inferior thyroid vessels.

Removal of the thymus (thymectomy) may be required because of tumour or as part of the treatment of myasthenia gravis. While an approach through the lower part of the neck may be possible, a wider exposure (described below) is obtained by splitting the sternum; this gives easier access and is necessary if there is enlargement of the organ.

Approach

The thorax is opened through a median sternotomy (page 94) (C).

Fatty retrosternal tissue is cleared to expose the pretracheal fascia that covers the thymus anteriorly.

The fascia is divided and the thymus separated from it and from the pericardium and great vessels behind (D). The organ is removed after the ligation of appropriate vessels.

Hazards and Safeguards

The thymus can be distinguished from fat in being slightly browner or pinker in colour, with lobules that are larger, smoother and denser than fat.

Haemorrhage must be carefully controlled, especially from veins. Thin-walled veins are easily torn, including the left brachiocephalic vein.

The phrenic nerves must not be damaged when clearing extrapleural fat, especially when the anterior part of the pericardium is being removed as well (as when dealing with a malignant thymic tumour).

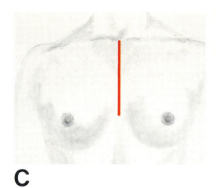

C

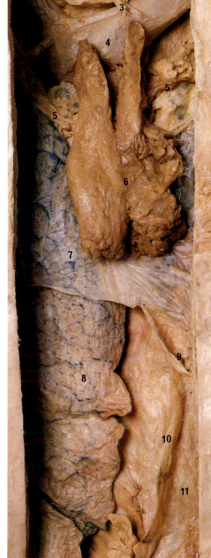

1 Right brachiocephalic vein
2 Right internal thoracic vein
3 Inferior thyroid vein
4 Left brachiocephalic vein
5 Thymic vein
6 Thymus
7 Pleura
8 Lung
9 Cut edge of left pleural sac
10 Cut edge of right pleural sac
11 Pericardium

D

A
Incision lines.

B
Right breast being elevated from the fascia over pectoralis major, showing some mammary vessels entering the deep surface of the gland.

C
Incision line for median sternotomy.

D
The thymus exposed after removal of the pretracheal fascia. In this dissection part of the right pleura has also been removed to emphasise that the right pleural sac has extended across the midline.

HEART

Background

The heart within its pericardial sac lies between the body of the sternum in front and the middle four thoracic vertebrae (fifth to eighth) behind. The greater part is to the left of the midline, with the apex and apex beat in the left fifth intercostal space about 9 cm from the midline. Much of the anterior (sternocostal) surface is right ventricle, with the right atrium forming the right border of the heart (underlying the third to the sixth costal cartilages at the right sternocostal margin), and the left ventricle forming most of the left border with the auricle of the left atrium at the upper end of this border (which runs from the second left costal cartilage at the sternocostal margin to the apex). The inferior border is mostly right ventricle with left ventricle at the apex, and this border is level with the xiphisternal joint. The base of the heart is its *posterior* surface (not the region where the great vessels are attached), and is formed by the left atrium with pericardium separating it from the oesophagus. The inferior surface formed by the ventricles is the diaphragmatic surface.

At the upper part of the heart viewed from the front, the superior vena cava, ascending aorta and pulmonary trunk are found in that order from the right to left. The pulmonary trunk divides under the arch of the aorta into right and left pulmonary arteries. The two pulmonary veins on each side run into the left atrium. The ligamentum arteriosum (or ductus arteriosus if it remains patent) runs from the upper surface of the left pulmonary artery to the under surface of the aortic arch. The right coronary artery arises from the front of the ascending aorta to run down the right atrioventricular groove; its origin is easily seen. The origin of the left coronary artery is behind the pulmonary trunk and so obscured by it when looking from the front; the artery continues as the circumflex branch in the atrioventricular groove posteriorly and gives off the anterior interventricular (descending) branch which is easily seen in the anterior interventricular groove and is the coronary vessel most commonly affected by arterial disease.

The position of the heart between the fixed vertebral column and the somewhat resilient sternum enables the heart to be squeezed in cases of cardiac arrest by rhythmic pressure on the lower sternum (external cardiac massage). Many operations on the heart and great vessels are carried out through a median sternotomy after opening the front of the pericardium but others require a left thoracotomy, including emergency internal cardiac massage.

In order to carry out operations inside the chambers of the heart (open heart surgery), e.g. to repair septal defects or replace diseased valves with artificial ones, blood must be diverted from the heart to be artificially oxygenated in a machine and then pumped back into the body so that circulation can be maintained. This is done by collecting venous blood from the superior and inferior venae cavae, passing it into an oxygenator and then pumping the warmed oxygenated blood into the aorta (or into a femoral artery so that the blood can run upwards into the aorta). This whole procedure is technically known as cardiopulmonary bypass, and it provides an 'extracorporeal circulation'; the apparatus is commonly called a heart-lung machine.

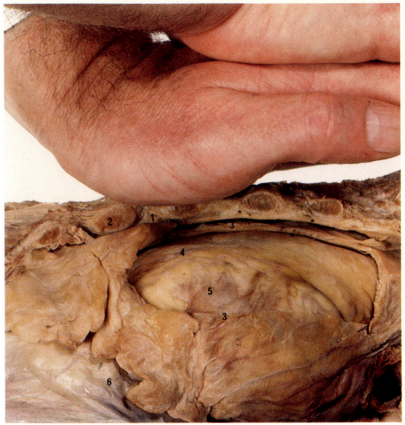

A

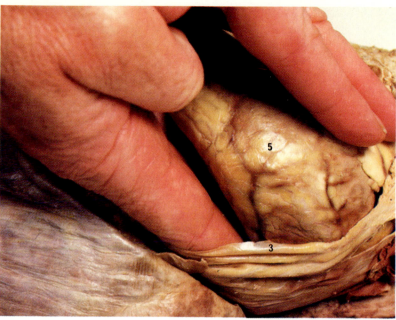

B

An indication of the routes by which some of the commoner cardiac operations are carried out is given below, and the anatomy of cardiac transplantation is also included.

External Cardiac Massage

Pressure is applied over the lower third of the sternum using the base of the palm of the outstretched hand, with the opposite hand on top to give added pressure (A).

The pressure is applied rhythmically at a rate of 70 per minute to simulate the normal heart rate, and should depress the sternum by 3–5 cm each time (relatively less in children), squeezing the ventricles between the sternum and the vertebral column and so maintaining blood circulation.

The respiratory failure which accompanies cardiac arrest should be treated by mouth-to-mouth ventilation.

Hazards and Safeguards

Over-enthusiastic pressure on the sternum has been known to cause fracture of ribs (especially in the elderly) and bruising of the liver.

Approach for Internal Cardiac Massage

The thorax is opened by a left anterolateral thoracotomy through the fourth or fifth interspace (page 94).

The pleura and pericardium are opened in front of the phrenic nerve and a hand is inserted behind the left ventricle so that the heart can be squeezed rhythmically against the fingers of the other hand placed in front of the ventricles (B).

Hazards and Safeguards

Since this procedure is taking place in an operating theatre, the accompanying respiratory problems can be dealt with by the anaesthetist.

A

External cardiac massage, demonstrated on a dissected left side of the thorax. The *lower* end of the sternum is rhythmically depressed, squeezing the ventricles between the sternum and the vertebral column.

B

Dissection showing the principle of internal cardiac massage, squeezing the ventricles between both hands.

1 Lower end of sternum
2 Sixth costal cartilage
3 Cut edge of pericardium
4 Right ventricle
5 Left ventricle
6 Diaphragm

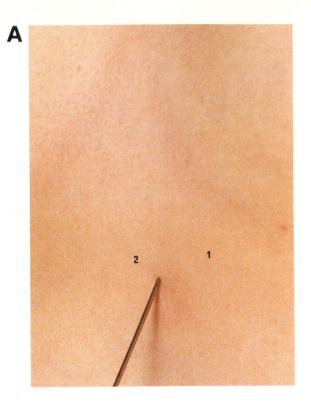

A

Pericardial Drainage

Through a wheal of local anaesthesia the needle is inserted in the angle between the xiphoid process and the left costal margin (seventh costal cartilage) (A), and is directed upwards, backwards and slightly medially through the central tendon of the diaphragm into the pericardial cavity (B).

For more permanent drainage by an in-dwelling tube, a transverse incision is made over the fifth costal cartilage. The perichondrium is incised and the cartilage resected. The internal thoracic vessels are divided and the pericardium is opened through a transverse incision in the bed of the cartilage.

Hazards and Safeguards

It is usually possible to feel when the needle passes through the diaphragm. If cardiac contractions are felt by the needle tip the needle is withdrawn slightly. The lung and the internal thoracic vessels should lie too far lateral to be damaged by this approach.

With open drainage after resecting the fifth costal cartilage, the left pleural cavity must not be entered.

Anterior Approach to the Heart

The thorax is opened by a median sternotomy (page 94).

The pericardium is incised using a vertical, cruciate or inverted T incision, the upper end of the longitudinal cut extending as high as the origin of the brachiocephalic artery (C).

Hazards and Safeguards

As for median sternotomy (page 94).

Any remains of the thymus can be divided vertically (between the two lobes), and particular care must be taken to avoid damage to the left brachiocephalic vein running obliquely across the three large arteries (brachiocephalic, left common carotid and left subclavian) that arise from the aortic arch, and to the phrenic nerves at each side.

Cardiopulmonary Bypass

After opening the thorax and pericardium through a median sternotomy, a cannula is passed upwards into the superior vena cava through an incision in the lateral wall of the right atrium, and another passed downwards into the inferior vena cava (D). The cannulae are held in position by ligatures on the outside of the vessels. (Alternatively, both cannulae may be inserted through the auricle of the right atrium, or even directly through the walls of the venae cavae themselves if it is desirable to avoid cannulae going through the atrial wall.) Through these cannulae venous blood is collected for delivery to the oxygenator.

A cannula is passed into the arch of the aorta proximal to the origin of the brachiocephalic artery (D). Through this cannula the warmed oxygenated blood is pumped into the aorta. Some of this blood will of course pass down into the ascending aorta and so get into the coronary arteries through their orifices just above the aortic valve cusps (which are kept closed by the pressure of the aortic blood).

A
Pericardial drainage, viewed from the left and in front. The needle passes between the xiphoid process and the seventh costal cartilage in an upward, backward and slightly medial direction.

B
Left half of a median sagittal section of the lower anterior part of the thorax, from the right, with a needle inserted for pericardial drainage.

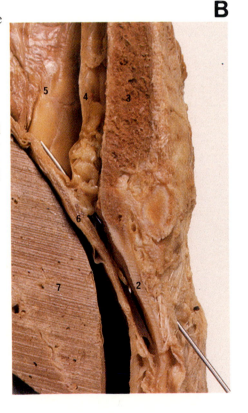

B

1 Seventh costal cartilage
2 Xiphoid process
3 Body of sternum
4 Pericardium
5 Right ventricle
6 Diaphragm
7 Liver

Hazards and Safeguards

Any atrial incisions must avoid the sinuatrial node, which is in the atrial and auricular wall just below the entry of the superior vena cava.

Some Open Heart Operations

As examples of operations that can be carried out on the heart and great vessels after setting up cardiopulmonary bypass, the following may be mentioned:

To repair atrial septal defects, the right atrium is entered by incising along its right border.

To repair ventricular septal defects, the right ventricle is incised either vertically or transversely.

For open operations on the mitral valve, the left atrium is entered *from the right* through an incision immediately behind the interatrial groove and in front of the two right pulmonary veins. (For closed operations on the mitral valve, see page 102.)

For operations on the aortic valves, the ascending aorta is opened vertically up to near the origin of the brachiocephalic artery. Coronary cannulae are passed into the orifices of the coronary arteries so that the myocardium can be adequately perfused.

For coronary artery bypass, a length of great saphenous vein from the lower leg can be anastomosed by one end to the ascending aorta and by the other end to the blocked vessel distal to the site of obstruction. Care must be taken to turn the vein graft upside down so that any valves within it do not obstruct the new arterial flow.

For pulmonary embolectomy (removal of emboli from the pulmonary trunk and right and left pulmonary arteries), the pulmonary trunk is opened by a vertical incision extending from above the pulmonary valve to the division of the trunk into the two arteries. Emboli can then be removed with forceps and by suction. In emergency the operation can be performed without cardiopulmonary bypass, using intermittent occlusion of the venae cavae.

Hazards and Safeguards

Incisions in the right atrium must avoid the sinuatrial nodal area below the superior vena cava.

Incisions in the right ventricle must avoid obvious major branches of the coronary arteries and cardiac veins.

C

The heart from the front, after opening the pericardium.

D

Diagram for cardiopulmonary bypass.

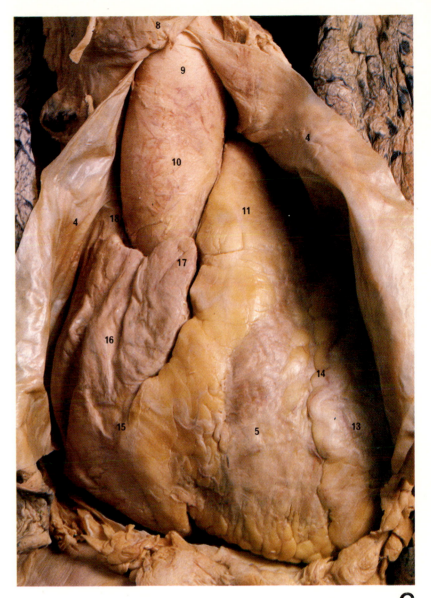

C

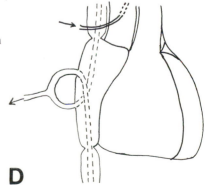

D

8	Left brachiocephalic vein
9	Arch of aorta
10	Ascending aorta
11	Pulmonary trunk
12	Auricle of left atrium
13	Left ventricle
14	Anterior interventricular branch of left coronary artery in interventricular groove
15	Right coronary artery in atrioventricular groove
16	Right atrium
17	Auricle of 16
18	Superior vena cava

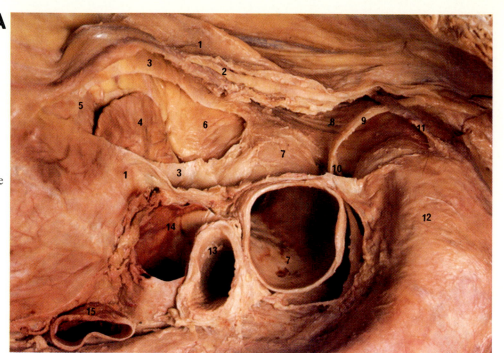

A

1 Pleura
2 Phrenic nerve
3 Pericardium
4 Auricle of left atrium
5 Left ventricle
6 Pulmonary trunk
7 Left pulmonary artery
8 Ligamentum arteriosum
9 Vagus nerve
10 Recurrent laryngeal nerve
11 Superior intercostal vein
12 Arch of aorta
13 Principal bronchus
14 Superior pulmonary vein
15 Inferior pulmonary vein
16 Left atrium
17 Right atrium
18 Inferior vena cava
19 Auricle of 17
20 Superior vena cava

Other Heart and Great Vessel Operations

The following are examples of heart or great vessel operations that are carried out through a left posterolateral thoracotomy:

For closed mitral valvotomy (enlarging a stenosed mitral valve without direct observation of the valve cusps), the chest is opened through the left fifth intercostal space. The pericardium is incised behind and parallel to the phrenic nerve (A) and an index finger is inserted into the left atrium through an opening made in the tip of the left auricle. The tip of the finger is pushed into the mitral valve orifice, enlarging it and breaking down the fusion between the cusps.

For closure of a patent ductus arteriosus or relieving coarctation (narrowing) of the aorta (which may be just proximal or distal to the ductus), the chest is opened through the left fourth interspace. The lung is retracted downwards and forwards to display the arch of the aorta and the left subclavian artery, pulmonary artery, superior intercostal vein, and the phrenic and vagus nerves (A). The pleura is incised over the aorta and just behind the vagus nerve, and the incision extended upwards to the origin of the subclavian artery. The pleural flap is reflected forwards with the vagus and recurrent laryngeal nerves so that the ductus and aortic arch can be fully exposed.

Hazards and Safeguards

The phrenic, vagus and recurrent laryngeal nerves must be carefully preserved, together with any obvious pulmonary branches.

For adequate mobilization of the aorta, some posterior intercostal arteries may have to be ligated.

A

Heart and great vessels, from the left, with the left lung removed and the pleura and pericardium incised for approaches to the auricle of the left atrium and the ductus arteriosus (here, ligamentum arteriosum).

B

Site for cardiac transplantation. The back and upper anterior part of the patient's right atrium remain so that the sinuatrial node is left intact. The back of the left atrium and the orifices of the four pulmonary veins are also left in situ.

C

Diagram indicating the mode of attachment of the donor heart. The donor's left atrium is trimmed through the orifices of the pulmonary veins and suturing begins at the left margin of the patient's left atrium. With the left atria joined, suture of the right atria begins at the left edge of the patient's right atrium. The margins of the donor's inferior vena caval orifice become part of the right atrial suture line; the donor's superior vena caval orifice remains closed by ligature. The aortae and pulmonary trunks are then joined.

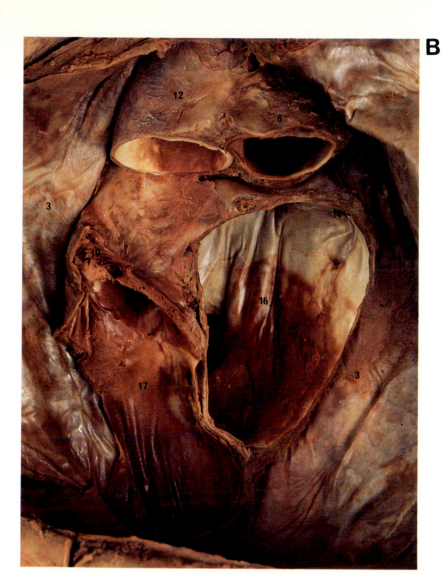

B

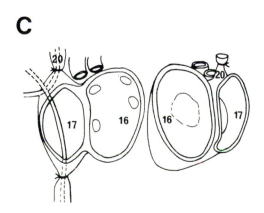

C

Cardiac Transplantation

After standard bypass cannulation of the venae cavae and aorta, the patient's heart is removed by incisions through the aorta and pulmonary trunk and through both atria. The incision line in the right atrium leaves both venae cavae and the posterior wall of the atrium intact; the uppermost part of the anterior wall is also retained so that the sinuatrial node is undisturbed. The left atrial incision leaves the posterior wall with the four pulmonary veins intact (B).

The donor heart is trimmed through the right and left atria so that their walls can match up with the remains of the patient's atria. The lowest part of the donor's superior vena cava is ligated and the atrial incision line avoids the sinuatrial donor area so that the donor heart includes the node. The patient will thus end up with his own normally innervated node and the denervated node of the donor heart.

The patient's and donor's left atria are anastomosed, followed by union of the right atria (C). The left atrium is cannulated through the auricle and infused to get rid of air.

The aortae and pulmonary trunks are sutured and the left atrial cannula removed, followed by removal of the bypass cannulae. Pacing wires are then attached to the donor right atrium.

Hazards and Safeguards

As with other transplanted organs, the problems of immunosuppression are greater than those of the anatomical and surgical techniques.

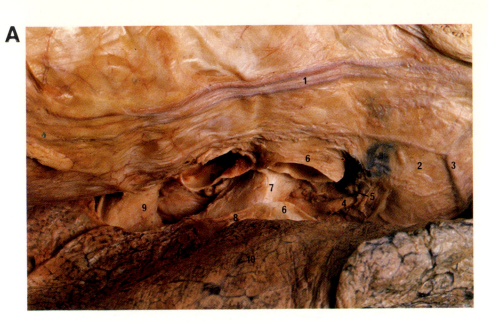

LUNGS

Background

Each lung is enveloped by pleura except at the hilum or lung root by which it is attached to the mediastinum (the central area within the thorax, between the two pleural sacs). The structures entering or leaving the lung at the hilum, and which therefore anchor it to the mediastinum, are the principal bronchus (and upper lobe bronchus on the right), pulmonary artery, superior and inferior pulmonary veins, bronchial arteries and veins, autonomic nerves, lymph nodes and lymphatic channels. The hilum of each lung is on a level with the third and fourth costal cartilages and the fifth, sixth and seventh thoracic vertebrae. The main structures of the lung root are arranged in the order vein, artery, bronchus from before backwards, with the inferior pulmonary vein being the lowest of all the structures. The pulmonary ligament is the double fold of pleura below the inferior pulmonary vein.

Removal of a lung (pneumonectomy) involves severing all the structures at the hilum, although the more localized removal of a lobe (lobectomy) or even individual segments can also be carried out. Here the approaches for right and left pneumonectomy are described; the method for each side is similar, the main difference (for technical reasons) being the order in which the main structures are dealt with, though this is subject to modification depending on the site and extent of disease.

Approach for Left Pneumonectomy

The left pleural cavity is entered by a posterolateral thoracotomy through the bed of the sixth rib (page 94).

The lung is displaced downwards and forwards to reveal the reflexion of the pleura behind the hilum, and the pleura is incised here.

The vagus nerve is divided distal to the origin of the recurrent laryngeal branch, and the pulmonary artery distal to the ligamentum arteriosum is dissected out and divided.

The lung is now displaced backwards and the superior pulmonary vein dissected out and divided (A).

With the lung displaced forwards again, the pulmonary ligament and inferior pulmonary vein at the lowest part of the hilum are dissected out and divided.

After transection of the main bronchus the lung can now be removed.

Hazards and Safeguards

Closure of the bronchus may be difficult due to the adjacent aortic arch.

If disease has involved lymph nodes and blood vessels it may be necessary to excise part of the pericardium in order to reach parts of the pulmonary vessels that are affected intrapericardially.

The recurrent laryngeal and phrenic nerves are preserved if possible but if they are seriously involved they must be sacrificed.

A

Root of the left lung, from the front and the left. The pulmonary artery and superior pulmonary vein are divided to show the principal bronchus that lies behind them. At operation for pneumonectomy the vagus nerve is cut distal to the recurrent laryngeal branch.

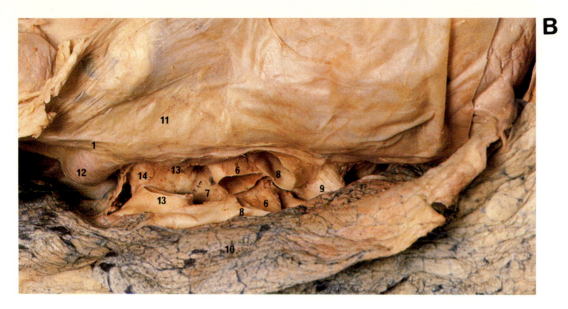

B

1 Phrenic nerve
2 Arch of aorta
3 Superior intercostal vein
4 Vagus nerve
5 Recurrent laryngeal nerve
6 Pulmonary artery
7 Principal bronchus
8 Superior pulmonary vein
9 Inferior pulmonary vein
10 Lung
11 Superior vena cava
12 Azygos vein
13 Superior branch of 6
14 Superior lobar bronchus

Approach for Right Pneumonectomy

The right pleural cavity is entered by a posterolateral thoracotomy through the bed of the sixth rib.

The lung is displaced downwards and backwards, and the pleura is incised at the front of the hilum.

The superior pulmonary vein and the pulmonary artery are dissected out and divided, including the branches to the upper lobe (B).

The lung is now retracted forward and the inferior pulmonary vein dissected out and divided.

Working from the front again, the main bronchus is divided and the lung removed.

Hazards and Safeguards

The arch of the azygos vein above the hilum is preserved if possible, as it affords collateral circulation in the event of obstruction of the superior vena cava.

The superior vena cava may have to be retracted forwards to assist in proper ligation of the pulmonary artery.

If vessels inside the pericardium have to be approached because of their involvement in disease, the pleural incision is made behind the hilum and the vagus and phrenic nerves may have to be sacrificed.

B
Root of the right lung, from the front and the right. The pulmonary artery, its branch to the upper lobe and the superior pulmonary vein are divided to show the principal bronchus giving off the superior lobe bronchus.

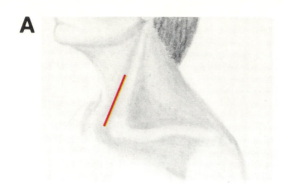

A

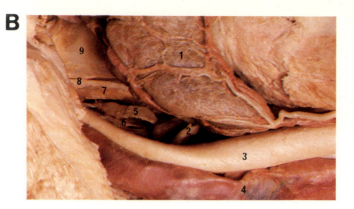

B

OESOPHAGUS

Background

The oesophagus begins as the continuation of the pharynx in front of the sixth cervical vertebra. Moving a few millimetres to the left as it enters the thorax, it regains the midline as it runs down in front of the thoracic vertebral column, usually inclining 2–3 cm to the left to pass through the oesophageal hiatus in the diaphragm and join the stomach. The cervical part of the oesophagus lies behind the trachea, with the thoracic duct running up behind the left oesophageal border before arching laterally at the level of the seventh cervical vertebra; the recurrent laryngeal nerve is in the tracheo-oesophageal groove on each side with the common carotid artery in the carotid sheath laterally and overlapped by the inferior pole of the lateral lobe of the thyroid gland. In the upper thorax the trachea remains in front until its bifurcation at the level of the lower border of the fourth thoracic vertebra. Below this the oesophagus is crossed by the *left* principal bronchus and the *right* pulmonary artery, and then the pericardium lies in front, separating the oesophagus from the left atrium. The aorta arches backwards across the left side of the oesophagus and the azygos vein arches backwards on the right side. Lower down the azygos vein is behind the right border and so is the thoracic duct, but this moves over to behind the left border at the fourth or fifth thoracic vertebral level. Posterior intercostal vessels run transversely behind. In the lower thorax viewed from the left, the oesophagus lies in a triangle formed by the heart and pericardium in front, the aorta behind and

the diaphragm below. After passing through the oesophageal hiatus, the 2 cm of abdominal oesophagus has a 'bare area' at the back in contact with the diaphragm; in front there is a covering of peritoneum of the greater sac, with a small part of the lesser sac at the right border. The vagal trunks lie in front and behind as they pass through the hiatus (page 120). The blood supply comes from several sources, mainly by branches from the inferior thyroid artery, from the aorta and from the left gastric artery, with minor contributions from the left subclavian, bronchial and inferior phrenic vessels. Veins correspond to some of the arteries and also drain to the azygos and hemi-azygos systems, but the most significant feature is that the left gastric veins belong to the portal system, so that the lower oesophagus is one of the sites of portal-systemic anastomosis. Lymphatic vessels pass to deep cervical, posterior mediastinal and left gastric nodes, but it is important to note that lymph may travel for long distances within channels in the oesophageal walls and there is no constant drainage pattern for any given part. Despite its close relation there is no direct drainage into the thoracic duct.

The oesophagus is 25 cm long, and since its commencement is 15 cm from the incisor teeth it follows that a tube or instrument being passed into the stomach must be at least 40 cm from the teeth before it is even in the upper part of the stomach. The narrowest parts are at its commencement, the regions where it is crossed by the aorta and the left bronchus, and at the oesophageal hiatus. It can be indented (as seen radiologically) by the aortic arch, the left bronchus and an enlarged left atrium of the heart.

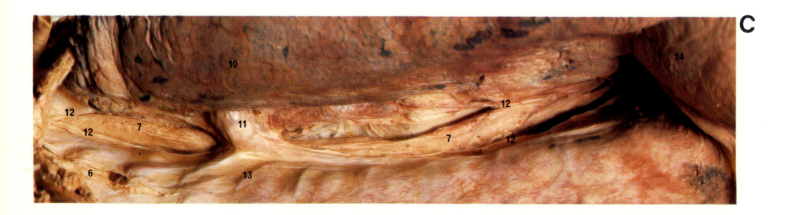

C

Tumours are the main reason for surgical approach to the oesophagus and most occur near the lower end although any part may be affected. The cervical part can be exposed in the neck by opening up the interval between the trachea and carotid sheath. In the thorax a long length is accessible from the right in front of the vertebral column after incising the pleura and especially after cutting the arch of the azygos vein, but for the lower part it may be easier to approach from the left, behind the heart and in front of the aorta. For reaching the abdominal part an upper abdominal or thoraco-abdominal incision (page 94) is required.

Approach to the Cervical Oesophagus

A skin incision (A) is made along the anterior border of sterno-cleidomastoid on the chosen side. The incision is deepened to include platysma, the investing layer of deep cervical fascia and the superior belly of omohyoid.

The middle thyroid vein and inferior thyroid artery are divided to expose the area between the trachea and oesophagus medially and the carotid sheath laterally. The oesophagus is seen behind the trachea (B).

Hazards and Safeguards

The recurrent laryngeal nerve must be avoided when ligating the inferior thyroid artery (page 22) and when dissecting out the oesophagus. So must the thoracic duct on the left side; it lies behind the left margin of the oesophagus and arches laterally (but not as high as the arch of the inferior thyroid artery) between the carotid and vertebral systems of vessels.

Approach to the Thoracic Oesophagus

A right posterolateral thoracotomy is carried out above the fifth, sixth or seventh ribs (page 94).

The lung is suitably retracted and the mediastinal pleura incised over the oesophagus (C). Division of the azygos vein allows a long continuous length to be exposed.

For the lower part, an alternative approach is through a left posterolateral thoractomy above the eighth rib. The oesophagus is identified in the triangle between the diaphragm below, the heart in the pericardium in front and the aorta behind, and the pleura over the front of the aorta is incised (D).

A left thoraco-abdominal approach can be used for access to the cardio-oesophageal junction.

Hazards and Safeguards

The posterior intercostal vessels and thoracic duct are candidates for injury when mobilizing the oesophagus posteriorly.

Having upper and lower ends that are relatively fixed, the removal of more than a few centimetres of oesophagus means that the cut ends cannot be joined together without undue tension and imperilling the blood supply, and it may be necessary to bring the upper end of the stomach up into the thorax or replace the oesophagus by a colonic transplant.

A

Incision line for cervical part.

B

Left side of the lower neck, from the front and the left, with the upper end of the oesophagus in view behind the trachea. A right-sided approach is often chosen to avoid possible damage to the thoracic duct.

C

Right side of the mediastinum, with the lung retracted forwards and the pleura incised to display the oesophagus. The azygos vein can be divided to give a long oesophageal exposure.

D

Lower left mediastinum with the pleura incised to show the lower part of the oesophagus in the triangle between the pericardium, diaphragm and aorta. The lung is retracted forwards.

1 Thyroid gland
2 Inferior thyroid artery
3 Common carotid artery
4 Internal jugular vein
5 Thoracic duct
6 Sympathetic trunk
7 Oesophagus
8 Recurrent laryngeal nerve
9 Trachea
10 Lung
11 Azygos vein
12 Cut edge of pleura
13 Posterior intercostal vessels
14 Diaphragm
15 Pericardium and heart
16 Anterior vagal trunk
17 Posterior vagal trunk
18 Aorta

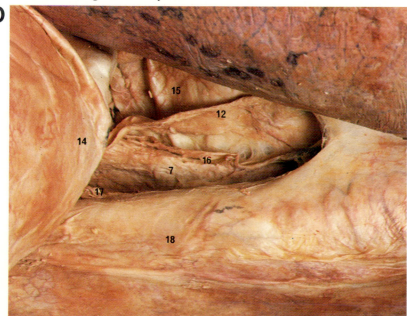

THORACIC SYMPATHETIC TRUNK

Background

In the upper thorax the sympathetic trunk is found deep to the parietal pleura; it crosses the neck of the first rib adjacent to the head, with laterally the supreme intercostal vein, superior intercostal artery and farther laterally still the part of the first thoracic nerve that contributes to the brachial plexus. The trunk lies in front of the heads of succeeding ribs and is lateral to the azygos vein. The first ganglion, at the level of the neck of the first rib, may be fused with the inferior cervical ganglion to form the stellate ganglion (page 19).

The lateral horn cells of the first three segments of the thoracic part of the spinal cord provide preganglionic sympathetic fibres for the innervation of head and neck structures, while for the upper limb the preganglionic fibres are derived from thoracic segments two to seven or even lower. Only 10% of subjects have any upper limb sympathetic innervation from the first thoracic segment, whose lateral horn fibres are therefore almost entirely destined for head and neck supply.

Sympathetic denervation (sympathectomy) of the upper limb to dilate blood vessels or inhibit sweat secretion can be achieved in most subjects by removing the part of the trunk that includes the second and third ganglia; the first is left intact to preserve sympathetic innervation to the head and neck and prevent the development of Horner's syndrome. The trunk can be approached from above the medial end of the clavicle, dividing scalenus anterior and stripping the pleura from the sides of the vertebral bodies and the adjacent ribs, or by a transaxillary route through the second interspace or the bed of the third rib. The operation through the lower neck is usually called *cervical* sympathectomy because of the position of the incision, although it is of course part of the *thoracic* sympathetic trunk that is being removed.

Supraclavicular Approach

A skin incision (A) is made just above and parallel to the medial half of the clavicle, and deepened to include platysma.

The external jugular vein, clavicular head of sternocleidomastoid and the inferior belly of omohyoid are divided.

The fat in the lower medial part of the posterior triangle is dissected with ligation of the superficial cervical and suprascapular veins to expose the prevertebral fascia overlying scalenus anterior and the phrenic nerve. The fascia is incised so that the phrenic nerve can be retracted medially towards the internal jugular vein which is at the medial border of scalenus anterior.

Scalenus anterior is divided transversely to display the subclavian artery and the suprapleural membrane. The artery is retracted upwards or downwards as convenient and the membrane is detached from the seventh cervical transverse process so that the pleura beneath it can be displaced from the sides of the upper thoracic vertebral bodies and the heads and necks of the adjacent ribs (B).

The sympathetic trunk is identified crossing the neck of the first rib and the heads of succeeding ribs. The second and third ganglia and the part of the trunk joining them are removed by severing the rami communicantes that connect them to their spinal nerves.

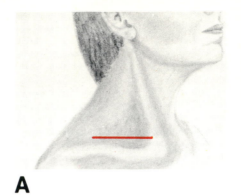

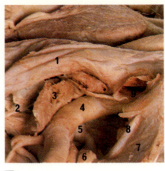

A **B**

Hazards and Safeguards

Pneumothorax will occur if the pleural sac is accidentally entered.

Haemorrhage from intercostal veins must be avoided.

Damage to the stellate ganglion may produce Horner's syndrome (page 19), and the phrenic nerve and lower part of the brachial plexus are at risk, as is the thoracic duct on the left side.

Transaxillary Approach

With the arm abducted to a right angle, a skin incision (C) is made over the third rib from the posterior to the anterior axillary fold.

Pectoralis major is retracted forwards and latissimus dorsi backwards, and serratus anterior and the periosteum of the third rib are incised so that the pleura can be divided through the bed of the rib (or a segment of rib resected). The long thoracic nerve on serratus anterior and the subscapular vessels and thoracodorsal nerve near the border of latissimus dorsi must be avoided (E).

The lung is displaced downwards and the sympathetic trunk identified (visually and by palpation) under the parietal pleura on the necks of the ribs.

The pleura over the sympathetic trunk is divided (D) so that a length of the trunk including the second, third and even fourth ganglia can be removed by severing the rami communicantes that attach them to intercostal nerves.

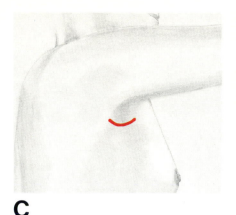

C

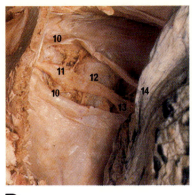

D

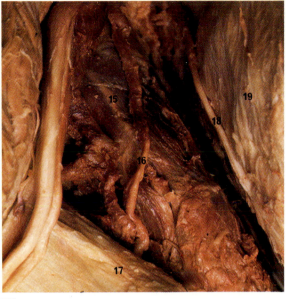

E

Hazards and Safeguards

The long thoracic nerve (to serratus anterior) runs vertically downwards on the outer surface of the muscle approximately in the midaxillary line, and should be retracted forwards when incising the muscle.

The thoracordorsal nerve (to latissimus dorsi) and subscapular vessels run along the posterior border of the axilla at the anterior margin of latissimus dorsi, and should be retracted backwards with the muscle.

Damage to intercostal vessels (and the azygos vein on the right) must be avoided to prevent haemothorax.

Damage to the stellate ganglion may produce Horner's syndrome (page 19). Such injury is more likely with the suprascapular than with the transaxillary approach, since exposure of the ganglion through the axilla is more limited.

On the left the aortic arch will be visible, and the thoracic duct lies anteromedial to the upper end of the sympathetic trunk.

A

Incision line for supraclavicular approach.

B

Right lower neck. Deep dissection with division of scalenus anterior and the suprapleural membrane, and with the pleura reflected laterally from the vertebral column to show the sympathetic trunk and inferior cervical ganglion. This is not the part of the trunk to be removed for sympathectomy, but from here the trunk can be followed down to the required level (second and third ganglia) by further stripping of the pleura from the vertebral bodies and ribs.

C

Incision line for transaxillary approach.

D

Right upper thoracic sympathetic trunk with the overlying pleura incised. The first and second ganglia are shown, and further pleural stripping and lung retraction will display the third which with the second and the intervening trunk can be removed from below upwards.

E

Right axilla, showing the long thoracic and thoracodorsal nerves. At operation, with the arm widely abducted, these nerves are retracted forwards and backwards respectively.

1 Internal jugular vein
2 Phrenic nerve
3 Scalenus anterior
4 Subclavian artery
5 Inferior cervical ganglion
6 Ventral ramus of first thoracic nerve
7 First rib
8 Cut edge of suprapleural membrane
9 End of subclavian vein
10 Cut edge of pleura
11 First thoracic sympathetic ganglion
12 Second rib and sympathetic trunk
13 Second thoracic sympathetic ganglion
14 Lung
15 Subscapularis
16 Thoracodorsal nerve
17 Latissimus dorsi
18 Long thoracic nerve
19 Serratus anterior over third rib

ABDOMEN AND PELVIS

ABDOMINAL WALL

Background

The anterolateral abdominal wall between the costal margin above and the iliac crests, inguinal ligaments and pubes below offers a variety of sites for incisions to gain access to abdominal organs. The pattern of incisions is dictated by the arrangement of muscles and their nerve supplies, and the need to ensure that when healed the wall will not be weakened. The rectus abdominis (with pyramidalis) lies within its sheath adjacent to the midline linea alba with the external oblique, internal oblique and transversus muscles laterally. The rectus sheath (A & B) is formed by the aponeurosis of the internal oblique, reinforced at the front and back by the aponeuroses of the external oblique and transversus respectively except below a level midway between the umbilicus and pubic symphysis where all three aponeuroses are in front of the rectus muscle. Between the skin and the muscles with their aponeuroses lies the superficial fascia, divided into an anterior fatty layer and a deep fibrous layer; there is no deep fascia in the abdominal wall. Behind the muscles and their aponeuroses are the transversalis fascia, extraperitoneal fat and peritoneum.

In general the lower six intercostal vessels and nerves run between internal oblique and transversus, supplying them. The lateral cutaneous branches of the nerves pierce internal oblique and then external oblique, supplying the latter before reaching the skin. After entering the rectus sheath by piercing the posterior layer of the internal oblique aponeurosis the nerves enter the rectus muscle near its midline to supply it and then emerge anteriorly to become the anterior cutaneous nerves. The ilio-hypogastric and ilio-inguinal nerves also lie in part of their course between internal oblique and transversus but they do not enter the rectus sheath and do not supply the rectus muscle or external oblique. At about the level of the anterior superior iliac spine they pierce the internal oblique and run forwards deep to the external oblique aponeurosis, the ilio-inguinal nerve entering the inguinal canal and then leaving it through the superficial ring. The iliohypogastric nerve is 2–3 cm higher and does not run into the canal. Both nerves supply the lowest fibres of internal oblique and transversus – the fibres that form the roof of the canal and which converge on to the conjoint tendon. If the nerves are damaged in the region of the anterior superior iliac spine these muscles fibres are denervated, leading to weakening of the normal canal controlling mechanism and predisposing to inguinal hernia. (Damage to the ilio-inguinal nerve *in the* canal does not cause paralysis – page 116.)

The largest vessels of the anterior abdominal wall are the superior and inferior epigastric, which enter the rectus sheath and then the rectus muscle, forming a profuse anastomosis within it. Other vessels include the posterior intercostals, lumbar and deep circumflex iliac. The inferior epigastric artery is of particular surgical relevance: its relation to the neck of an inguinal hernial sac determines whether the hernia is indirect or direct (page 116); it may give origin to an abnormal obturator artery (page 117); and if damaged (especially when arteriosclerotic and fractured) it may give rise to pain and diagnostic problems, simulating an acute abdominal emergency. The deep circumflex iliac artery runs laterally behind the inguinal ligament in a sheath formed by the transversalis and iliac fasciae, and near the anterior superior iliac spine it gives off an ascending branch that passes vertically upwards between internal oblique and transversus. All the vessels mentioned have anastomotic connexions with their near neighbours such that vascular deficiency is not normally a hazard of abdominal wall surgery.

An outline of the most common incisions is given below. The choice of any one often depends on the preference of the individual surgeon as well as the condition being treated.

Upper Midline (Epigastric) Incision

Commonly used for approach to the upper abdomen.

A skin incision (C) is made in the midline from the tip of the xiphoid process to above the umbilicus.

The skin and subcutaneous fat are dissected off the linea alba for about 1 cm either side of the midline.

The linea alba (A and B) is incised in the line of the skin incision to expose the transversalis fascia, extraperitoneal fat and peritoneum which in turn are incised as a single layer.

If required the incision can be extended upwards through or to one side of the xiphoid process, or downwards skirting to the right or left of the umbilicus and then regaining the midline.

Lower Midline (Subumbilical) Incision

Commonly used for approach to the lower abdomen and pelvis.

A skin incision (C) is made in the midline from below the umbilicus to above the pubic symphysis and the deeper layers are incised in the same line.

Hazards and Safeguards

These are the simplest and quickest of all abdominal incisions. Only very small vessels cross the midline and no major nerves are involved.

With the lower incision, the bladder must be empty; when distended it reaches up above the pubic symphysis and strips the peritoneum off the back of the abdominal wall (page 155).

The linea alba is narrower below the umbilicus than above it and the rectus muscles may lie very close together at their lower ends.

Peritoneal Drainage

Paracentesis (drainage of fluid from the peritoneal cavity) can be carried out by inserting a needle or trocar in the midline below the umbilicus.

Hazards and Safeguards

The point of entry must not be too near the pubic symphysis, to avoid a full bladder.

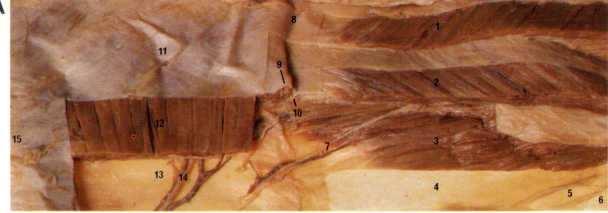

A

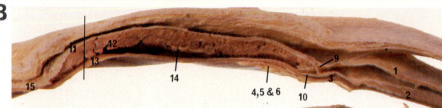

B

C

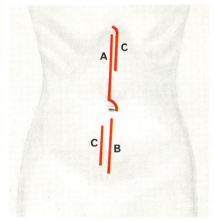

1	External oblique
2	Internal oblique
3	Transversus abdominis
4	Transversalis fascia
5	Extraperitoneal fat
6	Peritoneum
7	Intercostal vessels and nerve
8	Lateral margin of rectus sheath
9	Anterior lamina of internal oblique aponeurosis
10	Posterior lamina of internal oblique aponeurosis
11	Anterior layer of rectus sheath
12	Rectus abdominis
13	Posterior layer of rectus sheath
14	Inferior epigastric vessels
15	Linea alba
16	Tendinous intersection of 12

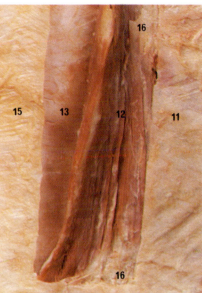

D

Paramedian Incision

Commonly used for access to all parts of the abdominal cavity depending on the side and length.

A skin incision (C) is made parallel to and 3 cm from the midline at an appropriate level. In the upper abdomen the upper end of the incision can be curved medially to follow the lower border of the costal margin.

The subcutaneous tissues are dissected off the anterior layer of the sheath (B) which is incised in the line of the skin incision.

The rectus muscle can either be retracted laterally or split in the line of the anterior sheath incision. At or below the umbilicus the tendinous intersections (D) must be freed from their adherence to the anterior layer of the sheath.

The posterior layer of the sheath is incised in the same line as the other incisions and the cut continued through to the peritoneum.

Hazards and Safeguards

If the rectus muscle is split instead of being retracted laterally, the line of the split must not be too far lateral, to avoid damage to the intercostal nerves that innervate the muscle by piercing it near its midline. The small part of the muscle medial to the split will be denervated and largely devascularized but this does not cause problems. An incision similar to the paramedian but near the *lateral* border of the muscle (pararectal or Battle's incision), with retraction of the muscle medially, was at one time in vogue but has fallen out of favour because of damage to the nerves entering the sheath laterally.

In the lower abdomen the inferior epigastric vessels must not be damaged as they lie on the posterior surface of the muscle (A and B). Above the pubis pyramidalis (page 115, C) can be dissected off the rectus and turned forward with the anterior layer of the sheath.

In the upper abdomen on the right, the line of incision passes lateral to the falciform ligament which may need to be divided if access towards the left side is required.

A

Layer dissection of the left rectus sheath and adjacent abdominal muscles. The vessels and nerves run between internal oblique and transversus, and enter the sheath by piercing the posterior lamina of the internal oblique aponeurosis.

B

Cross section of the left rectus sheath, with a line indicating the route of a paramedian incision.

C

Incision lines: midline epigastric (A), midline subumbilical (B), and left upper and right lower paramedian (C).

D

Tendinous intersections of the left rectus muscle, with part of the anterior layer of the sheath removed. Two intersections are seen, and the rectus is being displaced laterally to show the posterior layer of the sheath to which the intersections do not adhere; they are only attached to the anterior layer.

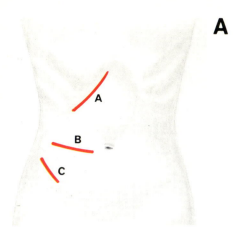

A

Right Subcostal Incision (Kocher's)

Commonly used for access to the biliary tract. A similar left-sided incision gives access to the spleen, but a combined right and left incision ('rooftop incision') is becoming increasingly used when wide access to the upper abdomen is required (e.g. for hepatic resection or difficult bile duct operations).

A skin incision (A) is made 3 cm below and parallel to the right costal margin, from the midline to beyond the lateral border of the rectus sheath.

The anterior layer of the rectus sheath and laterally the external oblique are divided in the line of the skin incision, followed by division of the rectus muscle in the same line with ligation of the superior epigastric vessels and their branches on the posterior surface of the rectus muscle. Intercostal nerves enter the sheath at its lateral margin, and one or even two may have to be cut.

The posterior layer of the sheath is divided, and the incision continued laterally into the internal oblique and transversus muscles. The transversalis fascia, extraperitoneal fat and peritoneum are then opened.

Hazards and Safeguards

Intercostal nerves enter the sheath laterally to supply the rectus muscle (B). The seventh nerve runs upwards immediately below and parallel to the costal margin but should be above the line of the incision. The eighth runs transversely and the ninth obliquely downwards, above the tenth which is directed towards the umbilicus. Sacrifice of two nerves (usually the ninth and tenth) will not significantly affect the rectus, but any further division should be avoided.

Vessels accompanying the intercostal nerves will require ligation, but the major haemorrhagic danger is from the superior epigastric vessels at the back of the rectus muscle.

Muscle fibres seen behind the upper part of the rectus muscle are those of transversus abdominis; the highest part of this muscle does not become aponeurotic until within two or three centimetres of the midline.

Oblique Muscle-Cutting Incision

Used on the right for draining an appendix abscess or for approaching the lower ureter or colon. Sometimes known as the iliac or Rutherford Morison's incision.

B

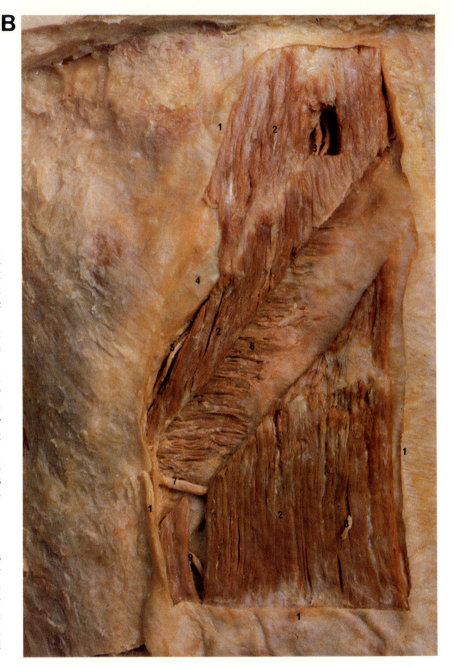

A skin incision (A) is made 3 cm above and parallel to the anterior part of the iliac crest and lateral part of the inguinal ligament.

The external oblique is incised in the line of its fibres, and the internal oblique and transversus are cut in the same line (not in the line of their own fibres as in the gridiron incision), followed by incision through to the peritoneum (which in the case of an abscess may be adhering to the abscess wall).

The lower part of the abdominal ureter (or nearby structures such as inferior vena cava or lumbar sympathetic trunk) can be approached retroperitoneally by reflecting the peritoneum instead of incising it (see below).

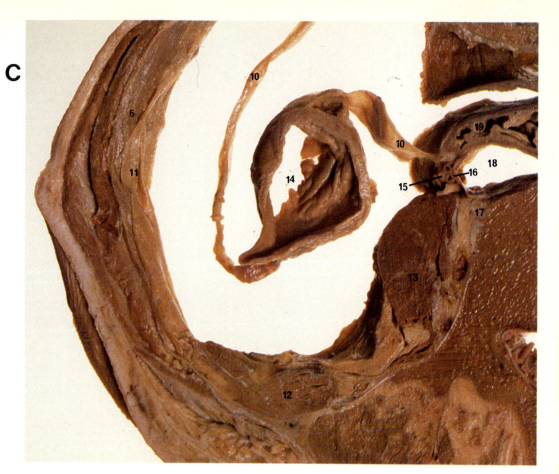

1 Cut edge of rectus sheath
2 Rectus abdominis
3 Superior epigastric vessels
4 Seventh costal cartilage
5 Seventh intercostal nerve
6 Transversus abdominis
7 Eighth intercostal nerve
8 Anterior cutaneous branch of 7
9 Ninth intercostal nerve
10 Peritoneum
11 Transversalis fascia
12 Quadratus lumborum
13 Psoas major
14 Ascending colon
15 Ureter
16 Gonadal vessels
17 Sympathetic trunk
18 Inferior vena cava
19 Duodenum

Hazards and Safeguards

The ascending branch of the deep circumflex iliac artery will be divided in the lateral part of the incision. If the incision has to be extended medially the inferior epigastric vessels will require ligation.

The iliohypogastric and ilio-inguinal nerves lie parallel to the incision and as with the gridiron incision (page 114) must not be damaged.

Transverse Muscle-Cutting Incisions

Transverse incisions can be made above or below the umbilicus, cutting through one or both rectus sheaths and muscles and extending laterally into the oblique and transversus muscles as required.

One type of transverse incision not involving the rectus muscle is used for gaining access to the lumbar sympathetic trunk (page 165) or inferior vena cava (page 142) extraperitoneally.

A skin incision (A) is made transversely on the appropriate side from the tip of the twelfth rib to the lateral border of the rectus sheath at the level of the umbilicus.

The external oblique is split in the line of its fibres followed by incision of the internal oblique and transversus and the transversalis fascia in the same line.

The peritoneum is not incised but stripped off the abdominal wall laterally and downwards and then medially across the posterior wall and over the psoas major (C).

A
Incision lines: right subcostal (A), right transverse muscle-cutting (B) and right oblique muscle-cutting (C).

B
Right costal margin, with removal of part of the rectus sheath and muscle, showing the position of intercostal nerves in this area.

C
Cross section of part of the right side of the abdomen, at the level of the fourth lumbar vertebra, from below, with peritoneum being stripped off the abdominal walls to give extraperitoneal access to such structures as the ureter, sympathetic trunk and inferior vena cava.

Hazards and Safeguards

Transverse incisions involving the rectus muscle may give considerable haemorrhage.

On the right above the umbilicus the falciform ligament will need to be cut.

Transverse incisions cross the paths of intercostal nerves which run mostly obliquely downwards in the lower abdomen, but more than one or two are not likely to be damaged.

When stripping peritoneum off the posterior abdominal wall it is important to remain in a plane anterior to psoas major and its sheath, and not to force a false passage behind the muscle; the very considerable forward projection of the vertebral column and psoas must be remembered.

The ureter adheres to the peritoneum, unless deliberately detached from it (as in C).

Gridiron Incision (McBurney's)

The right lower oblique muscle-splitting incision used for access to the appendix.

A skin incision (A) is made at right angles to a line drawn from the anterior superior iliac spine to the umbilicus, at the junction of the.outer and middle thirds of that line and parallel to the line of the iliac crest. An alternative is a more transverse incision starting above and medial to the anterior superior iliac spine.

The external oblique aponeurosis and more laterally its muscle fibres (B) are divided in the line of the skin incision (which is approximately the line of the external oblique fibres).

Then the internal oblique and transversus muscles are each split in the line of their own fibres, approximately transversely, to expose the peritoneum which can be opened transversely. At the position of the splitting the internal oblique is muscular, but the transversus is becoming aponeurotic so that the gap being made in it will be partly through muscle and partly aponeurosis. The transversalis fascia is thin at this level and will be divided with the transversus.

Hazards and Safeguards

The iliohypogastric or ilio-inguinal nerves may be seen between the internal oblique and transversus muscles (B) and should not be damaged. At this level in their course they supply the fibres of those two muscles that are attached to the conjoint tendon, and nerve injury here will weaken the protective effect the fibres exert on the inguinal canal.

Extension of the incision medially will involve the rectus sheath.

Extension of the incision laterally may cut the ascending branch of the deep circumflex iliac artery which lies between the internal oblique and transversus muscles in a vertical line above the anterior superior iliac spine.

B

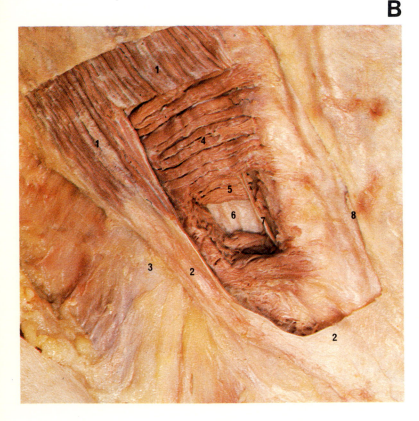

A

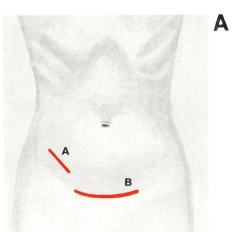

Lower Abdominal Transverse Incision (Pfannenstiel's)

Commonly used for approach to male and female pelvic organs.

A skin incision (A) is made transversely 3 cm above the pubic symphysis, curving slightly upwards on either side in the direction of the anterior superior iliac spine as far as the lateral borders of the rectus sheaths.

The anterior layers of the rectus sheaths are divided in the line of the skin incision and flaps dissected off the rectus muscles upwards and downwards. Midline tissue between the sheaths is included in the flaps and the pyramidalis muscles are included with the lower flaps.

The linea alba is incised *vertically* to expose extraperitoneal tissue, or the peritoneum can be incised if entry to the abdominal cavity is required.

Division of the rectus muscles transversely can provide wider exposure, or the incisions can be extended laterally into the flat muscles.

Hazards and Safeguards

The inferior epigastric vessels are behind the rectus muscles (or lateral to them low down) (C).

The bladder must be carefully avoided when incising the peritoneum suprapubically.

A

Incision lines: gridiron (A) and lower transverse (B).

B

Lower right anterior abdominal wall, with windows cut in the external oblique, internal oblique and transversus muscles. In a gridiron incision these muscles are all split in the line of their fibres, so avoiding any transverse incisions, and healing is good because the edges come together well.

C

Lower anterior abdominal wall, with the anterior layer of both rectus sheaths and the left pyramidalis removed and the rectus muscles separated; they are normally close together at this level. The left rectus muscle is split vertically to show the position of the inferior epigastric vessels behind it. In a lower transverse incision the linea alba is incised *vertically*; the incision gets its name from the line of the skin cut.

1   External oblique muscle
2   External oblique aponeurosis
3   Anterior superior iliac spine
4   Internal oblique
5   Transversus abdominis
6   Peritoneum
7   Ilio-inguinal nerve
8   Edge of rectus sheath
9   Linea alba
10   Rectus abdominis
11   Inferior epigastric vessels
12   Pyramidalis
13   Branch of subcostal nerve to 12

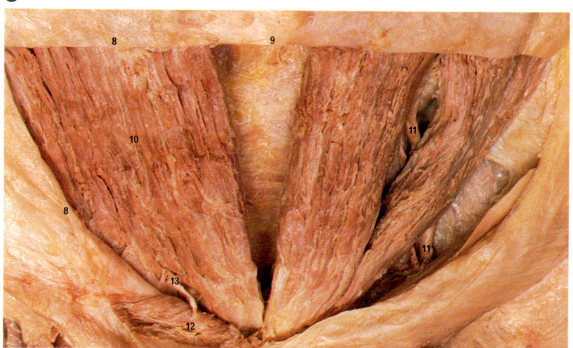

C

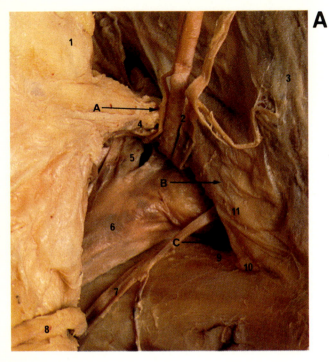

A

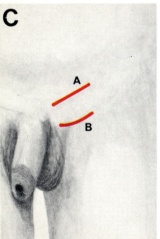

C

1	Peritoneum and fat reflected backwards
2	Inferior epigastric vessels
3	Posterior surface of rectus abdominis
4	Spermatic cord at deep inguinal ring
5	Deep circumflex iliac vein
6	External iliac vein
7	Abnormal obturator vein
8	Medial umbilical ligament
9	Pectineal ligament
10	Lacunar ligament
11	Inguinal ligament
12	Cut edge of external oblique aponeurosis
13	Internal oblique and transversus
14	Cut edge of spermatic cord coverings
15	Femoral artery
16	Femoral vein
17	Cut edge of superficial inguinal ring
18	Cribriform fascia

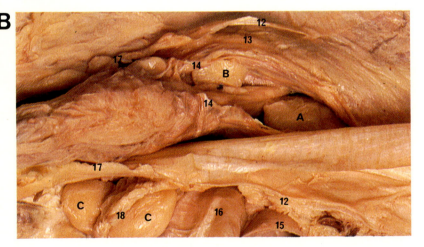

B

INGUINAL HERNIA

Background

In order to pass from the testis to the prostate, the ductus (vas) deferens must run through the inguinal canal which is an oblique gap in the lower anterior abdominal wall between the superficial inguinal ring (in the external oblique aponeurosis) and the deep inguinal ring (in the transversalis fascia). The floor of the inguinal canal is the medial end of the inguinal ligament and the lacunar ligament; resting on this floor in the male are the spermatic cord and the ilio-inguinal nerve (in the female, the round ligament of the uterus and the ilio-inguinal nerve). The anterior wall consists of the external oblique aponeurosis with laterally some of the fibres of the internal oblique that arise from the upper surface of the inguinal ligament. The posterior wall consists of the transversalis fascia with medially the conjoint tendon in front of the fascia. The roof is formed by fibres of the internal oblique and transversus muscles that arch medially and backwards from the inguinal ligament to the conjoint tendon.

The spermatic cord consists of its coverings and constituents. The coverings are the three spermatic fasciae: the external derived from the external oblique aponeurosis, the cremasteric from the internal oblique and transversus muscles, and the internal from the transversalis fascia. There is of course no external spermatic fascia around the cord where it lies in the inguinal canal, since this covering is a downward extension of the external oblique at the superficial inguinal ring. The principal constituent of the cord is the ductus deferens, together with the testicular, cremasteric and ductal arteries, the pampiniform plexus of veins, lymphatic vessels, the genital branch of the genitofemoral nerve and sympathetic nerves, and the obliterated processus vaginalis of peritoneum.

In an *indirect* inguinal hernia (A and B), the peritoneal sac enters the inguinal canal through the deep inguinal ring; the neck of the sac is therefore *in* the deep ring and lateral to the inferior epigastric vessels. In a *direct* inguinal hernia (A and B), the sac does not enter the canal through the deep ring but pushes part of the posterior wall of the canal forwards through an area bounded medially by the rectus muscle, laterally by the inferior epigastric

A
Lower left anterior abdominal wall, seen from the right and behind from within the abdomen, with peritoneum reflected backwards off the wall and pubis. The three hernial sites are indicated by the arrows: indirect inguinal (A), direct inguinal (B) and femoral (C). In this specimen there is an abnormal obturator vein; a similar artery would lie in the same position.

B
Left inguinal region, from the front and the left, showing the positions of three small hernial sacs, identified as in A. The femoral hernial sac is pushing through the cribiform fascia of the saphenous opening.

C
Incision lines: inguinal hernia (A) and femoral hernia (B).

vessels and below by the inguinal ligament (this area is the inguinal triangle). In this type of hernia the neck of the sac is medial to the inferior epigastric vessels. Until the precise location of the neck of the sac in relation to these vessels can be defined at operation it may not be possible to differentiate between these two types, but about 85% of inguinal herniae are indirect. In children the sac of an indirect hernia is formed by a patent processus vaginalis.

The repair of an inguinal hernia involves exposing the sac through the anterior wall of the canal and defining its neck so that the sac can be tied off there and removed. The weakened posterior wall of the canal is strengthened, with the aim of preventing recurrence of the hernia, principally by suturing the conjoint tendon to the inguinal ligament.

Approach

A skin incision (C) is made 1 cm above and parallel to the inguinal ligament, running medially from the deep inguinal ring (1 cm above the palpable femoral artery) to the pubic tubercle.

The subcutaneous tissue is cleared with the skin flaps to expose the external oblique aponeurosis, which is opened along the length of the inguinal canal including incision of the lateral margin of the superficial inguinal ring.

The cremasteric and internal spermatic fasciae are similarly divided to expose the constituents of the spermatic cord, and the indirect or direct hernial sacs can then be identified and dissected out (B).

The hernial sac is opened and any abdominal contents such as omentum or small intestine returned to the abdominal cavity after inspection to ensure that they are normal.

The neck of the sac is closed off with a ligature and the sac removed. Direct herniae often form a broad bulge with no distinct neck to the sac, in which case the contents are pushed back into the abdomen before proceeding with the abdominal wall repair.

The repair of the abdominal wall usually involves tightening up the transversalis fascia by incising it in a medial direction from the deep inguinal ring and stitching the upper flap to the front of the lower flap with a suitable overlap. The posterior wall is further reinforced by stitching the conjoint tendon to the inguinal ligament. There are many possible variations in the surgical technique involved.

Hazards and Safeguards

The bladder must be empty before operation; it can be injured if adherent to the peritoneum of a hernial sac.

Subcutaneous vessels in the incision line will need to be ligated but it is particularly important to avoid damage to major vessels such as the femoral, inferior epigastric and testicular.

The ilio-inguinal nerve passes through the superficial inguinal ring with the spermatic cord, lying deep to the external oblique aponeurosis and just below the cord at the level of the ring. It should be avoided when incising and stitching the aponeurosis, and so should the iliohypogastric nerve which probably lies 2–3 cm higher. Injury to these nerves at inguinal canal level may cause postoperative pain and anaesthesia in the inguinal region and scrotum. Injury at this level does *not* cause paralysis of the lowest parts of the internal oblique and transversus muscles; the motor

fibres have left the nerves farther laterally, where the nerves lie between the two muscles and are at risk from a gridiron incision (page 114).

The spermatic cord must not be constricted at any stage of the repair.

FEMORAL HERNIA

Background

The femoral canal is the most medial of the three compartments of the femoral sheath. The mouth of the canal is covered by transversalis fascia, extraperitoneal fat and peritoneum, and the boundaries of the mouth (the femoral ring) are: in front, the inguinal ligament; behind, the pectineus muscle; laterally, the femoral vein; and medially, the lacunar ligament. If an abnormal obturator artery is present, it usually lies along the lateral margin of the femoral ring, adjacent to the femoral vein; only rarely does such an artery lie at the medial margin of the ring, along the lateral border of the lacunar ligament.

In a femoral hernia, the peritoneal sac pushes through the femoral ring into the canal and may progress through the saphenous opening, with the fundus (tip) of the sac then turning *upwards* towards the inguinal ligament (because of the way the superficial fascia is attached to the deep fascia of the thigh). The repair of an uncomplicated femoral hernia involves an incision below the inguinal ligament, removal of the sac and the stitching of the inguinal ligament to the pectineal ligament to close over the abdominal opening of the canal. This is the standard 'low approach' and is described below; other methods will be found in surgical texts, including those going through the posterior wall of the inguinal canal above the inguinal ligament (high approach), which may be more appropriate when the hernia is strangulated (constricted) at the femoral ring, cutting off the blood supply to contents of the sac such as a loop of small bowel and where bowel resection may be necessary.

Approach

A skin incision (C) is made over the hernial swelling, 2 cm below and parallel to the inguinal ligament.

Subcutaneous tissue and the coverings of the sac are cleared to expose the sac, which can then be followed to its neck at the femoral ring. On its path through the femoral ring and canal and saphenous opening (B), the peritoneal sac will have acquired coverings of extraperitoneal fat, transversalis fascia, femoral sheath fascia and cribriform fascia.

The sac is opened and any abdominal contents returned to the abdominal cavity after ensuring that they are normal.

The sac is ligated at its neck and the rest of it removed.

The abdominal wall is repaired by suturing the part of the inguinal ligament lateral to the lacunar ligament to the pectineal ligament (along the pectineal line of the pubis).

Hazards and Safeguards

The bladder must be empty before operation. Extraperitoneal tissue normally adheres to the sac of a femoral hernia, and on the medial side the bladder may be adherent also.

Some of the superficial tributaries of the great saphenous vein may be in the incision line and will need to be ligated.

The femoral vein is on the lateral side of the femoral ring and therefore lateral to the neck of the hernial sac which must be carefully cleared from it. The vein is covered by the fascia of its own compartment of the femoral sheath and may not be easily seen. Palpation of the femoral artery which is immediately lateral to the vein will indicate the position of the vein. The vein must not be occluded when suturing the inguinal ligament to the pectineal ligament.

When opening the sac it is important to ensure that the sac proper has in fact been opened, and that opening up fascial planes outside the true sac is not mistaken for opening the sac itself.

If the lacunar ligament has to be cut to release constriction at the neck of the sac, the possible presence of an abnormal obturator artery must be remembered. However, an abnormal obturator artery is only rarely in the dangerous position on the lateral edge of the lacunar ligament; usually it runs beside the femoral vein at the lateral margin of the femoral ring.

DUCTUS (VAS) DEFERENS

Background

The ductus deferens, the more modern proper name for the vas deferens, passes from the epididymis (attached to the testis) in the scrotum, through the inguinal canal to enter the pelvis and join the duct of the seminal vesicle to form the ejaculatory duct which runs through the prostate gland to open into the urethra. From the epididymis to the deep inguinal ring it is one of the constituents of the spermatic cord, contained within the cord's fascial coverings (page 116). In the upper lateral part of the scrotum before entering the inguinal canal through the superficial inguinal ring, the spermatic cord is easily palpated and the ductus can be readily distinguished as a firm tubular structure. This is the site for removing a short length of ductus (on both sides) to produce male sterility; the operation is still known as vasectomy despite the tube's change of name, and can be carried out under local or general anaesthesia.

Approach

The upper part of the scrotum is palpated from the side between the thumb and two fingers, and the ductus identified as a firm cordlike structure.

A short transverse (1 cm) incision (A) is made in the scrotal skin to exposure the bundle of tissues that form the spermatic cord, including the ductus.

A length of ductus is dissected out from the surrounding spermatic tissues by incising the fascial coverings longitudinally; the ductus should be an unmistakeable white structure (B). A length of a centimetre or two is removed, and each remaining cut end of the ductus is folded back on itself and tied.

The operation is then carried out on the other side.

Hazards and Safeguards

The specimens of ductus removed must be sent for histological examination, to confirm that ductus has indeed been excised. The white tubular nature of the structure should make its identification easy, but lengths of dense connective tissue and blood vessels have been known to be removed in error!

Some swelling and haematoma formation may occur in the loose scrotal tissue.

Spontaneous reunion of the cut ends of the ductus is very rare.

A
Incision line for vasectomy.

B
Right ductus deferens exposed in the spermatic cord.

1   Cut edge of spermatic cord coverings
2   Ductus deferens

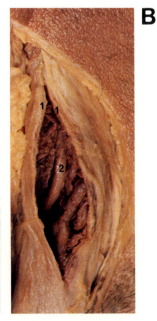

A

B

STOMACH

Background

The stomach lies in the left upper quadrant of the abdomen. Its lesser curvature is attached to the liver by the lesser omentum, while the greater omentum hangs down from the greater curvature and becomes fused with the underlying transverse colon and mesocolon. The left and right gastric arteries anastomose in the lesser omentum along the lesser curvature and give off numerous branches to the stomach. The left and right gastro-epiploic arteries lie in the greater omentum near the greater curvature; they do not directly anastomose with one another as frequently as textbook diagrams usually suggest, but they give off numerous branches both to the stomach and omentum. The upper part of the greater curvature and fundus receive the short gastric branches from the splenic artery. Veins and lymphatic channels accompany the above vessels. Lymph passes to four main groups of nodes – left gastric, pancreatico-splenic, right gastro-epiploic and pyloric.

The vagus nerves give important branches to the stomach, controlling motility and secretion. The anterior vagal trunk lies directly on the anterior wall of the abdominal part of the oesophagus, near its right margin; as it runs down in the lesser omentum near the lesser curvature with the left gastric artery (where it is often known as the anterior nerve of Latarjet), it gives branches to the anterior surface of the stomach, and a large hepatic branch which in turn gives a branch to the pyloric antrum. The posterior vagal trunk lies in loose tissue near the right margin of the abdominal oesophagus; as it passes down in the lesser omentum (as the posterior nerve of Latarjet) on a deeper plane than the anterior trunk, it gives off a large coeliac branch that runs backwards along the left gastric artery to reach the coeliac ganglion, and numerous branches to the posterior surface of the stomach.

The commonest operation on the stomach is its partial removal (partial gastrectomy) for peptic ulcer – to remove a gastric ulcer or to remove the acid-secreting pyloric area in cases of duodenal ulcer. More extensive (subtotal) or complete gastrectomy may be required for carcinoma. The approach for partial gastrectomy will be described here, together with that for vagotomy – sectioning the vagal trunks (truncal vagotomy) or their gastric branches (selective vagotomy) in order to diminish acid secretion in duodenal ulcer.

In view of its superficial position the stomach is easily visualised on opening the upper abdomen. For partial gastrectomy about two-thirds of the stomach is removed, the site of the distal transection being immediately beyond the pylorus. The remaining cut end of the duodenum is closed off, and the remaining cut end of the stomach is joined to the side of a loop of jejunum that has been brought up through an opening made in the greater omentum. For vagotomy the trunks are visualised by incising peritoneum at the lower end of the oesophagus and their branches can be ligated and cut with the branches of the gastric vessels in the lesser omentum.

Approach for Partial Gastrectomy

A midline epigastric or right paramedian incision is used.

The greater omentum at the greater curvature of the stomach is identified and the epiploic branches of the gastro-epiploic vessels that run along the greater curvature are ligated (page 120, A), beginning on the left below the short gastric vessels.

The stomach is now turned upwards and medially to free its posterior wall from the adherent transverse colon and mesocolon (B) and to visualise the gastro-duodenal artery and ligate further branches to the omentum and duodenum.

The right gastric vessels are exposed and divided by pulling the stomach upwards and to the left. The duodenum is cleared of vessels to just beyond the intended line of resection, and it is divided between clamps, the distal end being closed off.

The bile duct passing behind the superior (first) part of the duodenum should be farther to the right than the line of duodenal transection.

With the stomach held upwards and forwards the lesser omentum is examined and the left gastric artery identified, dividing branches to the gastric wall.

With the colon pulled downwards a line of resection can be selected below the short gastric vessels, and the required extent of the stomach removed.

Continuity between the remainder of the stomach and the small intestine is restored by suturing the cut end of the stomach to the side of a loop of jejunum that is brought up through a cut made in an avascular part of the greater omentum.

Hazards and Safeguards

The middle colic vessels which lie within the transverse mesocolon must not be damaged when freeing the posterior wall of the stomach. The greater omentum that hangs down from the greater curvature and the transverse mesocolon behind the omentum usually adhere to one another to a variable extent, and the plane of cleavage between them must be found (page 120, B). There is usually less adherence on the left, and this is where the separation should begin.

The left gastric artery is a much larger vessel than the right gastric, and for safety is doubly ligated.

An accessory hepatic branch arising from the left gastric artery should not be divided, nor should the branch of the left gastric that goes to the coeliac plexus (to avoid the posterior vagal trunk that runs with that branch).

The bile duct must not be damaged when closing off the duodenal stump.

When the loop of jejunum (about 50 cm from the duodenojejunal flexure) is brought up through a hole made in the greater omentum in order to anastomose it with the cut end of the stomach, care must be taken to ensure that the loop is sutured in place 'the right way round', i.e. that it is arranged isoperistaltically so that its contents are propelled distally.

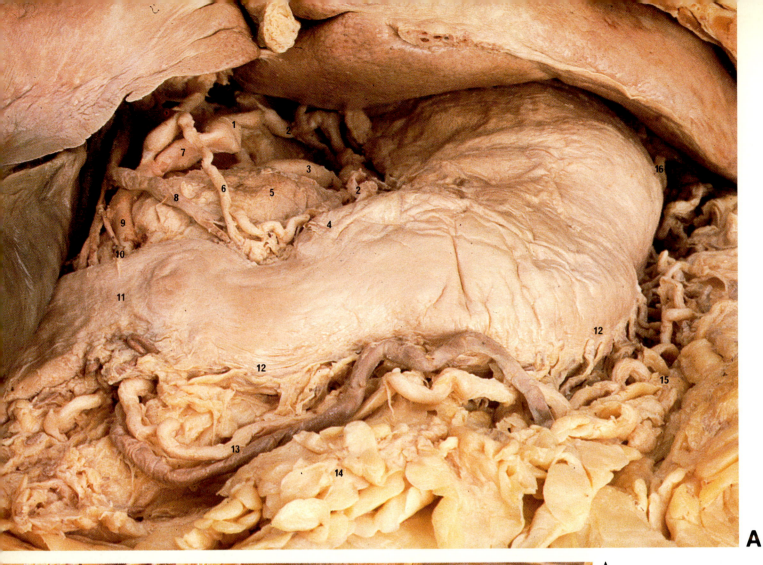

A

A

The stomach, with peritoneum removed, to show gastric vessels.

B

The greater omentum lifted up to show its adherence to the transverse colon. The plane between the two is opened up (as at the arrows) to approach the posterior surface of the stomach.

1	Coeliac trunk
2	Left gastric artery
3	Splenic artery
4	Lesser curvature
5	Pancreas
6	Right gastric artery
7	Common hepatic artery
8	Right gastric vein
9	Gastroduodenal artery
10	Prepyloric vein
11	Gastroduodenal junction
12	Greater curvature
13	Right gastro-epiploic vessels
14	Greater omentum
15	Left gastro-epiploic vessels
16	Short gastric vessels
17	Transverse colon

B

Approach for Vagotomy

A midline epigastric or right paramedian incision is used.

The left triangular ligament is incised so that the left lobe of the liver can be retracted to the right to give a clear view of the gastro-oesophageal junction.

For truncal vagotomy the peritoneum over the gastro-oesophageal junction is incised transversely and the anterior vagal trunk identified (C). A 2 cm length of it is excised.

The posterior trunk is identified and cut near the right oesophageal margin.

For selective vagotomy the trunks themselves are not cut, only their branches to the body of the stomach that run with or near the gastric vessels in the lesser omentum. Ligating vessels along the lesser curvature from below the gastro-oesophageal junction to the incisura angularis will inevitably include severing nerve branches, but any nerves that can be identified individually can also be cut. The peritoneum on the front of the stomach just below the gastro-oesophageal junction is incised down to muscle so that any anterior vagal branches coursing over the wall in this region can be dissected out and cut.

Branches from both vagal trunks can be dealt with from the front, but an alternative approach to the posterior trunk branches involves opening into the lesser sac below the greater curvature and turning the stomach upwards so that the posterior trunk can be exposed by cutting the peritoneum that forms the posterior layer of the lesser omentum (D).

Hazards and Safeguards

Given adequate exposure of the abdominal oesophagus, identification of the vagal trunks is not difficult. It must be remembered that the anterior trunk is in contact with the muscular wall of the oesophagus, whereas the posterior is not in contact but lies in loose tissue a little behind and to the right of the right oesophageal margin. The anterior trunk may be double (20%) but the posterior rarely so (1%).

The left inferior phrenic vein must not be damaged when cutting the left triangular ligament.

While the object in selective vagotomy is to cut only the branches to the body of the stomach and to leave pyloric, hepatic and coeliac branches intact, it is even more important to ensure that *all* the gastric branches are indeed severed; hence the need to clear any nerves on the front of the stomach wall below the gastro-oesophageal junction as well as those that run in from the lesser omentum.

Severing the gastric branches of the right and left gastric arteries in the lesser omentum does not imperil the blood suppy to the stomach since there is profuse anastomosis of vessels in the gastric wall.

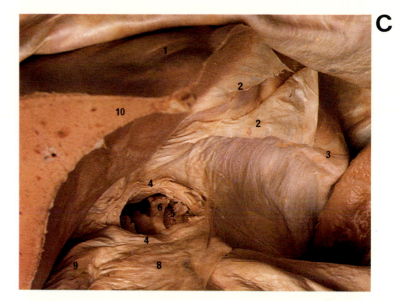

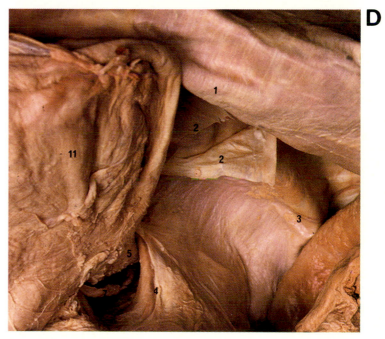

C

Anterior and posterior vagal trunks at the gastro-oesophageal junction. The peritoneum is incised over the junction to display the trunks. At operation the left lobe of the liver (here partly removed) is retracted by incising the left triangular ligament.

D

Posterior vagal trunk, exposed from behind through the lesser sac.

1	Diaphragm	**7**	Posterior vagal trunk
2	Left triangular ligament	**8**	Anterior surface of stomach
3	Inferior phrenic vessels	**9**	Lesser omentum
4	Cut edge of peritoneum	**10**	Left lobe of liver
5	Oesophagus	**11**	Posterior surface of stomach
6	Anterior vagal trunk		

DUODENUM AND PANCREAS

Background

The duodenum describes an approximately C-shaped curve that embraces the head of the pancreas, although the first part of the duodenum is in front of the pancreas. The first 2.5 cm is suspended, like the lesser curvature of the stomach, by the lesser omentum but the remainder of the organ is retroperitoneal. Above the superior (first) part, which is 5 cm long and passes from the pylorus not only to the right but *backwards*, is the right free margin of the lesser omentum, containing the portal vein with the hepatic artery in front of the vein but on its left, and the bile duct in front of the vein but on its right. The epiploic foramen (entrance to the lesser sac) is above this part of the duodenum and behind this part of the lesser omentum, and is bounded by two large veins – the portal in front and the inferior vena cava behind (page 130). The gastroduodenal artery and the bile duct run behind the superior part, the artery dividing at its lower border into the superior pancreaticoduodenal and right gastro-epiploic branches.

The descending (second) part overlaps the hilar region of the right kidney and is in contact with the right margin of the head of the pancreas. The root of the transverse mesocolon crosses the middle of this part, so that the upper half of this part is in the supracolic compartment (A) of peritoneum and the lower half in the infracolic compartment (B). The bile and pancreatic ducts enter this descending part on the posteromedial wall 8–10 cm from the pylorus at the hepatopancreatic ampulla (page 130). The accessory pancreatic duct enters about 2 cm more proximally. The superior pancreaticoduodenal artery anastomoses with its inferior namesake in the groove between this part of the duodenum and the head of the pancreas.

The transverse or horizontal (third) part of the duodenum is in contact with the lower border of the head and uncinate process of the pancreas. The superior mesenteric artery, with the companion vein on the right side of the artery, crosses in front of the uncinate process and this part of the duodenum to enter the root of the mesentery which itself crosses the left half of this region of the duodenum obliquely. The right psoas major, inferior vena cava and aorta are behind the duodenum here and are seen below its inferior border. The short ascending (fourth) part passes upwards and to the left at the left edge of the uncinate process to lie below the inferior surface of the body of the pancreas. Here the bowel turns forwards at the duodenojejunal flexure, marking the junction between the duodenum and the rest of the mall intestine, and where the root of the mesentery begins. The flexure is supported by a fibromuscular band, the suspensory muscle or ligament (of Treitz), which passes from the right crus of the diaphragm to the back of the flexure, running behind the pancreas and splenic vein and in front of the left renal vessels.

The clinically important first part of the duodenum is supplied by branches from several arteries – hepatic, gastroduodenal, superior pancreaticoduodenal, right gastro-epiploic and right gastric – with the remainder of the organ receiving branches from the superior and inferior pancreaticoduodenal, the latter anastomosing with jejunal vessels. Venous blood drains either directly into the portal vein or into its superior mesenteric or splenic tributaries.

Apart from peptic ulceration in the first centimetre or two, the duodenum is not often the site of disease, and the most proximal part is easily seen at gastric operations. The region that otherwise most commonly requires a surgical approach is the descending (second) part, in connexion with carcinoma of the head of the pancreas and for exploring the lower end of the bile duct and the hepatopancreatic ampulla. This part of the duodenum can be mobilized by cutting the peritoneum along its lateral margin and then peeling the organ forwards and medially. This kind of duodenal mobilization (known as Kocher's manoeuvre and de scribed here) can also be used for exposing the inferior vena cava for portacaval anastomosis, and for facilitating the anastomosis of duodenum to stomach after gastric operations.

The pancreas lies behind the peritoneum of the posterior abdominal wall, and is obliquely rather than transversely placed. A transverse section or CT scan will not normally pass through the whole length of the organ; the head is the right extremity and lies within the C-shaped curve of the duodenum at the level of the second lumbar vertebra, and the tail is at the left end between the two layers of peritoneum that form the lienorenal ligament and at the level of the first lumbar vertebra. The superior mesenteric vessels cross in front of the uncinate process of the head before running over the transverse (third) part of the duodenum and entering the root of the mesentery (B). The transverse mesocolon is attached to the lower border of the pancreas. The lower part of the head and the uncinate process are covered by peritoneum of the right infracolic compartment but the rest is behind the peritoneum of the posterior wall of the lesser sac. The beginning of the portal vein lies behind the neck of the pancreas and runs upwards and to the right to become enclosed by the peritoneum that forms the right free margin of the lesser omentum. The splenic vein, which unites with the superior mesenteric to form the portal vein, runs behind the tail and body of the pancreas.

Most of the pancreas receives its arterial blood from the splenic artery which runs a tortuous course behind the upper border of the body of the gland, but the head receives small branches from the superior and inferior pancreaticoduodenal vessels. Veins drain into the portal vein to its main tributaries.

The commonest reason for operative approach to the pancreas is the presence of carcinoma of the head of the pancreas causing obstruction to the lower end of the bile duct (with jaundice). It may be possible to remove the head of the pancreas together with the surrounding C-shaped loop of duodenum (pancreatoduodenectomy), and this approach will be described.

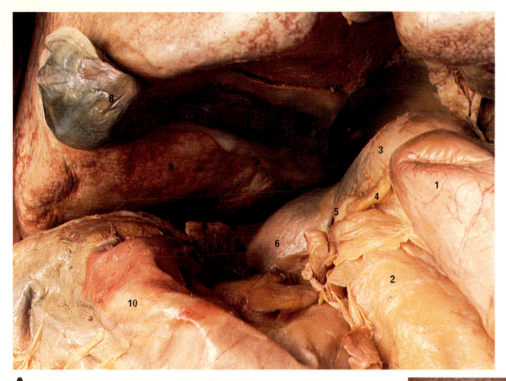

A

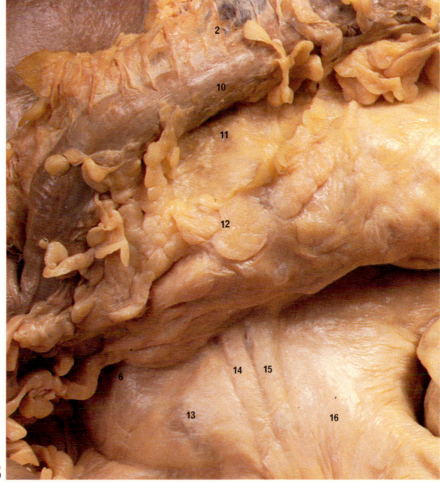

A

Right upper abdomen, showing the upper part of the C-shaped duodenal loop.

B

Upper abdomen, without dissection but with the greater omentum, transverse colon and mesocolon lifted up to show the transverse (third) part of the duodenum being crossed by the superior mesenteric vessels.

1 Pyloric end of stomach
2 Greater omentum
3 Superior part of duodenum
4 Gastroduodenal artery
5 Junction of 3 and 6
6 Descending part of duodenum
7 Hepatorenal pouch
8 Gall bladder
9 Right lobe of liver
10 Transverse colon
11 Transverse mesocolon
12 Posterior surface of stomach
13 Transverse part of duodenum
14 Superior mesenteric vein
15 Superior mesenteric artery
16 Root of mesentery

B

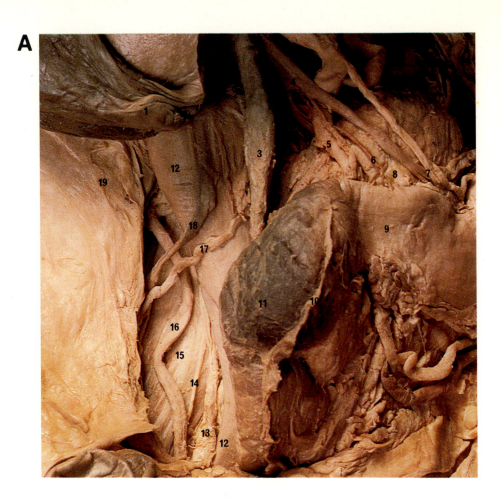

A

Mobilisation of the Duodenum

A right paramedian incision is used, extending from the xiphoid process to below the umbilicus.

The hepatic flexure of the colon is retracted downwards.

An incision in the peritoneum is made just to the right of the convex right border of the descending (second) part of the duodenum, where the peritoneum lies in front of the kidney. This part of the duodenum and the head of the pancreas can now be dissected off the kidney and the inferior vena cava and pulled forwards and to the left (A), enabling the lower end of the bile duct, the ampulla and the head of the pancreas to be palpated between the thumb and fingers (B). Further medial displacement will reveal the aorta with the coeliac trunk and the origin of the superior mesenteric artery.

Hazards and Safeguards

The inferior vena cava, ureter and the gonadal vessels must not be damaged when peeling the duodenum forwards. The sympathetic trunk is under cover of the right margin of the vena cava.

A

Right upper abdomen. Dissection after incising the peritoneum to begin mobilisation of the duodenum. In this specimen the duodenal loop is lower than in the usual textbook description and makes the gonadal vessels seem unusually high in relation to the duodenum.

B

Cross section of the abdomen at the level of the second lumbar vertebra, from below, showing the relationship of the descending part of the duodenum to the head of the pancreas bile duct and inferior vena cava.

C

Diagram of restoration of continuity.

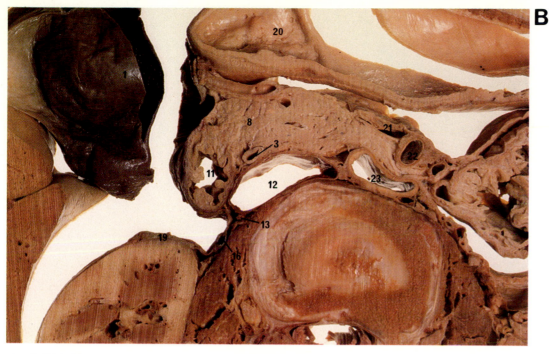

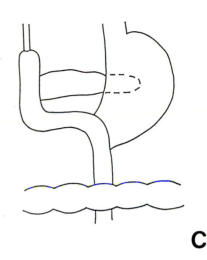

1	Gall bladder	13	Sympathetic trunk
2	Cystic duct	14	Genitofemoral nerve
3	Bile duct	15	Psoas major
4	Portal vein	16	Ureter
5	Gastroduodenal artery	17	Gonadal artery
6	Prepyloric vein	18	Gonadal vein
7	Right gastric vessels	19	Peritoneum over kidney
8	Pancreas	20	Stomach
9	Superior part of duodenum	21	Superior mesenteric vein
10	Cut edge of peritoneum	22	Superior mesenteric artery
11	Descending part of duodenum	23	Aorta
12	Inferior vena cava		

Approach to the Head of the Pancreas

A right paramedian incision extending from the xiphoid process to the umbilicus is commonly used.

The transverse colon is retracted downwards to reveal the descending (second) part of the duodenum, which is mobilised as described above. The head of the pancreas and the ampullary region of the bile and pancreatic ducts can now be palpated between the thumb and fingers. The gastroduodenal and right gastric arteries are divided above the pyloroduodenal junction so that the portal vein can be examined to see whether it can be freed from surrounding pancreatic tissue.

If the extent of disease is such that successful removal of the head of the pancreas is considered feasible, the stomach is transected so that its two ends can be reflected to give greater exposure of the pancreas.

The bile duct is transected above the duodenum, the pancreas is divided to the left of the portal and superior mesenteric vessels and dissected free from those vessels, and the jejunum is cut across distal to the duodenojejunal flexure. The whole C-shaped loop of gut with the head of the pancreas can now be removed.

Continuity is restored (C) by anastomosing the remaining cut end of the pancreas (with its duct) to the *side* of the jejunum, the bile duct to the cut *end* of the jejunum, and the stomach to the *side* of the jejunum.

Hazards and Safeguards

Resection of the head of the pancreas and adjacent structures is obviously a formidable undertaking that is usually carried out to alleviate rather than cure extensive malignant disease. As far as anatomy is concerned the portal vein is the commanding structure. If the disease has so involved the portal and superior mesenteric veins that they cannot be freed from the affected pancreatic tissue, it is not possible to proceed further with the operation. If resection is considered possible, ligation of small tributaries of these large vessels is important.

Going from right to left, the right renal vessels, the inferior vena cava and the aorta are behind the pancreas.

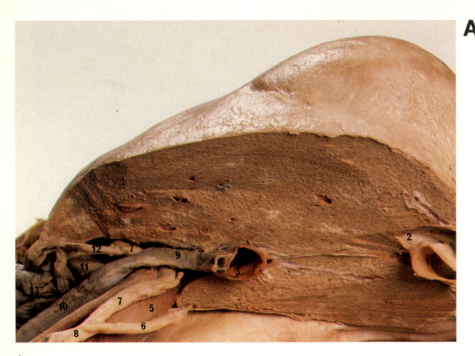

A

The liver after left lobectomy, from the left.

LIVER

Background

The liver is held in position below the diaphragm mainly by clasping the inferior vena cava in a deep groove, with the hepatic veins entering the vena cava while within the groove; the hepatic veins (usually three – right, middle and left) have no extrahepatic course. The peritoneum reflected from liver to diaphragm, forming the left triangular ligament on the left and the right triangular ligament and the upper and lower layers of the coronary ligament on the right, helps to anchor the liver to the diaphragm whose central tendon is firmly fused to the periphery of the vena cava. The main vessels and biliary ducts enter or leave at the porta hepatis and run in the right free margin of the lesser omentum, but the bare area between the two layers of the coronary ligament is in contact with the diaphragm and allows vascular communications between the two structures. These bare area anastomoses and connections with other phrenic vessels can provide a collateral arterial circulation that is sufficient to allow ligation of the hepatic artery in treating certain liver tumours; the tumour tissue appears to get its blood supply from branches of the hepatic artery and degenerates after ligation due to *local* ischaemia although normal liver tissue is not affected (but hepatic artery ligation in jaundiced patients causes *general* hepatic ischaemia).

Based on the way the main branches of the portal vein and hepatic artery divide and the course of bile drainage, functionally the left lobe of the liver includes the anatomical left lobe (to the left of the falciform ligament and the fissure for the ligamentum venosum) together with the quadrate and most of the caudate lobe. The right lobe is the part to the right of the groove for the inferior vena cava and the fossa for the gall bladder but includes a small part of the caudate lobe. The watershed between right and left lobes is approximately along a line drawn through the vena caval groove and gall bladder fossa. The anatomical left lobe forms the left lateral segment, while the quadrate and most of the caudate lobes constitute the left medial segment. The right lobe has anterior and posterior segments but externally the dividing line is not obvious; it extends approximately from the middle of the front of the right lobe to the vena caval groove.

Apart from treatment for abscesses and cysts, operations on the liver include removal of the right or left lobes (hepatic lobectomy), and these are described below, together with a brief account of liver transplantation. To obtain specimens of liver tissue for histological examination, it is easy to remove a small wedge from the inferior border during a laparotomy, but percutaneous biopsy is possible through an intercostal space, and this is also described.

Approach for Left Lobectomy

A right upper paramedian incision is used.

The left triangular ligament, ligamentum teres and the falciform ligament are divided.

The left hepatic duct and the left branches of the portal vein and hepatic artery are dissected out in the porta hepatis and divided (A).

The left lobe is retracted to the right so that the left hepatic vein can be dissected out and divided where it enters the vena cava.

Liver tissue is cut through, ligating vessels and ducts on the way, so that the left lobe together with most of the quadrate and caudate lobes can be removed, the line of resection at the back being level with the left edge of the vena cava. The gall bladder is not removed.

Approach for Right Lobectomy

A right thoraco-abdominal incision is used, in the line of the seventh or eighth rib.

The ligamentum teres, falciform ligament, right triangular ligament and the upper and lower layers of the coronary ligament are divided.

The porta hepatis is exposed and dissected so that the cystic duct and cystic artery, right hepatic duct and right branches of the portal vein and hepatic artery can be divided (B).

The liver is retracted to the left to expose the inferior vena cava so that the right hepatic vein can be dissected out and divided where it enters the vena cava.

Liver tissue is cut through along a line from the left of the gall bladder to the right edge of the vena cava, ligating vessels and ducts on the way, so that the right lobe including the gall bladder can be removed.

Hazards and Safeguards

Haemorrhage and bile leakage from the cut surface of the liver are major hazards and must be adequately controlled.

The right hepatic vein is short and wide and its ligation requires great care.

The thin-walled vena cava must not be torn and any anomalous vessels entering it must be identified and dealt with.

In right lobectomy it is important to preserve the left hepatic vein and vice versa.

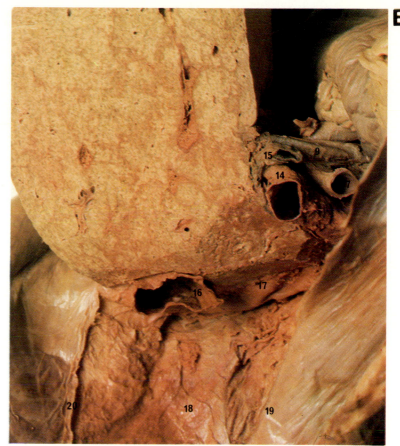

B
The liver after right lobectomy, from the right.

1 Left hepatic vein entering 17
2 Middle hepatic vein
3 Left branch of 5
4 Left hepatic duct
5 Portal vein
6 Left branch of 8
7 Right branch of 8
8 Hepatic artery
9 Common hepatic duct
10 Bile duct
11 Cystic duct
12 Cystic artery
13 Gall bladder
14 Right branch of 5
15 Right hepatic duct
16 Right hepatic vein
17 Inferior vena cava
18 Bare area of diaphragm
19 Lower layer of coronary ligament
20 Upper layer of coronary ligament

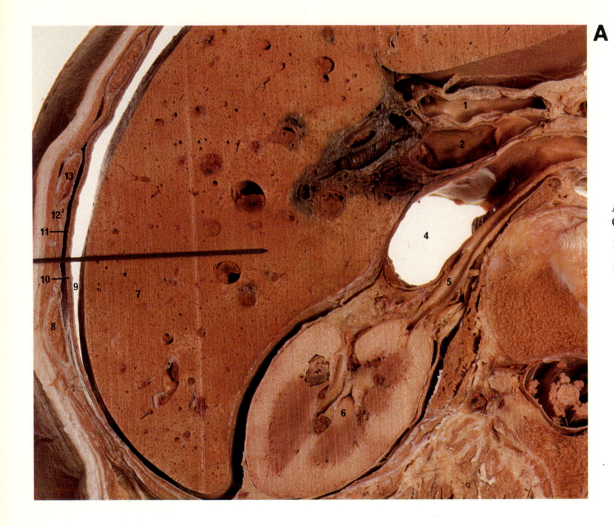

A
Cross section of the right side of the abdomen at the level of the first lumbar vertebra, showing the path of the needle for liver biopsy.

Needle Biopsy of the Liver

With the patient supine, the right ribs and intercostal spaces are identified by counting down from the second rib at the level of the manubriosternal junction. The interspace to be chosen is the one that gives maximum dullness on percussion, usually the eighth or ninth.

Through a wheal of local anaesthesia in the midaxillary line of the chosen space, the biopsy needle is inserted horizontally immediately above the rib at the lower boundary of the space. After skin the needle passes through the external oblique and the intercostal muscles into the costodiaphragmatic recess of the pleura (A). A small injection of saline clears any debris from the lumen of the needle, and then with slight suction on the attached syringe and while the patient stops breathing after an expiration, the needle is quickly plunged through to the liver for 4–5 cm. It goes through the diaphragm and the very narrow subdiaphragmatic compartment of peritoneum on its way into the liver, and is immediately withdrawn, the narrow cylinder of hepatic tissue remaining in the bore of the needle.

Hazards and Safeguards

The needle is inserted just above the rib at the lower border of the interspace to avoid the main intercostal vessels and nerve which run along the lower border of a rib (page 94).

The breath is held while the needle is in the liver substance to avoid lacerating it by movement of the diaphragm; the needle should only be in the liver for a fraction of a second.

By keeping below the eighth rib the lung will not be perforated; in the midaxillary line it does not extend below this level, and holding the breath in expiration at the moment of biopsy ensures that the lower limit of the lung remains as high as possible.

There may be some subsequent pain at the biopsy site, or even referred shoulder-tip pain (via the phrenic nerve) if the diaphragm has been irritated. Some minor haemorrhage is inevitable but penetration of a large vascular or biliary channel is rare.

A misplaced needle may damage the inferior vena cava, kidney, colon or pancreas, and a pneumothorax is a possible complication. The needle should not penetrate more than 6 cm from the skin surface to make sure of not reaching as far as the vena cava.

Transplantation of the Liver

The general principle of obtaining the liver from the donor is to remove the aorta and inferior vena cava from the diaphragm to the level of the common iliac arteries with the liver and kidneys remaining attached by their various vessels. The liver is perfused as soon as possible via the superior mesenteric vein, and the gall bladder is opened and washed out with saline. The liver (including the gall bladder) with supra- and infra-hepatic lengths of vena cava, the portal vein and the common hepatic artery (together with any anomalous hepatic vessels) is dissected out, further perfused and stored in ice-cold saline.

To remove the patient's liver, the bile duct is ligated and divided as high as possible, and the portal vein and hepatic artery defined (but not divided at this stage) (B). The triangular, falciform and coronary ligaments are divided and the bare area separated from the diaphragm. The inferior vena cava below the liver, the portal vein and the hepatic artery are now divided, followed by division of the vena cava above the liver so that the organ can be removed.

To install the donor liver, the suprahepatic vena cava is sutured to the same vessel of the donor liver but it remains clamped so that there is no blood flow. The patient and donor portal veins are joined, and portal blood is allowed to flow through the liver and out of the lower end of the donor vena cava before joining this to the patient's infrahepatic vena cava. The suprahepatic vena cava is now unclamped, and the patient and donor hepatic arteries joined, followed by reunion of the bile ducts. Finally the patient and donor falciform ligaments are sutured together.

Hazards and Safeguards

Enlarged retroperitoneal and bare area vessels may cause troublesome haemorrhage when removing the patient's liver.

After restoring portal vein continuity with the donor liver, the *suprahepatic* inferior vena cava must be kept clamped until blood has been allowed to drain out through the as yet unsutured *infrahepatic* vena cava. This is because potassium ions accumulate in the ischaemic liver and may cause cardiac arrest unless flushed out before hepatic blood enters the general circulation.

If the donor liver has any anomalous hepatic arteries they must be preserved with any appropriate parent vessel so that they can become part of the restored arterial circulation. For example, a right hepatic artery arising from the superior mesenteric may entail removing it from the donor in continuity with the adjacent part of the superior mesenteric so that the latter can be anastomosed with the patient's splenic artery.

The viability of the bile duct of the transplant is important; its cut end should bleed when the hepatic circulation is restored if anastomosis with the patient's duct is to be successful.

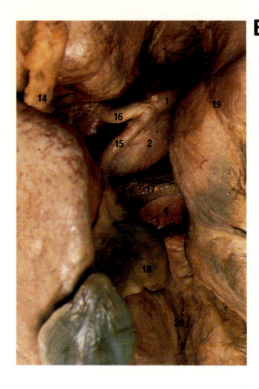

B

B

Portal vein, hepatic artery and bile duct, from the right, after removal of peritoneum. These major structures, together with the inferior vena cava above and below the liver, must be divided for transplantation.

1 Hepatic artery
2 Portal vein
3 Right hepatic duct
4 Inferior vena cava
5 Right renal artery
6 Kidney
7 Right lobe of liver
8 Tenth rib
9 Peritoneal cavity
10 Diaphragm
11 Pleural cavity
12 Intercostal muscles
13 Ninth rib
14 Falciform ligament in fissure for ligamentum teres
15 Right branch of 1
16 Left branch of 1
17 Bile duct
18 Gall bladder
19 Gastroduodenal junction
20 Hepatorenal pouch

PORTAL VEIN

Background

After being formed by the union of the superior mesenteric and splenic veins behind the neck of the pancreas, the portal vein courses upwards and to the right to reach the porta hepatis. It passes behind the superior (first) part of the duodenum and then runs in the right free margin of the lesser omentum with the bile duct in front and on the right of the vein and the hepatic artery in front and on the left of the vein. The vein within its peritoneal covering here forms the anterior boundary of the epiploic foramen. The inferior vena cava is immediately behind the epiploic foramen at this level, and the portal vein crosses the vena cava obliquely rather than running parallel with it.

The portal vein can be anastomosed to the inferior vena cava (portacaval anastomosis) in order to reduce the pressure of blood in dilated oesophageal varices. The two veins are conveniently close to one another where they form the anterior and posterior boundaries of the epiploic foramen, and when freed from their peritoneal coverings they can be joined in this region.

Approach

A right subcostal (Kocher's) incision is used.

The duodenum is mobilised (Kocher's manoeuvre – page 124) and turned to the left to expose the vena cava.

The peritoneum of the lesser omentum below the porta hepatis is incised to identify the bile duct which is retracted to the left so that the portal vein can be fully exposed, retracting also if necessary the hepatic artery (page 129, B).

The portal vein is transected near the porta hepatis so that the distal end of it can be anastomosed to the side of the vena cava.

Hazards and Safeguards

Damage to the biliary tract or hepatic arteries must be avoided, with care being taken to recognise any anomalies of the duct system or aberrant vessels.

When making the anastomosis with the portal vein the vena cava must not be drawn away from the posterior abdominal wall, otherwise lumbar veins may be torn.

GALL BLADDER AND BILE DUCT

Background

The essential relations of the gall bladder are the liver, anterior abdominal wall, transverse colon and duodenum. The fundus normally lies beneath the right ninth costal cartilage where the lateral border of the rectus sheath reaches the costal margin. At the opposite end of the gall bladder the cystic duct is continuous with the neck of the gall bladder and joins the common hepatic duct 1–2 cm above the duodenum to form the bile duct (formerly known as the common bile duct) (A and B). The bile duct runs downwards in the right free margin of the lesser omentum, anterolateral to the portal vein and with the hepatic artery on the left of the duct. Here the epiploic foramen is behind the portal vein. The duct then passes behind the superior (first) part of the duodenum to run in a groove or tunnel in the pancreas and enter the posteromedial wall of the descending (second) part of the duodenum, usually joining the main pancreatic duct at the hepatopancreatic ampulla whose opening into the duodenum is about 10 cm beyond the pylorus.

The hepatic artery divides below the porta hepatis into right and left branches. In the standard textbook description the right branch passes behind the common hepatic duct and gives off the cystic artery, which should normally be found running to the gall bladder in the triangle formed by the liver, common hepatic duct and cystic duct (Calot's triangle). The many variations in the arterial and duct systems constitute the main hazards in biliary tract surgery.

A diseased gall bladder can be removed (cholecystectomy) or it can simply be opened (cholecystostomy) to remove stones without being itself removed. The bile duct can also be opened (choledochotomy) for the removal of stones or the cystic duct opened for the insertion of a cannula for performing operative cholangiography.

The fundus of the gall bladder is easily visualised after opening the abdomen below the right costal margin, but to display the rest of it and the duct system the surrounding structures must be retracted and the peritoneum of the right free margin of the lesser omentum incised.

Approach

A right subcostal (Kocher's) incision is commonly used.

The liver, transverse colon and duodenum are suitably retracted to expose the gall bladder. If it is to be opened (not removed) for removal of gallstones it is first drained of bile by inserting a trocar and cannula into the fundus; the same opening can then be enlarged as required for removing the stones.

For cholecystectomy, the peritoneum over the cystic duct and the upper end of the lesser omentum is incised transversely so that the anatomy of the cystic duct, bile duct, cystic artery and other vessels can be defined.

The cystic duct and cystic artery are ligated, allowing the gall bladder to be dissected from its hepatic bed from the neck down towards the fundus and removed.

To open the bile duct it is incised longitudinally as it lies above the superior (first) part of the duodenum.

For operative cholangiography the cannula is inserted into the cystic duct and then led down into the bile duct.

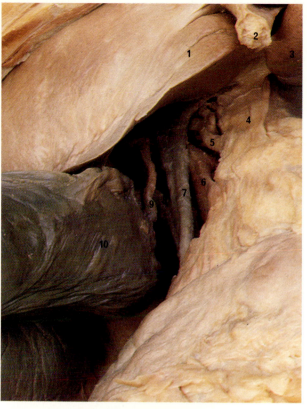

A

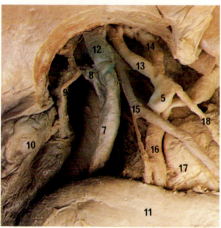

B

Hazards and Safeguards

About 15% of patients have some variation from the standard textbook description of the duct system but arterial anomalies are much commoner.

Of duct anomalies the commonest are a long cystic duct running parallel to a long common hepatic duct before they join together behind the duodenum or pancreas (instead of above the duodenum), and a cystic duct that spirals round behind the common hepatic duct to join it on its left side (instead of the right side).

In 20% of subjects the right hepatic artery passes in front of the common hepatic duct instead of behind it, and instead of arising from the right hepatic artery the cystic artery may come from any other adjacent vessel such as the hepatic artery itself, the left hepatic or the gastroduodenal.

The right hepatic artery may accompany the cystic duct and be mistaken for the cystic artery.

Other aberrant or accessory hepatic arteries may be present, and before ligating what is considered to be the cystic artery it must be positively identified, especially when there are vessels in unusual positions.

A

The bile duct is being dissected in the right free margin of the lesser omentum.

B

A more extensive dissection of the bile duct and related structures.

1	Right lobe of liver
2	Falciform ligament
3	Quadrate lobe
4	Lesser omentum
5	Hepatic artery
6	Portal vein
7	Bile duct
8	Cystic duct
9	Cystic artery
10	Gall bladder
11	Superior part of duodenum
12	Common hepatic duct
13	Right branch of 5
14	Left branch of 5
15	Right gastric vein
16	Gastroduodenal artery
17	Pancreas
18	Right gastric artery

SPLEEN

Background

The spleen lies in the lateral angle between the stomach and left kidney, in the long axes of the ninth to eleventh ribs and separated from them posterolaterally by the diaphragm and pleural cavity. It is attached to the kidney, which is medial to it, by the two layers of peritoneum that form the lienorenal ligament and that contain the splenic vessels and the tail of the pancreas which lies against the splenic hilum where the vessels enter and leave (A). It is attached to the stomach, which is in front of it, by the two layers of peritoneum that form the gastrosplenic ligament and contain the short gastric vessels. The spleen is thus at the left lateral margin of the lesser sac. The left flexure of the colon (splenic flexure) is in front of the lower end of the spleen. A normal spleen cannot be felt; it must be at least twice its normal size before becoming palpable at the costal margin.

The spleen may have to be removed because of rupture and dangerous haemorrhage following abdominal or thoracic injuries, or for specific diseases of the organ especially in tropical areas. It is also removed as part of the therapy of various blood disorders, in Hodgkin's disease and as part of extensive abdominal operations such as total gastrectomy. The operation of removing the spleen (splenectomy) essentially involves cutting through the lienorenal and gastrosplenic ligaments.

Approach

A left paramedian incision is commonly used, extending from the xiphoid process to below the umbilicus.

The spleen is drawn medially and the left (outer) layer of the lienorenal ligament incised to expose the splenic vessels and the tail of the pancreas. The pancreas is dissected free and the splenic vessels ligated (the artery first, then the vein).

The right (inner) layer of the lienorenal ligament is divided, so entering the lesser sac and freeing the spleen from the kidney and diaphragm. The splenic flexure of the colon may be adherent to the spleen and is separated from it.

The spleen now remains attached to the stomach by the gastrosplenic ligament containing the short gastric vessels. These are ligated and the spleen removed by cutting through the rest of the ligament.

An alternative method of splenectomy, especially after traumatic rupture with haemorrhage, is first to enter the lesser sac by cutting the gastrosplenic ligament, incise the peritoneum of its posterior wall and ligate the splenic artery. Then the lienorenal ligament is dealt with, dissecting out the tail of the pancreas and ligating further splenic vessels.

Hazards and Safeguards

Damage to the pancreas and stomach must be avoided when ligating vessels, especially the short gastrics when the upper part of the stomach is adherent to a large spleen; inadvertent perforations can be easily made in the stomach wall.

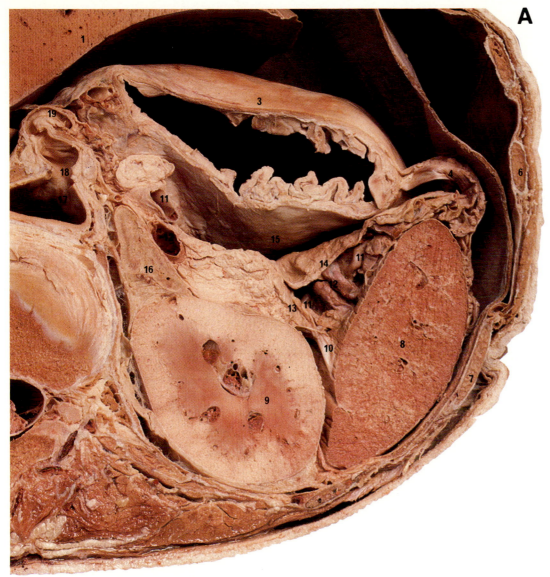

A

Cross section of the left upper abdomen, at the level of the disc between the twelfth thoracic and first lumbar vertebrae, to show the relations and peritoneal attachments of the spleen.

1 Left lobe of liver
2 Diaphragm
3 Stomach
4 Gastrosplenic ligament
5 Pleural cavity
6 Ninth rib
7 Tenth rib
8 Spleen
9 Kidney
10 Posterior layer of lienorenal ligament
11 Splenic artery
12 Splenic vein
13 Tail of pancreas
14 Anterior layer of lienorenal ligament
15 Lesser sac
16 Suprarenal gland
17 Aorta
18 Coeliac trunk
19 Left gastric artery

SUPRARENAL GLAND

Background

The right suprarenal gland rests above the upper pole of the right kidney, within its own compartment of the renal fascia and to the right of the inferior vena cava but on a deeper plane (due to the forwards projection of the vertebral column) (page 165, B). It is mostly covered anteriorly by peritoneum of the greater sac but its upper extremity has no peritoneal covering and is in contact with the bare area of the liver. It is supplied by many small arteries derived from the aorta and the inferior phrenic and renal arteries but there is usually only one vein that drains directly into the vena cava.

The left suprarenal gland lies along the medial side of the upper pole of the left kidney, within its own compartment of the renal fascia and to the left of the aorta but on a deeper level (page 133, A). It is mostly covered anteriorly by peritoneum of the lesser sac but its lower tip is usually overlapped by the pancreas. The arterial supply is similar to that of the right gland and there is one longer vein draining to the left renal vein. The left greater splanchnic nerve is usually behind the left gland.

The suprarenal glands may require to be removed because of tumours in the glands themselves, or as treatment of other endocrine disorders or certain cases of carcinoma of the breast. Both glands can be approached from the front through the peritoneal cavity. The right gland is exposed by incising the peritoneum over the upper pole of the kidney; on the left the stomach and spleen are retracted medially and the peritoneum incised so that the part that forms the posterior wall of the lesser sac can be stripped medially with the splenic vessels and the tail of the pancreas until the gland is exposed. A single anterior abdominal wall incision is used if both glands are to be dealt with at the same operation, as described here, but for approaching a single gland a posterior retroperitoneal route can be used as for the kidney (page 138).

Approach

For the anterior approach to both glands, a left paramedian incision is made from the xiphoid process to below the umbilicus.

To approach the right gland through the anterior abdominal incision, the falciform ligament is divided.

With the liver retracted upwards and the hepatic flexure of the colon and the duodenum drawn downwards, the peritoneum over the upper pole of the right kidney is incised transversely towards the inferior vena cava. Peritoneal flaps are raised to expose the gland (A). The short right suprarenal vein is ligated close to the vena cava and the gland can be removed after detaching the numerous small arteries.

To approach the left gland the spleen and intestines are held out of the way and the peritoneum on the posterior abdominal wall between the splenic flexure and the oesophageal hiatus is incised. A flap of peritoneum is peeled towards the right together with the spleen and its vessels and the tail of the pancreas. The peritoneum is stripped medially until the gland is exposed on the medial side of the upper pole of the kidney (B).

The suprarenal vein is ligated before dealing with the numerous small arteries and the gland can then be removed.

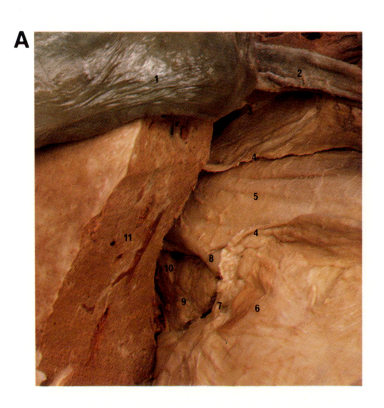

A

The retroperitoneal approach to either gland is made through the bed of the eleventh rib on the appropriate side.

The kidney is identified and the renal fascia incised so that the suprarenal gland can be exposed and removed after ligating the vessels.

Hazards and Safeguards

The right suprarenal vein is only 0.5cm or less in length and it or the vena cava itself can be easily torn. Sometimes there are two or three smaller veins instead of one large one.

The left suprarenal vein is usually single; it is always longer than the right and so easier to ligate. The gland must be subjected to as little handling as possible before venous ligation to prevent surges of hormone release; the veins are ligated before the arteries.

The pleura is at risk in posterior approaches.

A

Right suprarenal gland, from the right. Part of the right lobe of the liver is removed (at operation it is retracted) and the peritoneum is incised over the inferior vena cava and at the reflexion of the inferior layer of the coronary ligament from liver to kidney. This gland is unusually close to the renal vein.

B

Left suprarenal gland, from the left. The left lobe of the liver is removed, together with peritoneum of the lesser omentum and lesser sac, and the stomach is retracted to the subject's left. In this specimen the inferior phrenic vein joins the suprarenal vein instead of entering the inferior vena cava directly.

1   Gall bladder
2   Bile duct
3   Epiploic foramen
4   Cut edge of peritoneum
5   Inferior vena cava
6   Right kidney
7   Cut edge of inferior layer of coronary ligament
8   Right renal vein
9   Right suprarenal gland
10 Right suprarenal vein
11 Right lobe of liver
12 Left lobe of liver
13 Aorta
14 Left inferior phrenic artery
15 Left gastric artery
16 Left coeliac ganglion
17 Left inferior phrenic vein
18 Left suprarenal gland
19 Left suprarenal vein
20 Left renal vein
21 Splenic artery
22 Pancreas
23 Cut edge of lesser omentum at lesser curvature of stomach

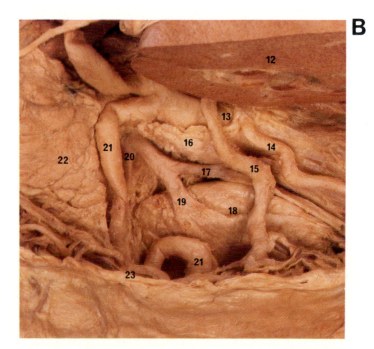

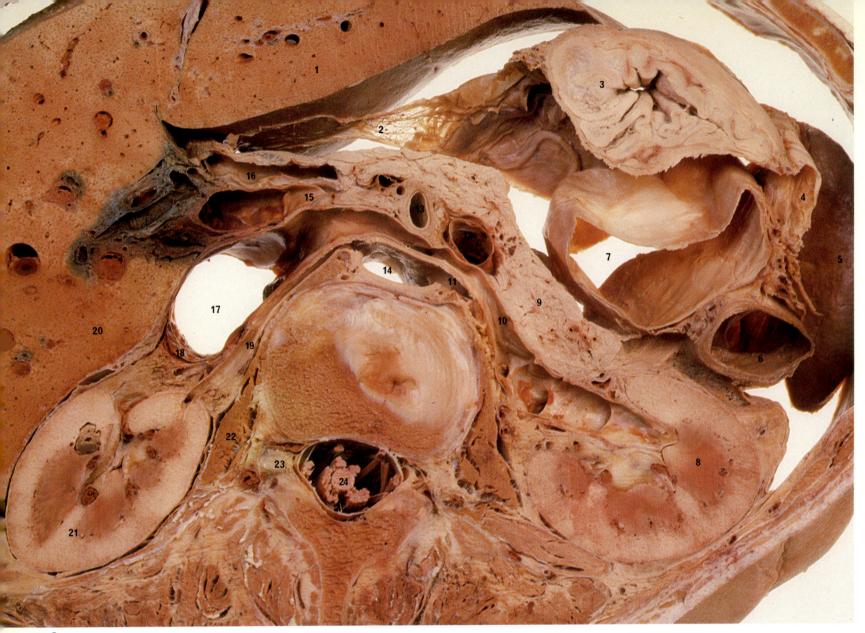

A

KIDNEY

Background

The kidneys lie behind the peritoneum of the upper posterior abdominal wall (A). Their essential posterior relations are the pleura, diaphragm, psoas major, quadratus lumborum and transversus abdominis. The upper pole of the left kidney rises as high as the eleventh rib but on the right only the level of the twelfth rib is reached. The hilum on the right is just below, and on the left just above, the transpyloric plane (which passes through the lower part of the first lumbar vertebra). Part of the colon overlaps the kidney anterolaterally.

At the front, the medial part of the right kidney is overlapped by the descending (second) part of the duodenum with the transverse mesocolon crossing transversely. The right suprarenal gland is at the top of the upper pole, where the peritoneum of the greater sac is reflected on to the liver as the inferior layer of the coronary ligament, so forming the hepatorenal (Morison's) pouch. On the left the pancreas crosses the central part of the kidney with the spleen

Cross section of the abdomen at the level of the disc between the first and second lumbar vertebrae, from below, showing the kidneys and renal vessels.

B

Cross section of the abdomen through the lower pole of the right kidney, from below, with dissection of the renal fascia. In this specimen the perirenal fat (between the renal capsule and renal fascia) is scanty and does not form a complete layer, and there is negligible extraperitoneal fat (outside the renal fascia).

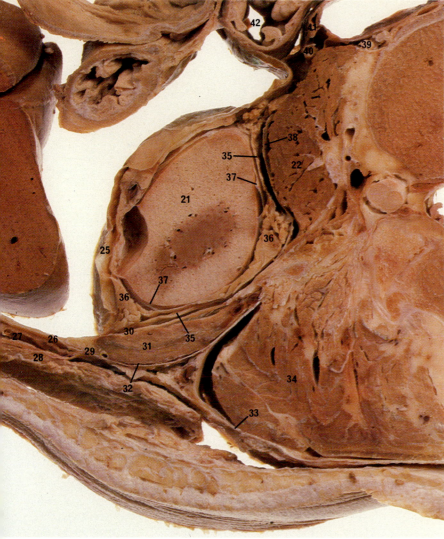

B

1	Left lobe of liver
2	Lesser omentum
3	Pyloric part of stomach
4	Greater omentum
5	Lower end of spleen
6	Descending colon
7	Transverse colon
8	Left kidney
9	Pancreas
10	Left renal vein
11	Left renal artery
12	Splenic vein
13	Superior mesenteric artery
14	Aorta
15	Portal vein
16	Hepatic artery
17	Inferior vena cava
18	Edge of right renal vein
19	Right renal artery
20	Right lobe of liver
21	Right kidney
22	Psoas major
23	First lumbar nerve
24	Conus medullaris and cauda equina
25	Peritoneum
26	Transversus abdominis
27	Internal oblique
28	External oblique
29	Lumbar fascia
30	Anterior layer of 29
31	Quadratus lumborum
32	Middle layer of 29
33	Posterior layer of 29
34	Erector spinae
35	Renal fascia
36	Perirenal fat
37	Renal capsule
38	Sheath of 22
39	Sympathetic trunk
40	Ureter
41	Gonadal vessels
42	Descending part of duodenum

lying against the upper lateral side and attached by the lienorenal ligament. The left suprarenal gland is on the *medial* side of the upper pole which is here covered by peritoneum of the lesser sac. The renal vein, artery and pelvis (which continues into the ureter) are in the hilum of the kidney in that order from front to back, although branches of the main vessels may alter this general pattern. The kidney has its own capsule, outside which is the perirenal fat which in turn is surrounded by the renal fascia (B). The suprarenal gland is enclosed in its own compartment of this fascia.

Many operations on the kidney are performed through a posterolateral approach so that the procedure can be carried out retroperitoneally without opening the peritoneal cavity, and a typical lumbar approach for kidney removal (nephrectomy) is described. An outline is also given of the procedures necessary for transplanting a kidney, and for obtaining a percutaneous biopsy of renal tissue.

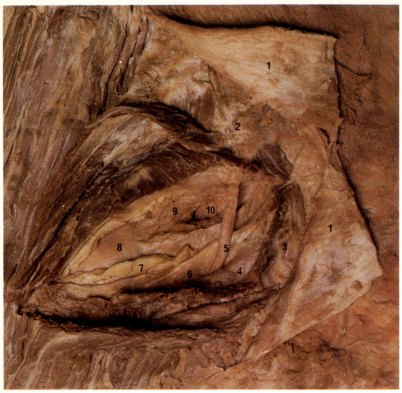

B

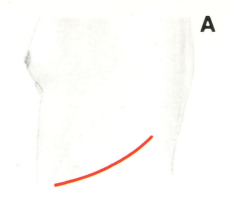

A

Hazards and Safeguards

It is essential to identify correctly the twelfth rib by correlating palpation with radiography, otherwise an unusually short rib may lead to the incision being made below the eleventh rib with inadvertent entry into the pleural cavity. Extending the normal incision medially into erector spinae also puts the pleura at risk since the lower limit of the pleura does not follow the oblique line of the rib but runs *horizontally*, crossing the rib at the outer border of erector spinae. Special care is required if an alternative approach is used by excising the twelfth rib after stripping it from its periosteum and incising through the bed of the rib.

Latissimus dorsi has a lateral free margin which overlaps the posterior free margin of the external oblique. The internal oblique and transversus, having an origin from the lumbar fascia, do not have free margins although the most posterior fibres of internal oblique do not always appear to have a fascial attachment.

The subcostal nerve and vessels lie below the tip of the twelfth rib between internal oblique and transversus (although the distinction between these two muscles here is often indistinct). The nerve should be preserved and retracted downwards but the vessels can be ligated. The iliohypogastric and ilio-inguinal nerves are at a lower level but if seen must also be preserved. Postoperative pain may be caused if any of these nerves are accidentally damaged by sutures or forceps.

After the muscle incisions have been made care must be taken not to open the peritoneal cavity. The amount of extraperitoneal fat (between the transversalis fascia and peritoneum and outside the renal fascia) is very variable and it must not be mistaken for the *perirenal* fat which is *inside* the renal fascia (page 137, B). The initial opening in the renal fascia should be made towards the medial end of the incision to lessen the risk of entering the peritoneal cavity.

When mobilising the kidney the related retroperitoneal structures and their vessels must be remembered, especially when disease has caused undue adherence: on the right the colon, ureter, duodenum, inferior vena cava and suprarenal gland, and on the left the colon, ureter, spleen, tail of the pancreas and suprarenal gland.

Abberant renal vessels and small vessels passing to the suprarenal gland require careful identification and ligature. Normally the renal artery divides into anterior and posterior branches; the anterior lies superior to the main tributary of the renal vein, and the posterior is superior and posterior to its companion vein, but

Lumbar Approach for Nephrectomy

With the patient lying on the opposite side, the skin incision (A) extends from the lateral border of erector spinae just below the twelfth rib to a point 2 cm above the anterior superior iliac spine.

The skin flaps are raised to expose the lateral part of latissimus dorsi overlapping the posterior border of external oblique. Both muscles are cut in the line of the skin incision (B).

The cut muscle edges are retracted so that the underlying internal oblique and transversus merging with the lumbar fascia medially can also be incised. The subcostal nerve deep to internal oblique should be preserved (B).

The transversalis fascia is incised and the extraperitoneal fat in the posterior part of the incision separated to expose the renal fascia. This in turn is incised to expose the perirenal fat which is separated to reveal the kidney (B).

The upper pole of the kidney is freed from fascia and fat, leaving the suprarenal gland within its own compartment of the fascia. The overlying peritoneum is pushed away forwards and medially without incising it.

Pulling the upper pole gently downwards exposes the renal artery and vein running to the hilum. The artery or its main divisions are ligated, followed by ligation of the vein.

With the vessels cut, the kidney can be moved further forwards and downwards to reveal the renal pelvis and ureter which can be ligated and cut so that the organ can be removed.

there can be many variations. Aberrant vessels, especially those to the lower pole, must not be torn.

It is of course necessary to ligate arteries before veins; in such a highly vascular organ this is a physiological necessity rather than an anatomical one!

The descending part of the duodenum overlaps the front of the right kidney and must not be perforated. On the left the pancreas is less liable to damage.

The right renal vein is only 2.5 cm long, so the inferior vena cava is very near the operation area.

Needle Biopsy of the Kidney

The object in percutaneous renal biopsy is to obtain a sample of tissue from the outer part of the lower pole of the kidney, usually on the right. The use of an exploratory needle is often advised to determine the depth required for the biopsy needle.

The patient lies prone and the position of the kidney has been identified radiologically.

A thin exploratory needle is inserted perpendicular to the skin surface 2.5 cm below the twelfth rib, at a distance from the midline determined by measurement on the radiograph to ensure that the lower pole will be entered. Because of the curvature of the body lateral to erector spinae, the needle will be directed somewhat medially.

After skin the needle passes through the lateral margin of quadratus lumborum (enclosed by layers of the lumbar part of the thoracolumbar fascia), retroperitoneal fat, renal fascia, renal fat and finally the renal capsule into the substance of the kidney (C). The needle is advanced by stages with the patient holding the breath in inspiration between each advance and breathing freely between each advance. As the kidney is being entered, a vertical swinging movement is imparted to the needle by the kidney movements that follow diaphragmatic excursion, and a final advance into the depth of the lower pole is made during another held inspiration.

The depth to which the fine exploratory needle has been inserted is noted, and the larger biopsy needle is then inserted in the same line to the same depth.

Hazards and Safeguards

The needle is only advanced when the patient's breath is held, and the needle must not be held when the patient is breathing, so that the kidney is not torn by its respiratory movement against the needle tip.

Damage to a renal vessel or calyx is a potential hazard.

A
Incision line.

B
Lumbar approach to the left kidney. After incising the muscles and transversalis fascia, the extraperitoneal fat is separated to display the renal fascia which is then incised to expose the perirenal fat and the kidney. The dissection shows the initial exposure, towards the medial end of the incision, and it is made wider by broadening the renal fascia opening in a lateral direction.

C
Cross section of the abdomen through the lower pole of the right kidney, from below, showing the route for needle biopsy of the kidney.

1	Latissimus dorsi	9	Perirenal fat
2	Tip of twelfth rib	10	Kidney
3	External oblique	11	Psoas major
4	Internal oblique	12	Ureter
5	Subcostal nerve	13	Erector spinae
6	Transversus abdominis	14	Quadratus lumborum
7	Extraperitoneal fat	15	Liver
8	Renal fascia		

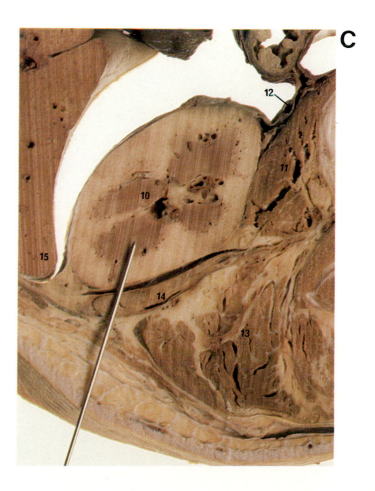

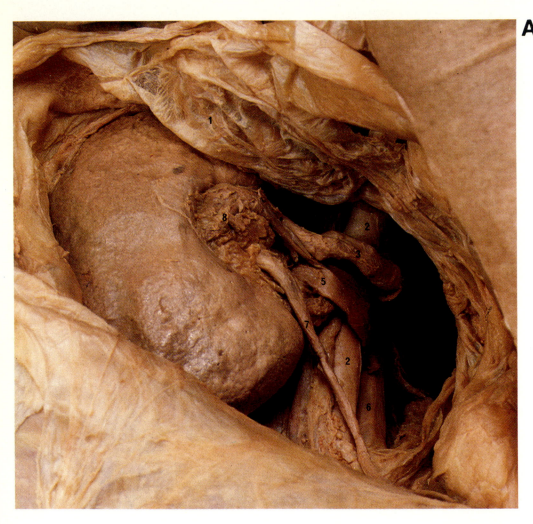

A

Approach for Kidney Transplantation

To obtain a donor kidney from a living donor, the kidney is removed through a lumbar incision as for a standard nephrectomy but the vessels are ligated near the aorta and inferior vena cava, leaving the hilum undisturbed. On the left the suprarenal and gonadal veins which normally drain into the renal vein will require ligation. The ureter is dissected out to the level of the bony pelvic brim and transected there; the immediate periureteric connective tissue is preserved round the ureter so that the longitudinal ureteric blood vessels remain intact.

To obtain donor kidneys from a cadaver (normally maintained on a ventilator after established brain death), a wide abdominal exposure is necessary, either through a cruciate incision from the xiphoid process to the pubic symphysis and transversely at umbilical level, or through an inverted V incision with the apex at the xiphoid process and the bases at the anterior superior iliac spines. The caecum and ascending colon are mobilised to the left by incising the peritoneum in the right paracolic gutter, the duodenum and pancreas are freed, and the descending colon mobilised by incising in the left paracolic gutter. The aorta and inferior vena cava are transected at the level of the fourth lumbar vertebra, and the ureters divided at the pelvic brim, with upper transections of the aorta at the aortic opening in the diaphragm and of the vena cava as it enters the groove on the back of the liver. The whole mass of kidneys and major vessels can then be removed for suitable preservation and dissection of each kidney with its vessels and ureter.

For transplantation of the kidney into the recipient, the object is to place the kidney retroperitoneally in an iliac fossa, anastomosing the renal vessels to iliac vessels and implanting the ureter into the bladder. Because of the lengths of the renal vessels it is usually convenient to place a left kidney in the right iliac fossa and vice versa but each case must be judged individually.

A lower oblique muscle-splitting incision is used on the appropriate side. The peritoneum is not incised but reflected off the anterior and posterior abdominal walls as far as the iliac vessels and the pelvic brim.

The kidney is placed in the iliac fossa so that the hilum lies above and parallel to the external iliac vessels (A).

The renal vein is anastomosed end-to-side with the external iliac vein.

The renal artery is anastomosed end-to-end with the proximal end of the internal iliac artery that has been transected at a convenient level below the common iliac bifurcation and above the origin of its first branch (normally the superior vesical). An alternative is an end-to-side anastomosis with the external iliac artery.

The ureter is implanted into the anterior surface of the bladder.

Hazards and Safeguards

Among the many preliminary investigations required for a living kidney donor, it is anatomically important to include an aortogram to confirm that the donor kidney has a normal single renal artery; most kidneys with aberrant vessels (or ureters) are not suitable.

Although the left gonadal and suprarenal veins normally drain into the left renal vein, the right gonadal vein does not always drain into the inferior vena cava directly as most textbooks suggest; as many as 25% in males may enter the right renal vein.

Fat in the hilum of the donor kidney is not removed, in order not to imperil the blood supply of the renal pelvis which (like that of the ureter) depends on small vessels running through the immediately surrounding connective tissue.

The problems of immunosuppression, suture technique and kidney preservation outweigh the anatomical hazards of transplantation.

A

Transplantation of a left kidney into the right iliac fossa. The renal artery is in place for anastomosis to the proximal cut end of the internal iliac artery, and the renal vein will be joined to the side of the external iliac vein. The ureter is transplanted into the front of the bladder (not shown).

1	Peritoneum	5	Renal vein
2	External iliac artery	6	External iliac vein
3	Renal artery	7	Ureter
4	Proximal cut end of internal iliac artery	8	Fat in hilum

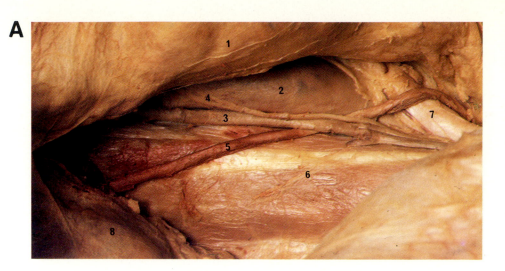

ABDOMINAL AORTA, INFERIOR VENA CAVA AND URETER

Background

In the abdomen the inferior vena cava is on the right of the aorta, both lying retroperitoneally in front of the vertebral column. The vena cava begins opposite the fifth lumbar vertebra by the union of the two common iliac veins and the upper end passes through the tendinous part of the diaphragm at the level of the disc between the eighth and ninth thoracic vertebrae. The aorta enters the abdomen behind the median arcuate ligament opposite the twelfth thoracic vertebra and ends at fourth lumbar level by dividing into the two common iliac arteries.

The part of the aorta above the renal vessels can be exposed through a left thoraco-abdominal incision by retracting the stomach, spleen and pancreas forwards and incising the peritoneum to reveal the kidney, aorta and suprarenal gland (as on page 135). Part of the vena cava above renal vessel level is embedded in the groove on the back of the liver and is not visible, but below the liver it can be seen behind the portal vein (page 129) and the duodenum and pancreas (page 124). Approaches to the infrarenal parts of the two great vessels can be made transperitoneally or retroperitoneally; here a transperitoneal approach to the aorta and a retroperitoneal approach to the vena cava are described. For the aorta, the peritoneum on its left side is incised after opening the peritoneal cavity and displacing the gut to the right. The vena cava is approached from the right through the anterior abdominal wall without entering the peritoneal cavity but by stripping the peritoneum off the wall until the vena cava is reached.

Each ureter runs down the posterior abdominal wall beneath the peritoneum and *adhering* to it. On psoas major it lies between the genitofemoral nerve which is behind it and the gonadal vessels which are in front. Right or left colic vessels cross superficial to the gonadal vessels, as does the root of the mesentery on the right. The ureter enters the pelvis at the bifurcation of the common iliac artery; it crosses the external iliac artery and runs down *in front of*

the internal iliac. On the left the apex of the sigmoid mesocolon overlies the ureter where it crosses the external iliac artery – a useful identification point. The ureter obtains its blood supply from small branches from the aorta and the renal, gonadal and iliac vessels. The branches form fine longitudinal anastomotic channels in the connective tissue immediately surrounding the ureter; for this reason the ureter must not be stripped clean of connective tissue for more than 2 cm otherwise the blood supply may be imperilled.

The pelvic course of the ureter is considered on page 155 (male) and page 159 (female).

The commonest reason for exposing the ureter is to remove renal stones that have become stuck in the abdominal part during their passage from kidney to bladder. The narrowest parts of the ureter are at its upper end (at the junction with the renal pelvis), at the pelvic brim and where it enters the bladder, and these are the commonest sites for stones to lodge. The general plan for removal is to incise the ureter retroperitoneally through lumbar or lower abdominal wall incisions depending on the site involved.

Approach to the Infrarenal Inferior Vena Cava

A right transverse muscle-cutting incision is used and the peritoneum stripped off the abdominal walls (as described on page 113):

The peritoneal stripping is continued over psoas major until the vena cava is reached (A).

Hazards and Safeguards

The ureter adheres to overlying peritoneum and should be detached to remain on the front of the psoas sheath where it is crossed by the gonadal vessels (A). To preserve its blood supply it must not be cleanly stripped from surrounding connective tissue.

The sympathetic trunk is under cover of the lateral margin of the vena cava.

The right gonadal artery crosses the upper part of this region of the vena cava, with the gonadal vein entering the anterolateral surface.

If the vena cava has to be displaced, the lumbar veins entering it must not be torn, nor the lumbar arteries behind it.

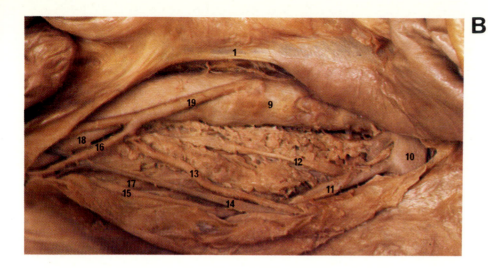

B

Approach to the Ureter

For exposure of the upper part of the ureter, the lumbar route to the kidney is used (page 138), and the ureter identified so that it can be incised (retroperitoneally) longitudinally over the stone.

To reach the ureter in the region of the pelvic brim, a gridiron incision (page 114) is made on the appropriate side to expose the peritoneum which is not incised but retracted medially after enlarging the incisions in the internal oblique and transversus muscles in the line of the fibres of the external oblique.

If the site of the stone is not obvious, the ureter is identified at the bifurcation of the common iliac artery and followed upwards.

Hazards and Safeguards

The ureter adheres to overlying peritoneum. If it cannot be found easily on psoas major it may have been displaced with the peritoneum when elevating that sheet from the posterior abdominal wall.

The ureter can be distinguished from nerves and vessels by the fact that it is a whitish cord that is non-pulsatile and which shows peristaltic movements when gently pinched with forceps.

It must not be stripped clean of surrounding connective tissue to avoid destroying the blood supply.

Approach to the Infrarenal Aorta

A long midline incision is used, from below the xiphoid process to above the pubic symphysis, skirting to the left of the umbilicus.

The greater omentum and transverse colon and mesocolon are lifted up, and the mesentery with coils of small intestine displaced to the right.

The peritoneum on the posterior abdominal wall is incised from the left of the duodenojejunal flexure and down over the aorta on to the beginning of the right common iliac artery. Flaps of peritoneum are raised to expose the required length of aorta (B). The inferior mesenteric vein can be divided if necessary at the upper end of the peritoneal incision.

Hazards and Safeguards

The inferior mesenteric vein normally runs into the splenic vein behind the body of the pancreas but it may lie more medially and so get in the way of the upper end of the peritoneal incision.

The left renal vein crosses the aorta deep to the inferior mesenteric vein (but sometimes the renal vein or its tributaries pass behind the aorta). The vein and its gonadal tributary must not be damaged when reflecting the peritoneum. To gain higher aortic exposure, the renal vein can be divided at its entry into the vena cava, leaving the gonadal and suprarenal tributaries to provide collateral circulation.

The inferior mesenteric artery is retracted to the right but it can be displaced to the left when dealing with the aortic bifurcation (B).

If the aorta has to be mobilized, the lumbar arteries and veins behind it must be remembered and not torn.

The sympathetic trunk is adjacent to the left margin of the aorta (B).

A
Inferior vena cava and right ureter, from the right, after reflecting the peritoneum forwards and medially off the posterior abdominal wall. In this view the sympathetic trunk is obscured by the gonadal vessels.

B
Aorta and left ureter, from the left, after incising peritoneum along the line of the aorta. The sympathetic trunk is being dissected out from retroperitoneal fat, and the gonadal artery (not seen) and ureter are displaced with the lateral peritoneal flap.

1	Peritoneum	11	Left gonadal vein
2	Inferior vena cava	12	Sympathetic trunk
3	Right gonadal vein	13	Upper left colic artery
4	Right gonadal artery	14	Inferior mesenteric vein
5	Right ureter	15	Left ureter
6	Psoas sheath	16	Lower left colic artery
7	External iliac artery	17	Genitofemoral nerve
8	Kidney	18	Left common iliac artery
9	Aorta	19	Inferior mesenteric artery
10	Left renal vein		

APPENDIX

Background

The opening of the (vermiform) appendix into the posteromedial wall of the caecum is 2 cm below the ileocaecal junction. Following the taeniae coli downwards over the wall of the caecum will always lead to the base of the appendix (A). The organ varies in length from 2 to 23 cm; on average it is about 9 cm long. Its position is very variable and although it is commonly visualized as lying over the pelvic brim, it more often lies behind the caecum. It may also be found behind the lower ascending colon (in which case it is retroperitoneal), on the lateral side of the ascending colon (not retroperitoneal), or close to the inguinal ligament. Its blood supply from the appendicular artery, usually a branch of the posterior caecal, runs at first in the free border of the mesoappendix and then along the side of the appendix (A). Inflammatory disease (appendicitis) may cause obstruction of the vessel and ischaemia of the distal end of the viscus, leading to perforation and peritonitis or abscess formation.

Appendicitis is the commonest abdominal surgical emergency in the Western world and in all but the mildest cases requires removal of the appendix (appendicectomy in English; appendectomy in American).

Approach

A right gridiron incision is commonly used.

The caecum is identified and the taeniae on its surface followed to the base of the appendix from which the rest of it can be traced (A).

The appendix is freed from adherence to surrounding structures and then transected at its base together with the mesoappendix so that it can be removed. The caecal stump is closed off and buried into the caecum with a surrounding purse-string suture.

Hazards and Safeguards

If the position of the appendix is not readily apparent on opening the abdomen, the taeniae coli must be followed downwards over the caecum to lead to the base of the appendix.

Great care must be taken to prevent perforation of an inflamed appendix, especially when it is adherent to surrounding organs.

A
Appendix, caecum and terminal ileum, from behind, with dissection of peritoneum to show the appendicular artery which runs at first near the free margin of the mesoappendix and then close to the wall of the appendix. The taeniae coli, two of which are seen in this posterior view (the other is anterior), lead to the base of the appendix.

B
Right part of the large intestine, with the transverse colon and greater omentum lifted upwards and peritoneum dissected to show branches of the superior mesenteric artery. The stump of the corresponding vein remains on the right side of the artery. In this specimen the right colic artery is a small branch of the ileocolic which is double, arising from a common stem; the more usual position for a right colic artery is indicated by the interrupted line.

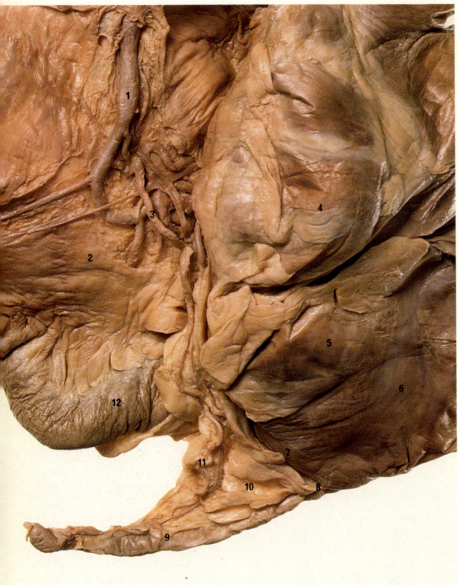

A

B

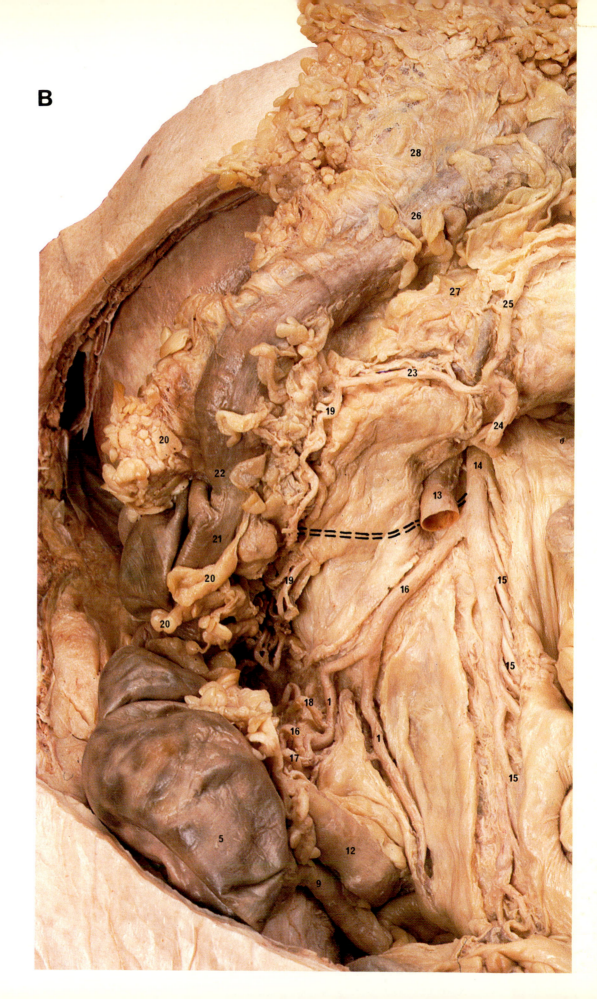

1 Ileocolic artery
2 Mesentery
3 Posterior caecal artery
4 Ascending colon
5 Caecum
6 Posterolateral taenia coli
7 Posteromedial taenia coli
8 Base of 9
9 Appendix
10 Mesoappendix
11 Appendicular artery
12 Terminal ileum
13 Superior mesenteric vein
14 Superior mesenteric artery
15 Jejunal and ileal branches
16 Common trunk of ileocolic and right colic branches
17 Anterior caecal artery
18 Right colic artery
19 Marginal artery
20 Some appendices epiploicae
21 Anterior taenia coli
22 Right colic (hepatic) flexure
23 Right branch of 24
24 Middle colic artery
25 Left branch of 24
26 Transverse colon
27 Transverse mesocolon
28 Greater omentum

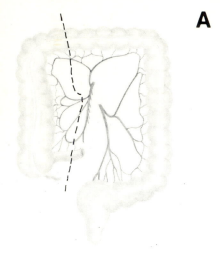

A

COLON

Background

On opening the abdomen much of the colon can be seen easily after retracting the greater omentum or coils of small intestine. The colon is identified from small intestine because of its taeniae and appendices epiploicae.

The ascending and descending colon adhere to the posterior abdominal wall behind the peritoneum but the transverse and sigmoid parts are suspended by their own mesenteries, the transverse and sigmoid mesocolons. The transverse mesocolon adheres to the greater omentum (page 120, B) so that the transverse colon appears to have a peritoneal attachment to the stomach that is sometimes called the gastrocolic omentum (although strictly speaking this is an alternative term for the greater omentum). The various colonic blood vessels run either behind the peritoneum or within the mesocolons. The ileocolic, right colic and middle colic branches of the superior mesenteric artery supply the colon as far as the left third of the transverse part, beyond which the left colic and sigmoid branches of the inferior mesenteric take over. Anastomoses between these various vessels form a usually prominent 'marginal artery' near the inner colonic border. The potentially weakest spot in this continuous arterial link is near the left colic (splenic) flexure, where the superior and inferior mesenteric areas of supply may have a rather small and inadequate union. It is the vascular patterns that determine the extent of colonic resections for carcinoma and other diseases, not only because of the distribution of the main arteries but because lymph vessels and nodes accompany the blood vessels.

Although the whole colon can be removed (total colectomy) it is more common to undertake partial removals. For a right hemicolectomy the resection extends from the terminal ileum to the proximal part of the transverse colon. In a transverse colectomy the transverse colon and the right and left colic flexures are removed together with the transverse mesocolon and the greater omentum. For a left hemicolectomy the resection is from the left end of the transverse colon to a part of the sigmoid colon, and for sigmoid colectomy from the lower descending colon to the begin-ning of the rectum. The precise extent of any removal depends on the site of the disease and the local pattern of vessels. The general principle for a malignant tumour is to remove the tumour together with a length of normal bowel on either side and all the associated peritoneum, vessels and nodes.

Approach for Right Hemicolectomy

A right paramedian incision is used, extending for 10 cm above and below the umbilicus.

The caecum and ascending colon are mobilised by incising the peritoneum of the posterior abdominal wall along the lateral border of the colon and then lifting the colon medially (with the peritoneum still attached to the medial border), avoiding any damage to the underlying duodenum, kidney, ureter and gonadal vessels as the peritoneum is lifted off these structures.

The greater omentum is separated from the right side of the transverse colon and mesocolon, and the transverse colon and mesocolon are lifted upwards so that the right branch of the middle colic artery can be cut.

The right colic and ileocolic vessels are divided close to their origins from the right side of the superior mesenteric vessels (page 145, B) and any mesentery between the ligation points is also divided.

The ileum is transected 10 cm or more from the ileocaecal junction.

The gastrocolic omentum and transverse colon are transected near their midpoint so that the terminal ileum, caecum, ascending colon, hepatic flexure and adjacent transverse colon can be removed en bloc with their attached peritoneum (A).

The remaining cut end of the transverse colon is closed off and the continuity of the gut is restored by anastomosing the cut end of the ileum end-to-side with the colonic stump.

Hazards and Safeguards

The gonadal vessels, kidney, ureter and duodenum must not be damaged when stripping the peritoneum and colonic vessels from the posterior abdominal wall.

The ileocolic and right colic arteries are ligated close to their parent superior mesenteric trunks so that as much as possible of their companion lymph vessels and nodes can be removed. The lymph channels cannot usually be seen but are inevitably included when ligating the blood vessels. The main trunk of the middle colic artery is left intact so that the remaining part of the transverse colon retains a good blood supply and does not have to rely on the anastomosis with the inferior mesenteric along the marginal artery. It is only the right branch of the middle colic artery that is cut.

A

Diagram of the amount of bowel removed in a right hemicolectomy (between the interrupted lines).

B

Transverse colon, lifted upwards with the transverse mesocolon and greater omentum, with peritoneal dissection to show the branches of the middle colic artery. In its normal position the middle colic artery of course passes downwards; only with the transverse colon lifted upwards does the artery appear to run

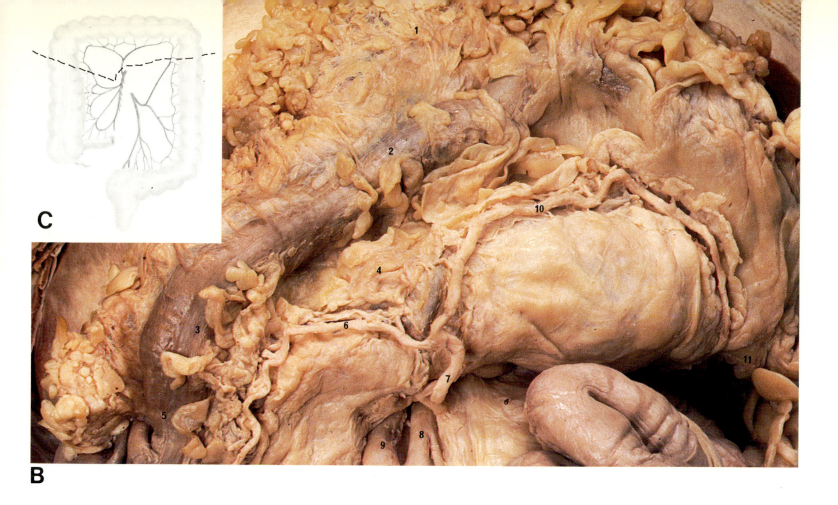

C

B

upwards. The right and left branches of this artery themselves form the marginal artery here.

C

Diagram of the amount of bowel removed in a transverse colectomy (between the interrupted lines).

1 Greater omentum
2 Transverse colon
3 Anterior taenia coli
4 Transverse mesocolon
5 Right colic (hepatic) flexure
6 Right branch of 7
7 Middle colic artery
8 Superior mesenteric artery
9 Superior mesenteric vein
10 Left branch of 7
11 Left colic (splenic) flexure

Approach for Transverse Colectomy

A right paramedian incision is used, extending for 10 cm above and below the umbilicus.

The stomach and greater omentum are identified, and the gastric branches of the gastro-epiploic vessels are divided so that the transverse colon and mesocolon can be detached from the stomach.

The transverse colon and mesocolon are lifted upwards and the middle colic artery is divided at its origin from the superior mesenteric (B), together with its accompanying vein.

The transverse mesocolon is divided by a V-shaped incision, with the extremities of the V at least 8 cm on either side of the tumour and the apex at the ligated origin of the middle colic artery (C).

The appropriate length of transverse colon is then removed with its mesocolon and the greater omentum.

Bowel continuity is restored by joining together the remaining cut ends of the colon by an end-to-end anastomosis.

Hazards and Safeguards

The gastro-epiploic arteries are removed as part of the greater omentum. It is their *gastric* branches that are severed here, in contrast to partial gastrectomy where the *epiploic* branches are cut (page 119).

If the tumour is near either of the colic flexures, a length of ascending or descending colon must be included in the resection.

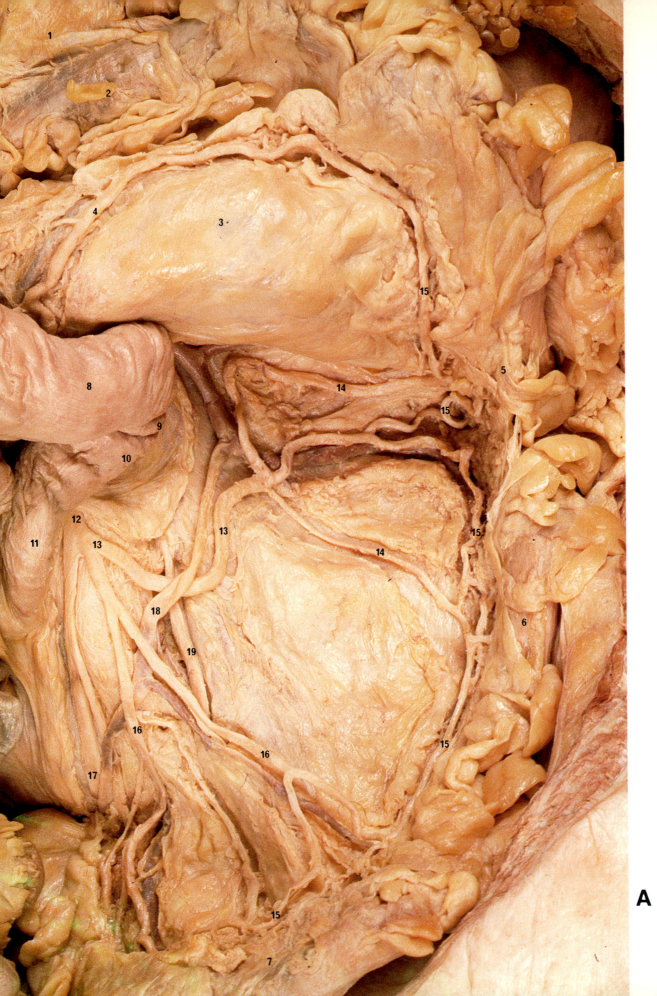

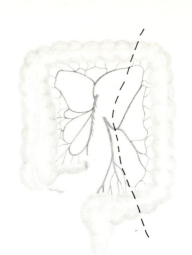

B

A

Approach for Left Hemicolectomy

A left paramedian incision is used, extending for 10cm above and below the umbilicus.

The descending colon is mobilised by incising the peritoneum of the posterior abdominal wall along its lateral margin and lifting it medially (with the peritoneum still attached to its medial border) off the posterior abdominal wall and kidney, avoiding damage to the duodenojejunal flexure, kidney, ureter and gonadal vessels.

The inferior mesenteric artery is divided at its origin from the aorta (A) by incising the peritoneum at the lower border of the duodenum over the aorta so that the origin can be visualised. But depending on the extent of disease it may be possible to preserve the inferior mesenteric artery itself and simply ligate left colic and sigmoid branches.

The inferior mesenteric vein is divided at the lower border of the pancreas.

The peritoneum over the front of the aorta is incised vertically and the incision carried down and to the left into the sigmoid meso-colon to the point chosen for transection of the colon, with ligation of sigmoid vessels as required.

The middle of the transverse colon with its mesocolon is transec-ted with division of the left branch of the middle colic artery, and the phrenicocolic ligament is divided enabling the splenic flexure to be mobilised.

The left half of the transverse colon, splenic flexure, descending colon and part of the sigmoid colon, together with the inferior mesenteric vessels and the associated peritoneum and lymphatics, can now be removed en bloc (B).

Continuity of the gut is restored by anastomosing the remaining cut end of the transverse colon to the sigmoid colon; to do this the right half of the transverse colon must be mobilised by division of the gastrocolic omentum.

Hazards and Safeguards

The duodenojejunal flexure, kidney, ureter and gonadal vessels are at risk when mobilising the descending and sigmoid colon.

A

Left part of the large intestine, with the transverse colon and meso-colon and greater omentum lifted upwards and peritoneum dissec-ted to show the inferior mesenteric artery and branches. Note how the vessels anastomose to form a continuous marginal artery.

B

Diagram of the amount of bowel removed in a left hemicolectomy (between the interrupted lines).

1	Greater omentum	11	Transverse (third) part of duodenum
2	Transverse colon		
3	Transverse mesocolon	12	Inferior mesenteric artery
4	Left branch of middle colic artery	13	Left colic artery
5	Left colic (splenic) flexure	14	Branch of 13
6	Descending colon	15	Marginal artery
7	Sigmoid colon	16	Sigmoid artery
8	Jejunum	17	Superior rectal artery
9	Duodenojejunal flexure	18	Inferior mesenteric vein
10	Ascending (fourth) part of duodenum	19	Ureter

1 Descending colon
2 Sigmoid colon
3 Sigmoid mesocolon
4 Attachment of 3 over external iliac vessels
5 Ureter
6 Attachment of 3 over posterior pelvic wall
7 Uterine tube
8 Ovary
9 Rectum
10 First piece of sacrum
11 Superior rectal vessels
12 External iliac artery
13 External iliac vein
14 Ovarian vessels
15 Superior vesical artery
16 Uterine artery
17 Internal iliac artery
18 Internal iliac vein
19 Common origin of inferior vesical,
   vaginal and middle rectal arteries
20 Middle rectal artery
21 Common origin of inferior gluteal
   and internal pudendal arteries
22 Superior gluteal artery
23 A lateral sacral artery
24 Waldeyer's fascia
25 Uterosacral ligament
26 Vagina
27 Uterus
28 Bladder

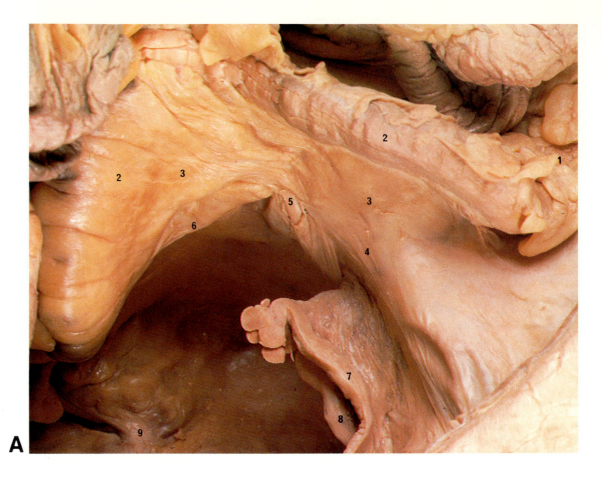

A

Approach for Sigmoid Colectomy

A midline subumbilical incision is used.

The sigmoid colon and mesocolon (A) are identified and the inferior mesenteric artery is ligated at its origin (as in left hemicolectomy) by incising the peritoneum over the aorta at the lower border of the duodenum so that the origin can be defined clearly. For non-malignant disease the main artery may be left intact and only colic and sigmoid branches divided. The inferior mesenteric vein is divided as high as necessary depending on the level chosen for colonic resection.

An appropriate length of descending colon is mobilised by incising the peritoneum along its lateral border, and the colon transected.

The cut end of the colon is reflected medially by stripping the peritoneum and colic vessels off the posterior abdominal wall, and both limbs of the sigmoid mesocolon (B) are detached from the abdominal and pelvic walls.

The lower end of the bowel is transected at a convenient point in the region of the rectosigmoid junction and the resected portion removed with all its attached peritoneum and vessels (C).

Continuity is restored as in left hemicolectomy.

Hazards and Safeguards

The ureter lies under the apex of the sigmoid mesocolon (B).

The gonadal vessels lie deep to the branches of the colic vessels but superficial to the ureter.

A
Sigmoid colon in the female, lifted up out of the pelvis to show the line of attachment of the sigmoid mesocolon. A small window is cut at the apex of the mesocolon over the ureter.

B
Left half of a median sagittal section of the female pelvis, from the right and in front, with most of the bowel and peritoneum removed, but with the attachment of the sigmoid mesocolon left in place.

C
Diagram of the amount of bowel removed in a sigmoid colectomy (between the interrupted lines).

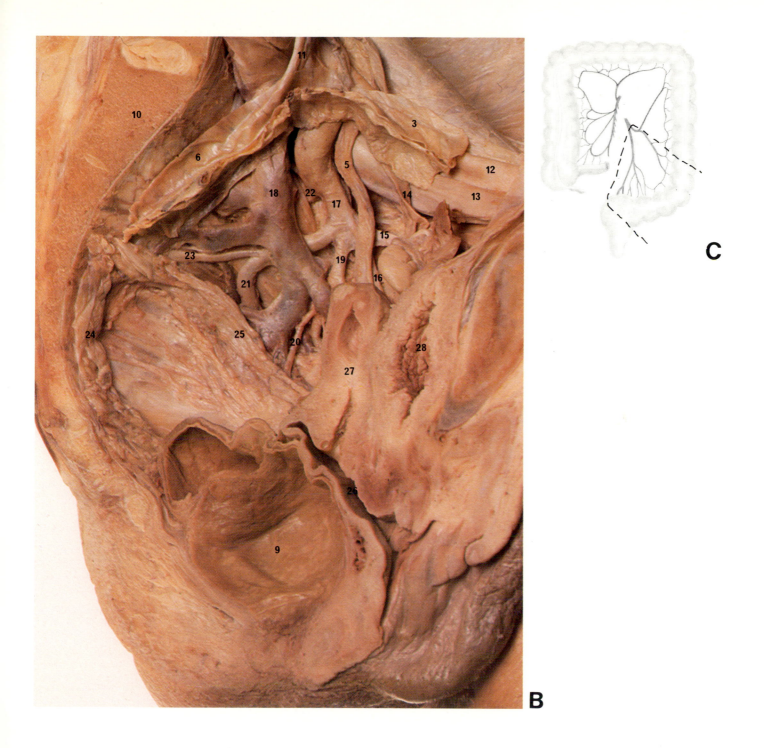

B

C

RECTUM AND ANAL CANAL

Background

The change of name from sigmoid colon to rectum occurs at the level of the third piece of the sacrum. The rectum ends at the ano-rectal junction which is about 3 cm below and in front of the tip of the coccyx. The peritoneum covers the front and sides of the upper third of the rectum and the front of the middle third (A), but the lower end in the male is below the level of the rectovesical pouch of peritoneum and is separated from the seminal vesicles, bladder and prostate by connective tissue that forms the rectovesical fascia (of Denonvilliers). In a similar position in the female, the lowest part of the peritoneum is called the recto-uterine pouch (of Douglas) although it is in fact reflected from the rectum to the posterior fornix of the vagina, and below the pouch there is corresponding connective tissue between the rectum and vagina. In both sexes the posterior surface of the rectum adheres to the pelvic surface of the sacrum by rather dense connective tissue commonly called the fascia of Waldeyer, while similar tissue under the peritoneum passing to the side walls of the pelvis constitutes the lateral rectal ligaments. At the anorectal junction the 90° angulation between rectum and anal canal is maintained by the puborectalis fibres of the levator ani muscles which here unite in slinglike fashion and fuse with the anorectal wall at the sides and back. The two levator ani muscles together with the small coccygeus muscles (which are really the muscular parts of the sacrospinous ligaments) form the pelvic floor or pelvic diaphragm; the terms are synonymous. The lowest fibres of puborectalis fuse with the upper end of the external anal sphincter (skeletal muscle) which surrounds the internal anal sphincter (visceral muscle) formed by the downward continuation of the inner circular layer of rectal muscle. These two sphincters form the muscle of the anal canal which is the terminal 4 cm of the alimentary tract.

The blood supply of the rectum is mainly from the superior rectal artery, which is the continuation of the inferior mesenteric after it has crossed the pelvic brim, supplemented on each side by the middle rectal vessels (from the internal iliac) which run through the lateral ligaments. As the superior rectal approaches the upper end of the rectum it divides into two branches that run down either side, the one on the right also dividing into two, giving with their accompanying veins an arrangement of vessels in positions at 3, 7 and 11 o'clock as viewed from the lithotomy position. The median sacral artery supplies a very small area at the anorectal junction posteriorly. There are veins corresponding to all the arteries, the important feature being that the superior rectal vein belongs to the portal system whereas the others are systemic. The *inferior* rectal vessels do not directly supply the rectum despite their name; they supply the lower part of the anal canal, and the anastomoses with other vessels occur in the anal columns of the upper third of the canal (the site of haemorrhoids or piles), not in the rectum. The lymphatic drainage of the rectum is essentially upwards to iliac and aortic nodes; there is negligible downward spread, but the lower part of the anal canal drains to inguinal nodes.

On rectal examination in either sex (by the index finger inserted through the anal canal), the coccyx and lower sacrum can be detected behind, with the ischial spines and ischiorectal fossae at the sides. In the male at the front the prostate can be felt, while in the

1 Sigmoid colon
2 Rectum
3 Fundus of uterus
4 Bladder
5 Uterine tube
6 Round ligament
7 Broad ligament
8 Ligament of ovary
9 Mesovarium
10 Ovary
11 Ovarian vessels in suspensory ligament
12 Appendix

A

Central and right parts of the female pelvic cavity, from above and in front. Coils of intestine have been lifted out to show the rectum on the posterior pelvic wall and other pelvic viscera.

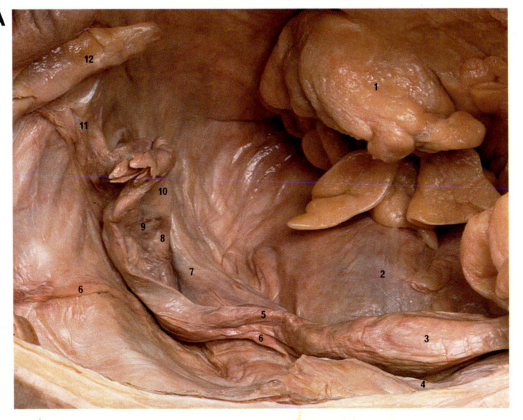

A

female the cervix can be palpated through the vaginal wall.

Surgical access to the rectum may be required for carcinoma and certain inflammatory diseases. If disease includes the lower part of the rectum, removal may have to include the anal canal, in which case an artificial bowel opening (colostomy) will have to be made in the anterior abdominal wall. For higher lesions preservation of the anal canal may be possible. The two procedures described below are the more conservative operation – anterior resection – and the more extensive removal commonly called combined abdomino-perineal resection. With access to the pelvis through the anterior abdominal wall, the rectum can be freed by cutting through peritoneum and dissecting away from surrounding structures. The abdomino-perineal operation additionally involves cutting through the pelvic diaphragm, and often two surgeons work at the same time, one in the abdomen and the other on the perineum. A variable amount of sigmoid colon is removed with the rectum, depending on the extent of the disease, the vascular patterns and the length requirements for anastomosis or colostomy.

Approach for Anterior Resection

A lower left paramedian incision is used, from the pubis to above the umbilicus.

Coils of small intestine are held out of the way, upwards and to the right.

The sigmoid colon is identified and retracted to the right so that the left limb of the sigmoid mesocolon (page 150, A) can be detached from the posterior abdominal wall (along the line of the external iliac vessels) (page 151, B). The gonadal vessels must be identified and preserved.

The inferior mesenteric artery is divided at or near its origin from the aorta (page 148, A), the exact position depending on the disease, the pattern of its branches and the site chosen for transection. The companion vein to the left of the artery is divided at the same level.

The sigmoid colon and mesocolon are transected at the chosen site, ensuring that sufficient length is left for the later anastomosis.

The peritoneum on each side of the rectum is incised as far down as the rectovesical (or recto-uterine) pouch (page 154, A), and the lower ends of the incisions joined transversely across the front of the rectum.

The rectum is freed from the sacrum behind by incising Waldeyer's fascia, and from the seminal vesicles, bladder and upper part of the prostate (or from the vagina) in front. On each side the lateral ligaments containing the middle rectal vessels are divided, avoiding damage to the ureters which cross the upper part of the ligaments.

The rectum is transected at the chosen level and the length of bowel removed. The remaining cut ends of sigmoid colon and rectum are joined.

Approach for Abdomino-perineal Resection

The abdominal part of the operation proceeds as for anterior resection, as far as mobilising the rectum from the sacrum and from the structures in front of it (page 154, A). Depending on the extent of disease and the vascularity of the colon it may be necessary to mobilise the descending colon by incising the peritoneum along its left border so that it can be raised from the posterior abdominal wall on a 'mesentery' formed by the peritoneum along its right margin.

While the above is being carried out, the second surgeon begins the perineal part of the operation.

An elliptical skin incision is made on either side of the anus from the tip of the coccyx to the bulb of the penis.

The ischiorectal fossa (page 154, B) on each side is entered through the fat and the tissues attached to the tip of the coccyx released so that the space containing Waldeyer's fascia can be opened up from below.

The posterior (iliococcygeus) part of levator ani on each side is divided and the inferior rectal vessels ligated. The abdominal and perineal surgeons can now make contact behind the rectum.

In front of the anal canal the superficial and deep transverse perineal muscles, the external anal sphincter and the anterior (pubococcygeus) parts of levator ani are divided.

The plane between the rectum and prostate is defined by opening up the lower part of the rectovesical fascia (page 157, A), and the tissue connecting the rectum to the apex of the prostate and perineal body is transected. In the female the corresponding fascial plane between the rectum and vagina can be opened up, but alternatively part of the posterior vaginal wall can be removed with the rectum. The abdominal and perineal surgeons can now make contact in front of the rectum.

The puborectalis is divided together with any remaining parts of the lateral ligaments. The now free length of bowel can be withdrawn through the perineum.

The colostomy is usually made in the left iliac fossa, at the junction of the lateral and middle thirds of a line from the anterior superior iliac spine to the umbilicus. A 2 cm circle of skin is removed followed by a similar trephine of the rest of the abdominal wall. The mucous membrane of the cut end of the sigmoid colon is sutured to the circular skin edge.

Hazards and Safeguards

The bladder must be completely emptied by catheter before the operation starts, both to protect it and to give as much room as possible in the pelvis.

The blood supply of the remaining colon must be assured. It may be necessary to divide the inferior mesenteric artery distal to the origin of the left colic branch to give an adequate input to the marginal artery (page 146).

The left ureter at the apex of the sigmoid mesocolon and both ureters at the back of the bladder are vulnerable. As they approach the bladder in the pelvis the ureters should lie anterolateral to the peritoneal incision lines and they cross the top of the lateral rectal ligaments. Apart from peritoneum, only the ductus (vas) deferens in the male or the uterine artery in the female lie superficial to the ureter in the pelvis.

A

Left half of a median sagittal section of the female pelvis, to show the anterior and posterior relations of the rectum.

B

Right ischiorectal fossa in the right half of a median sagittal section of the female pelvis, from below and slightly right so that the lower part of the rectum and vagina can be seen. Some of the ischio-rectal fat and inferior rectal vessels and nerves are removed, and so is part of the bulbospongiosus muscle, to show the underlying bulb of the vestibule and the greater vestibular (Bartholin's) gland.

MALE BLADDER, URETHRA AND GENITAL ORGANS

Background

In the adult the bladder is a pelvic organ, lying centrally behind the pubic symphysis and the bodies of the pubic bones (in contrast to the newborn where it is above the pubic symphysis). Peritoneum covers the upper surface and the adjacent part of the base which is the *posterior* surface, and as the bladder becomes distended it rises upwards behind the anterior abdominal wall, stripping the peritoneum off the wall (page 157, A). The ductus (vas) deferens (page 117) and seminal vesicle on each side lie up against the base, and the peritoneal reflexion from the upper part of the base to rectum is the rectovesical pouch. Below peritoneal level connective tissue called the rectovesical fascia (of Denonvilliers) intervenes between bladder and rectum. The upper and inferolateral surfaces of the bladder meet at the front to form the apex, from which the obliterated remains of the urachus run upwards in the midline of the anterior abdominal wall as the *median* umbilical ligament. The superior vesical artery, the highest branch of the internal iliac, leaves the side wall of the pelvis in a small 'mesentery' of peritoneum to reach the upper part of the bladder; the distal part of the vessel becomes obliterated and continues forwards on to the abdominal wall as the *medial* umbilical ligament. The inferior vesical branch arises much lower and runs below the peritoneal floor of the pelvis. The veins do not accompany the arteries; they converge on the vesicoprostatic plexus, found principally in the

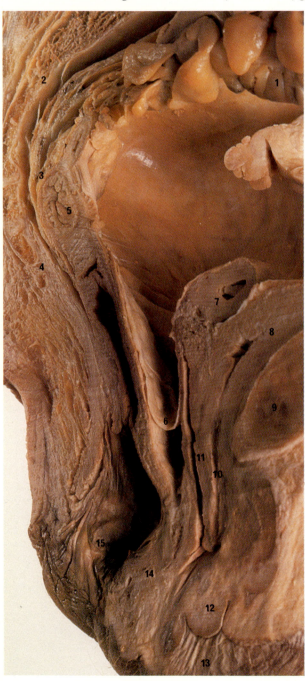

A

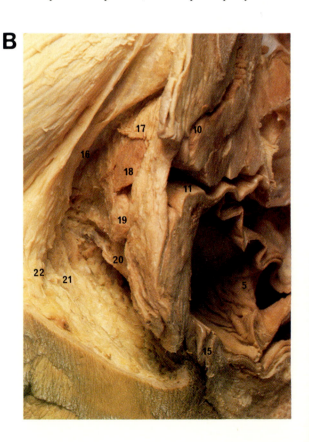

B

1	Sigmoid colon
2	Third piece of sacrum
3	Waldeyer's fascia
4	Tip of coccyx
5	Rectum
6	Recto-uterine pouch
7	Uterus
8	Bladder
9	Pubic symphysis
10	Urethra
11	Vagina
12	Labium minor
13	Labium majus
14	Perineal body
15	Anal canal
16	Ischiopubic ramus
17	Bulbospongiosus
18	Bulb of vestibule
19	Greater vestibular gland
20	Levator ani
21	Pudendal canal
22	Medial side of ischial tuberosity

groove between bladder and prostate and draining backwards to the internal iliac veins. Lymphatics also pass backwards to internal iliac nodes. The ureters enter at the upper corners of the base (after being crossed superficially by the ductus deferens) and run obliquely through the wall for 2 cm before opening internally at the upper angles of the trigone, at whose lower angle (neck of the bladder) the urethra leaves to pass through the prostate.

The prostate gland is too deeply placed to have any peritoneal covering. Its base is the *upper* surface, beneath the neck of the bladder, and is penetrated by the urethra which runs through for 3 cm to emerge just in front of the apex of the prostate and became the membranous part of the urethra (see below). The inferolateral parts of the prostate are cradled by the medially-sloping levator ani muscles, the most medial fibres being known as levator prostatae. A few fibres pass behind the membranous urethra forming a 'pubourethral sling' like puborectalis (page 152) but smaller. Some retropubic connective tissue may be condensed between the prostate (and bladder) and pubic bones as the puboprostatic ligaments but these are sometimes very indefinite structures. On each side the ejaculatory ducts, formed by the union of the ductus deferens and the duct of the seminal vesicle, pass through the gland to open into the prostatic urethra on the seminal colliculus at the side of the opening of the prostatic utricle. The prostate's own secretion enters by numerous small ducts. The blood supply is mainly from the prostatic branch of the inferior vesical artery, with veins draining to the vesicoprostatic plexus. The veins lie between the prostate's own capsule and a 'false capsule' of surrounding fascia. Benign growths (adenomata – see below) can be 'shelled out' of the surrounding glandular tissue without entering the plane of the plexus. The anterior lobe of the prostate is the part in front of the urethra and has hardly any glandular tissue. The triangular part between the two ejaculatory ducts and behind the upper part of the urethra is the middle lobe; it is the part commonly involved in 'enlargement of the prostate' (benign hypertrophy, adenomata) and causes urethral obstruction. In contrast, carcinoma usually occurs in other parts – in the posterior lobe (behind the median lobe) or lateral lobes.

After leaving the prostate, the next 1 cm of urethra is its membranous part. This part and the distal end of the prostatic urethra (distal to the seminal colliculus or verumontanum) are both surrounded by the sphincter urethrae, which consists of an inner layer of visceral muscle and an outer layer of skeletal muscle. The sphincter is tubular, *not* a flat sheet as described and drawn in most anatomy texts. The urethra then pierces the connective tissue that forms the perineal membrane and changes direction forwards as the spongy or penile part, about 15 cm long running through the corpus spongiosum of the penis. On each side the duct of the bulbo-urethral (Cowper's) gland opens into the bulb of the urethra, the dilated posterior part of the spongy portion. This continues into the pendulous part which contains a dilated area, the navicular fossa, just before the external urethral opening on the tip of the glans penis. Clinically the spongy part is called the anterior urethra, while the membranous and prostatic parts form the posterior urethra. The narrowest parts of the urethra are at the external opening, the proximal end of the navicular fossa, the membranous part, and at the bladder neck. It is dilated at the fossa, the bulb of the spongy part and in the prostatic part. There

are small blind-ending pockets of mucous membrane in the fossa and pendulous parts with some mucous glands (of Littré) in the anterior and lateral walls. There are no glands in the membranous part; although the bulbo-urethral glands are deep to the perineal membrane their ducts pierce the membrane to enter the bulb of the spongy part.

The commonest procedure on the bladder is catheterisation – inserting a catheter through the urethra. Where catheterisation is not possible, as with a grossly enlarged prostate gland, a temporary drainage tube can be inserted retroperitoneally through the lower anterior abdominal wall (suprapubic cystostomy). For inspection of the internal surface of the bladder a cystoscope can be passed through the urethra and some operations such as removal of stones and small tumours or removal of parts of the prostate can be carried out through this instrument. If the bladder has to be opened for more extensive procedures it is usually done retro-peritoneally (retropubic approach) as for suprapubic cystostomy but it may be necessary to open the peritoneal cavity.

The prostate can be approached by four routes – retropubically, through the bladder (transvesical approach), through the urethra (transurethral approach) or rarely through the perineum (perineal approach) – the choice depending on the nature and extent of the disease, but the transurethral route is now the commonest.

Catheterisation

In the uncircumcised the prepuce (foreskin) is retracted.

The penis is held upwards towards the anterior abdominal wall and the tip of a suitably lubricated catheter inserted into the penile urethra. It is gently pushed onwards with slight traction on the penis.

Hazards and Safeguards

In the absence of prostatic disease the urethra is most likely to be damaged at the normal constrictions in the navicular fossa, and at the beginning of the membranous part where it changes direction on passing through the perineal membrane. To prevent the tip of a fine catheter becoming lodged in a mucosal fold in the roof of the navicular fossa, it is directed downwards on entering the external meatus.

If the prostate is grossly enlarged it may be difficult or even impossible to pass the catheter through the prostatic urethra, and it is important not to create a false passage by force.

The retracted foreskin must be restored to its normal position to avoid any possible constricting effect.

Retropubic Approach to the Bladder and Prostate

If not already distended by urinary retention, the bladder is filled via a urethral catheter to ensure that it extends well above the pubic symphysis and lifts the peritoneum off the anterior abdominal wall (A).

For suprapubic cystostomy:

A short vertical midline suprapubic incision is made in the anterior abdominal wall.

The bladder wall is identified beneath the incised linea alba and can be opened as required, after confirming that the peritoneum is suitably displaced above the level of the incision.

For retropubic approach to the prostate:

A lower midline or lower transverse (Pfannenstiel's) incision is used.

The loose tissue of the retropubic space (A) is opened up to expose the midline of the prostatic capsule which is incised transversely, ligating any necessary vessels.

The plane between the false capsule and the pathological tissue mass is identified and opened up so that by finger dissection the mass can be shelled out.

The urethra is divided at the apex of the prostate and at the neck of the bladder, and a wedge of tissue is removed from the lower part of the trigone to ensure that there will be free drainage from the bladder. A catheter is inserted through the urethra into the bladder so that the prostatic bed can contract around it when the capsule has been sutured and so form a new portion of urethra.

Hazards and Safeguards

The peritoneum must be out of harm's way above the level of all incisions.

Some bleeding when cutting the capsule and from the prostatic bed is inevitable, and comes from branches of the prostatic artery as well as from veins. The vesicoprostatic venous plexus is most profuse in the groove between the bladder and prostate laterally, and tributaries of the dorsal vein of the penis may run into it over the anterior surface of the bladder.

When removing the wedge of trigonal tissue the ureteral orifices must be identified and not damaged.

Transvesical Approach to the Prostate

The retropubic space is opened up as for retropubic prostatectomy.

The bladder is opened by a transverse incision extraperitoneally.

The pathological glandular mass is enucleated from the prostate, mostly by finger dissection once the correct plane has been found; this process can be assisted by a finger of the operator's other hand inserted into the rectum and applying counterpressure in a forward direction.

Hazards and Safeguards

The main hazards are from haemorrhage and finding the correct plane between normal and pathological tissue. Benign adenomata shell out easily once this plane is found.

Transurethral Approach to the Prostate

With the patient in the lithotomy position, the resectoscope is passed through the urethra so that the appropriate parts of the gland can be snipped away, flushed into the bladder and evacuated.

Hazards and Safeguards

The resection of tissue takes place *proximal* to the seminal colliculus (verumontanum) in order to avoid damage to the sphincter urethrae which is distal to it.

A
Right half of a median sagittal section of the male pelvis, with some peritoneum removed over the ureter and ductus deferens. In this specimen the bladder and prostate are higher than usual, and there is slight enlargement of the middle lobe of the prostate (a common occurrence after the age of 50). The arrows indicate the routes for retropubic (A), transvesical (B) and perineal (C) approaches to the prostate. Although not usually a midline structure, one of the ejaculatory ducts is seen in this section.

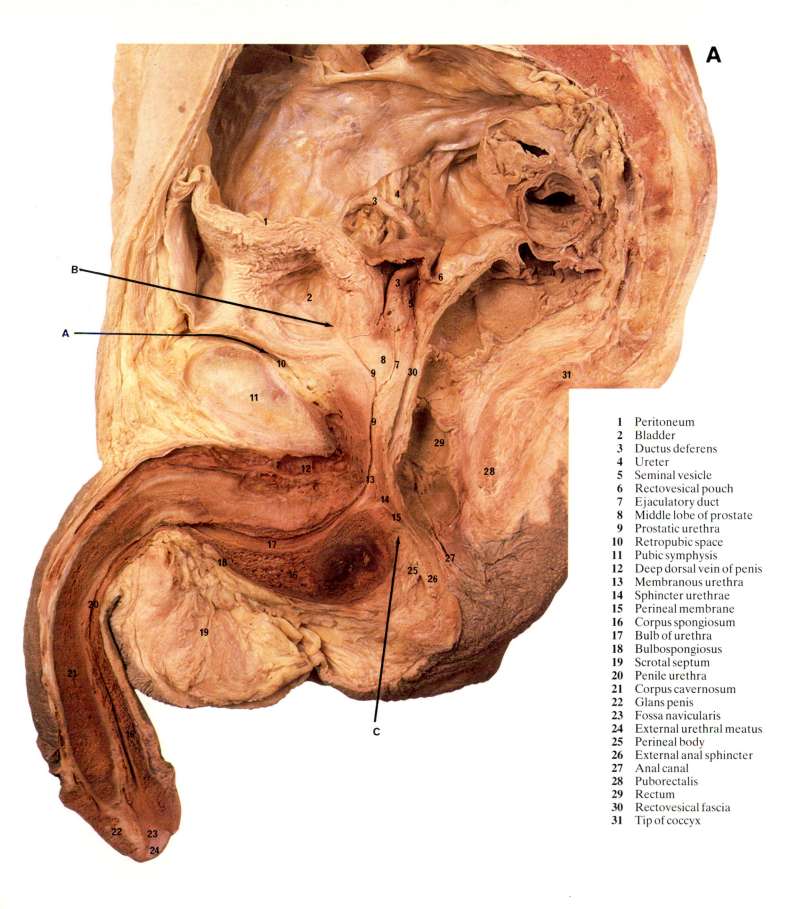

A

1	Peritoneum
2	Bladder
3	Ductus deferens
4	Ureter
5	Seminal vesicle
6	Rectovesical pouch
7	Ejaculatory duct
8	Middle lobe of prostate
9	Prostatic urethra
10	Retropubic space
11	Pubic symphysis
12	Deep dorsal vein of penis
13	Membranous urethra
14	Sphincter urethrae
15	Perineal membrane
16	Corpus spongiosum
17	Bulb of urethra
18	Bulbospongiosus
19	Scrotal septum
20	Penile urethra
21	Corpus cavernosum
22	Glans penis
23	Fossa navicularis
24	External urethral meatus
25	Perineal body
26	External anal sphincter
27	Anal canal
28	Puborectalis
29	Rectum
30	Rectovesical fascia
31	Tip of coccyx

TESTIS

Background

The testis is surrounded by the fibrous tunica albuginea and also by a serous covering, the tunica vaginalis, except at the back where the epididymis is attached to the testis posterolaterally. When fluid accumulates within the tunica vaginalis (hydrocoele), the swelling lies in front of the testis; swellings of the epididymis are posterolateral to the testis. Hydrocoeles may be tapped by needle puncture through the front of the scrotum but they recur, and when operation is required the tunica vaginalis can be opened, turning the tunica inside out and stitching the cut edges together behind the epididymis. Tumours of the testis require removal (orchidectomy), but open operation may also be required for biopsy of the testis, since needle biopsy is often unreliable.

Biopsy

The scrotal skin is stretched over the anterior surface of the testis.

A short longitudinal incision is made through the scrotal wall down to the tunica vaginalis, which is opened to display the tunica albuginea (A).

The tunica albuginea is incised transversely, and *gentle* pressure is exerted on the testis to squeeze out a little testicular tissue which can then be cut off.

Hazards and Safeguards

The posterolateral position of the epididymis must be confirmed before incising what is believed to be the tunica vaginalis.

A

Right testis, with the tunica vaginalis opened from the front and the tunica albuginea incised to show testicular tissue.

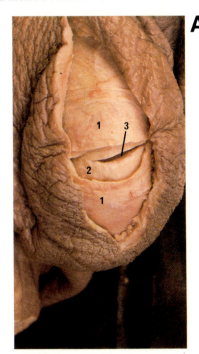

A

1 Tunica vaginalis
2 Tunica albuginea
3 Testicular tissue

FEMALE BLADDER, URETHRA AND GENITAL ORGANS

Background

The adult female bladder occupies a similar retropubic position to that in the male (B). The peritoneum on its upper surface does not reach as far as the posterior surface but is reflected on to the cervix and body of the uterus as the vesico-uterine pouch. The bladder's posterior surface is in front of the vagina with connective tissue intervening, and the ureters cross the lateral and anterior fornices before entering the bladder. The urethra, which leaves at the neck below the trigone and at first lies in front of the vagina, soon becomes embedded within the anterior vaginal wall. Normally 4cm long, the urethra can be distended by the pressure of the pregnant uterus to as much as 10cm. There are small mucous glands in its wall; the largest, at the lower end, are the paraurethral glands (of Skene) and are the female homologue of the prostate. The external urethral orifice opens in front of the vaginal orifice and 2.5cm behind the clitoris. Compared with the male, catheterisation is comparatively simple in view of the short straight urethra but urethral elongation in the later stages of pregnancy must be remembered. As in the male the bladder can be approached cystoscopically or through the anterior abdominal wall.

The body of the uterus is enclosed by peritoneum and rests on the upper surface of the bladder. At the sides of the uterus the two layers of peritoneum come together to form the broad ligament which attaches to the side wall of the pelvis. The upper margin of the broad ligament forms the mesosalpinx and contains the uterine tube, while a fold of peritoneum just below and *in front of* the tube encloses the round ligament of the uterus which enters the inguinal canal through the deep inguinal ring. The round ligament thus pursues a course that resembles that of the ductus deferens (although the two structures are developmentally different). A fold of peritoneum below and *behind* the tube forms the mesovarium; it contains the ovary and the ligament of the ovary which runs to the angle between the body of the uterus and tube. The ovary lies adjacent to the peritoneum of the lateral pelvic wall, between the medial umbilical ligament (obliterated umbilical artery) above and the ureter behind, with the obturator nerve deep to the peritoneum. The ovarian vessels cross the external iliac vessels to reach the ovary in a fold of peritoneum known as the suspensory ligament of the ovary.

The cervix of the uterus projects into the vagina. The supravaginal part anteriorly has no peritoneal covering and is connected to the bladder by connective tissue, but at the back peritoneum from the body of the uterus passes over this part of the cervix on to the fornix of the vagina, and then on to the front of the rectum forming the recto-uterine pouch (of Douglas). The subperitoneal tissue in the region of the cervix and upper vagina is condensed to form so-called ligaments; the uterosacral ligaments pass backwards on either side of the rectum to the sacrum, and the lateral cervical ligaments (otherwise known as lateral, cardinal or Mackenrodt's ligaments) pass to the lateral pelvic wall below the leaves of peritoneum that form the broad ligament. These connective tissue condensations are of prime importance in keeping

B

Right half of a median sagittal section of the female pelvis, with the peritoneum intact and coils of bowel removed.

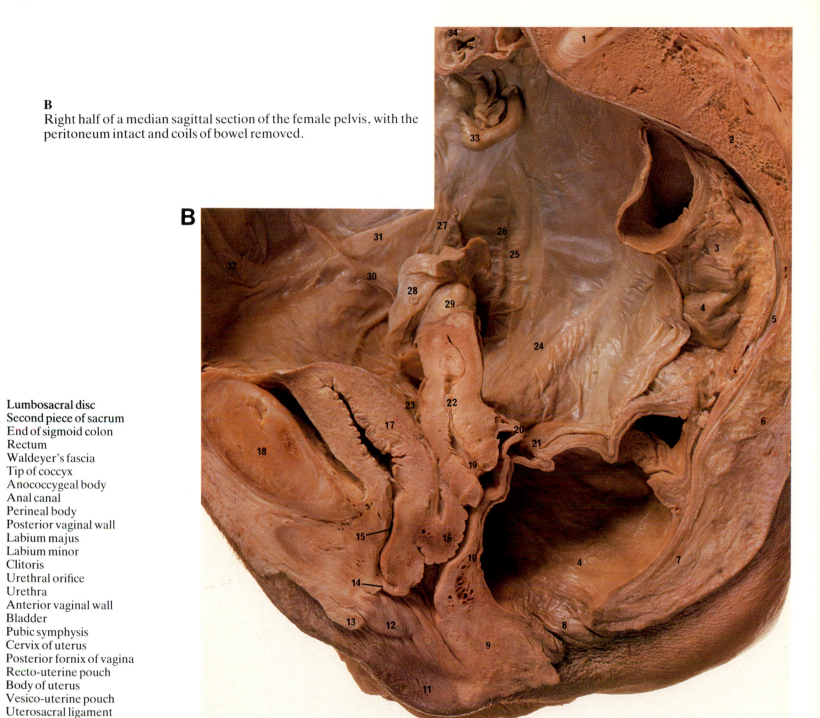

1   Lumbosacral disc
2   Second piece of sacrum
3   End of sigmoid colon
4   Rectum
5   Waldeyer's fascia
6   Tip of coccyx
7   Anococcygeal body
8   Anal canal
9   Perineal body
10 Posterior vaginal wall
11 Labium majus
12 Labium minor
13 Clitoris
14 Urethral orifice
15 Urethra
16 Anterior vaginal wall
17 Bladder
18 Pubic symphysis
19 Cervix of uterus
20 Posterior fornix of vagina
21 Recto-uterine pouch
22 Body of uterus
23 Vesico-uterine pouch
24 Uterosacral ligament
25 Ureter
26 Uterine artery
27 Suspensory ligament with ovarian vessels
28 Uterine tube
29 Ovary
30 Round ligament of uterus
31 Obliterated umbilical artery
32 Medial umbilical fold
33 Appendix
34 Terminal ileum

the uterus in its normal position by helping to anchor the cervix; in addition, the round and broad ligaments keep the body of the uterus angled forwards at its junction with the cervix (angle of anteflexion), and the cervix angled forwards at its junction with the vagina (angle of anteversion). The uterine artery, from the internal iliac, approaches the uterus under the posterior leaf of the broad ligament on the upper surface of the lateral cervical ligament. It crosses superficial to the ureter – the only structure in the pelvis to do so – and runs up the side of the uterus between the two layers of the broad ligament to anastomose with the ovarian artery. Veins do not necessarily run with the arteries; they join the profuse plexus that drains to the internal iliac vein.

In view of its close relationship to the cervix of the uterus and vagina, the ureter has been called the gynaecologist's nightmare. It lies in the base of the broad ligament, adhering to its posterior peritoneal layer and being crossed superficially by the uterine artery. It is at first on the upper surface of, and then penetrates, the condensed connective tissue of the lateral cervical ligament before crossing the lateral part of the vaginal fornix about 1–2 cm from the cervix. It then enters the bladder wall in front of the fornix.

Lymph from the body of the uterus passes mainly to external iliac nodes, but some channels reach paraaortic nodes via the ovarian vessels and others reach inguinal nodes (which are readily palpable) by running with the round ligament. From the cervix drainage is to external and internal iliac nodes and to sacral nodes (but not to the inguinal group). The ovary drains mainly to paraaortic nodes along the ovarian vessels, and some lymph passes to inguinal nodes along the round ligament, but it is also possible for it to reach the opposite ovary by channels that run along the ligament of the ovary, across the fundus of the uterus to the opposite ligament of the ovary. The lower vagina and external genitalia drain to inguinal nodes (like the lower anal canal).

Vaginal examination using the index and middle fingers can detect the uterine cervix in the vaginal vault, with the bladder, urethra and pubic symphysis at the front. The rectum is at the back while at the side the ovary and uterine tube may be palpated. The recto-uterine pouch (of Douglas) is above and behind the posterior part of the vaginal fornix, through which it may be possible to detect cancerous deposits that have gravitated to this lowest part of the peritoneal cavity.

Some common operations on the uterus such as 'D and C' (dilatation of the cervix and curettage of the endometrial lining for diagnostic and therapeutic purposes) and evacuation of the uterus (abortion) are carried out through the vagina and cervix, but other pelvic operations require an abdominal approach. After loops of bowel have been lifted out of the pelvis the true pelvic organs can be identified. The general approach is described below with specific reference to removal of the uterus (hysterectomy), ligation of the uterine tubes for sterilisation (tubal ligation), and removal of the ovary (ovariectomy or oophorectomy).

Approach to the Uterus, Uterine Tube and Ovary

A lower midline or lower transverse (Pfannenstiel's) incision is used and loops of bowel are retracted so that the other pelvic viscera can be seen.

For total hysterectomy (removal of body and cervix), the broad ligaments on each side are divided near the uterus, together with division of the round and ovarian ligaments and the uterine tubes.

The peritoneum of the uterovesical pouch is incised transversely so that the bladder and lower ends of the ureters can be pulled away from the body of the uterus, cervix and fornix of the vagina, and the uterine arteries are divided (A and B).

The uterosacral ligaments are transected and the anterior and posterior vaginal walls cut across below the cervix so that the whole specimen can be removed.

For subtotal hysterectomy (leaving the lower part of the cervix and the vagina intact), the procedure is similar to the above as far as the division of the uterine arteries. Thereafter the cervix is cut across at the level of the lateral ligaments without opening into the vagina.

For tubal ligation, the uterine tube is identified and from a point 2.5 cm from the body of the uterus a 1 cm length of it is removed. Vessels in the mesosalpinx are ligated but the ovarian artery itself should be preserved.

For ovariectomy, the ovary is removed by appropriate transection of the mesovarium and vessels, with preservation of the uterus and tube. For benign cysts, only the cyst itself need be removed since for endocrine reasons it is usually desirable to leave as much ovarian tissue as possible, provided it is normal.

Hazards and Safeguards

In operations on female pelvic organs the ureters are the structures at greatest risk, especially when disease has distorted the normal anatomy. Each ureter lies under the posterior layer of the broad ligament and is crossed by the uterine artery before entering the bladder by running along the side and front of the vaginal fornix.

The essential secret of success in tubal ligation is the proper identification of the tube from the round ligament. The ligament passes laterally to reach the deep inguinal ring while the tube runs farther back to its fimbriated end.

The profuse plexus of pelvic veins can cause troublesome bleeding.

A

Left half of a median sagittal section of the female pelvis, from the right and above.

B

As A, with the vesico-uterine pouch being opened up and the uterus and vagina separated from the bladder.

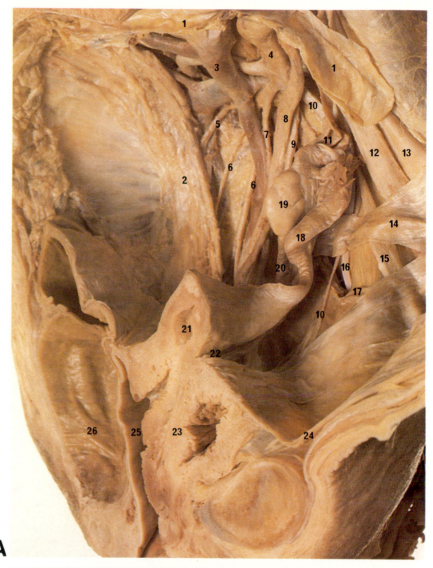

A

1 Sigmoid mesocolon
2 Uterosacral ligament
3 Internal iliac vein
4 Internal iliac artery
5 Middle rectal artery
6 Vaginal artery (double in A)
7 Inferior vesical artery
8 Ureter
9 Uterine artery
10 Superior vesical artery
11 Ovarian vessels
12 External iliac vein
13 External iliac artery
14 Round ligament of uterus
15 Obliterated umbilical artery
16 Obturator nerve and vein
17 Abnormal obturator artery
18 Uterine tube
19 Ovary
20 Ligament of ovary
21 Uterus
22 Vesico-uterine pouch
23 Bladder
24 Median umbilical fold and urachus
25 Vagina
26 Rectum
27 Lateral cervical ligament
28 Upper surface of lateral fornix

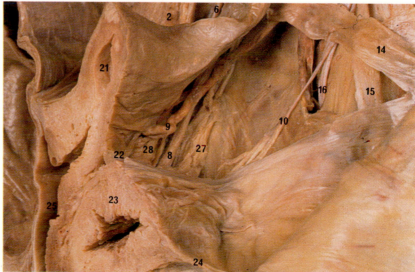

B

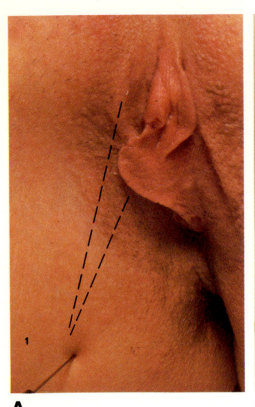

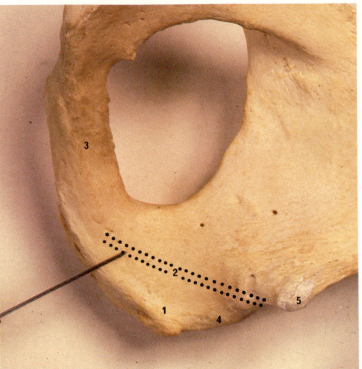

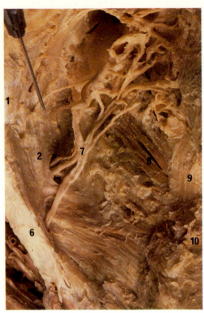

A

B

C

PUDENDAL NERVE

Background

From its origin from the ventral rami of the second, third and fourth sacral nerves, the pudendal nerve leaves the pelvis below piriformis and crosses the ischial spine medial to the internal pudendal vessels to enter the perineal region and run in the pudendal canal on the side wall of the ischiorectal fossa. It gives off inferior rectal branches, and at the anterior end of the canal it divides into the perineal nerve and the dorsal nerve of penis or clitoris.

For anaesthetising much of the perineum, the pudendal nerve can be blocked at the ischial spine by the vaginal route or in the pudendal canal by the perineal route. These blocks will not affect the most anterior part of the vulva, which is supplied by the ilio-inguinal and genitofemoral nerves.

Perineal Approach for Nerve Block

With the patient in the lithotomy position, the ischial tuberosity is palpated.

The needle is introduced just medial to the tuberosity (A and B) to a depth of 2.5 cm which should place the tip in the region of the pudendal canal (C), and the injection is made here.

For anaesthetising the anterior part of the vulva, the needle is partly withdrawn and redirected medially into several areas of the labia (A) so that the soft tissues innervated by the ilio-inguinal and genitofemoral nerves are infiltrated.

Vaginal Approach for Nerve Block

With the patient in the lithotomy position, the ischial spine is palpated through the vagina.

Using the two palpating fingers as a guide, the needle is introduced through the vaginal wall to the region of the spine and the injection made here (D).

Hazards and Safeguards

As usual, aspiration is essential to ensure that the needle is not in a vessel.

1   Ischial tuberosity
2   Pudendal canal (dotted in B)
3   Ischiopubic ramus
4   Lesser sciatic notch
5   Ischial spine
6   Sacrotuberous ligament
7   Inferior rectal vessels and nerves
8   Levator ani
9   External anal sphincter
10 Anococcygeal body
11 Internal iliac artery
12 Internal iliac vein
13 First sacral ventral ramus
14 Second sacral ventral ramus
15 Third sacral ventral ramus
16 Piriformis
17 Uterosacral ligament
18 Coccygeus
19 Inferior gluteal artery
20 Pudendal nerve
21 Internal pudendal artery
22 Middle rectal artery
23 Vaginal artery
24 Ureter
25 Uterus
26 Vagina
27 Rectum

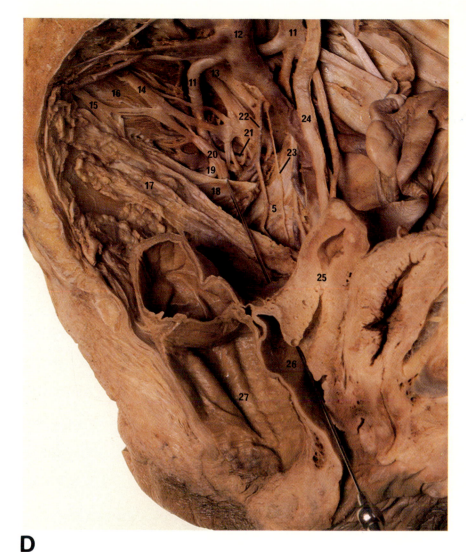

D

A
Right pudendal nerve block in the perineum, on the medial side of the ischial tuberosity. After injection here to block the nerve in the pudendal canal, the needle is partially withdrawn and directed in several more anterior directions (indicated by interrupted lines) towards the labia in order to infiltrate the front of the vulva which is supplied by ilio-inguinal and genitofemoral nerves, not by the pudendal.

B
Medial surface of the lower part of a right hip bone, with the needle position for nerve block in the pudendal canal (dotted lines), on the medial side of the ischial tuberosity.

C
Right ischiorectal fossa, from below and behind, with the needle adjacent to the pudendal canal. Note that this is a more postero-inferior view than in A and B.

D
Left half of a median sagittal section of the female pelvis, showing the vaginal route for pudendal nerve block. The needle passes through the fornix of the vagina to lie adjacent to the ischial spine (identified by a palpating finger through the vagina), so anaesthetising the nerve as it leaves the pelvis.

LUMBAR SYMPATHETIC TRUNK

Background
Removal of lumbar sympathetic ganglia, usually the second and third with the intervening part of the trunk (lumbar sympathectomy) to improve circulation in the lower limb by abolishing vasoconstriction, can be carried out by an anterior extraperitoneal approach. On the right the sympathetic trunk is overlapped by the inferior vena cava along the line of junction between the vertebral column and the psoas major (page 142, A) On the left it is level with the lateral border of the aorta rather than being overlapped by it (page 143, B). An appropriate length of trunk with its ganglia can be dissected out from behind the peritoneum and removed. It is also possible to achieve lumbar sympathetic block by injection from behind, sliding the needle along the side of the first lumbar vertebra.

Approach for Lumbar Sympathectomy
A transverse muscle-cutting incision is made on the appropriate side.

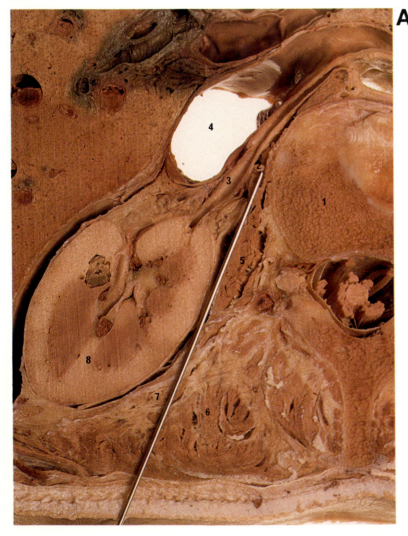

A

The peritoneum is *not* incised but stripped off round the abdominal walls as far as psoas major and the vertebral column (page 113, C).

The trunk and its ganglia are identified below the level of the renal vessels, and two ganglia with the intervening length of trunk are removed.

Hazards and Safeguards
The abdominal incision must not penetrate the peritoneum.

As the peritoneum is stripped from the anterior surface of psoas major the ureter is carried with it.

The sympathetic trunk is a cord-like structure (but not necessarily a single trunk) running vertically with ganglionated swellings. It must not be confused with the genitofemoral nerve which emerges through the anterior surface of psoas, has no swellings and runs downwards and slightly laterally, deep to the ureter (page 142, A). The trunk usually lies in front of the lumbar arteries and veins but some of the veins may cross the trunk and damage to any of these vessels must be avoided.

Approach for Lumbar Sympathetic Block
A skin wheal is raised 8 cm from the midline just below the twelfth rib.

The needle is inserted in a slightly medial direction towards the first lumbar vertebral body; it passes through erector spinae, quadratus lumborum and psoas major (A). When it strikes bone it is withdrawn slightly and redirected more deeply until it slips off the side of the vertebral body. After aspiration and a radiological check the injection can be made.

Hazards and Safeguards
The trunk lies outside the psoas sheath, where the sheath meets the vertebral column, and so the needle tip must pass out of the sheath to be in the correct position. The injection of a small amount of contrast medium under radiological control will demonstrate by the spread of the medium whether it is inside or outside the sheath.

The left trunk lies behind the left margin of the aorta, and the right trunk is overlapped by the inferior vena cava; it is essential that the needle does not enter them, nor any renal or lumbar vessels.

A
Cross section of the right side of the abdomen at the level of the disc between the first and second lumbar vertebrae, showing the route for lumbar sympathetic block.

B
Cross section of the posterior abdominal wall at the level of the disc between the twelfth thoracic and first lumbar vertebrae, showing the route for coeliac plexus block on the left.

1	First lumbar vertebra	8	Kidney	14	Splenic artery
2	Sympathetic trunk	9	Twelfth	15	Splenic vein
3	Renal artery		thoracic vertebra	16	Suprarenal gland
4	Inferior vena cava	10	Stomach	17	Pancreas
5	Psoas major	11	Left gastric artery	18	Crus of diaphragm
6	Erector spinae	12	Coeliac trunk	19	Aorta
7	Quadratus lumborum	13	Coeliac ganglion		

COELIAC PLEXUS

Background

The coeliac plexus consists of a mass of mostly sympathetic nerve fibres on the front of the abdominal aorta around the origins of the coeliac trunk and superior mesenteric artery at the level of the first lumbar vertebra. It includes the two coeliac ganglia on either side of the base of the coeliac trunk and in front of the crura of the diaphragm; the right ganglion is overlapped by the inferior vena cava. Many pain fibres pass through the plexus from abdominal viscera on their way to spinal nerves via lumbar and thoracic spinal nerves and white rami communicantes.

Coeliac plexus block may be used in the control of chronic abdominal pain, usually from cancerous lesions in the pancreatic area. The needle is introduced from the back at the side of the vertebral column, similar to the approach to the lumbar plexus (page 186) but going deeper. (A direct injection can be made during an abdominal operation.)

Approach for Coeliac Plexus Block

With the patient lying prone, the left twelfth rib and twelfth thoracic spine are identified.

At a point just below the rib and 7 cm from the midline, the needle is introduced at an angle of 60° to the sagittal plane and slightly upwards in the direction of the twelfth thoracic spine, to strike the body of the first lumbar vertebra. It is partially withdrawn and reinserted to slip off the side of the vertebral body and then pushed forward (B). When suitably placed the needle should show transmitted pulsation from the aorta. The skin to plexus distance varies from 7–10 cm. The injection is made after aspiration to ensure that the needle is not in a vessel. If radiological control is available, injection of contrast medium should indicate a spread round the aorta and vena cava when the needle is in the correct position.

Hazards and Safeguards

The twelfth rib must be properly identified and checked radiologically to avoid entering the pleural sac.

Aspiration is essential to avoid a vascular injection. There should be no resistance to injection; if there is, it suggests penetration of periosteum, the psoas major muscle, pancreas or suprarenal gland. By paralysing sympathetic activity, satisfactory block will cause vasodilatation and pooling of blood in the intestines with hypotension.

1   Sartorius
2   Tensor fasciae latae
3   Ascending branch of lateral circumflex femoral artery
4   Rectus femoris
5   Reflected head of rectus femoris
6   Gluteus minimus
7   Gluteus medius
8   Gluteus maximus
9   Piriformis
10 Obturator internus and gemelli
11 Quadratus femoris
12 Sciatic nerve
13 Posterior femoral cutaneous nerve
14 Adductor magnus
15 Adductor brevis
16 Pectineus
17 Medial circumflex femoral artery
18 Obturator externus
19 Capsule
20 Head of femur
21 Iliacus

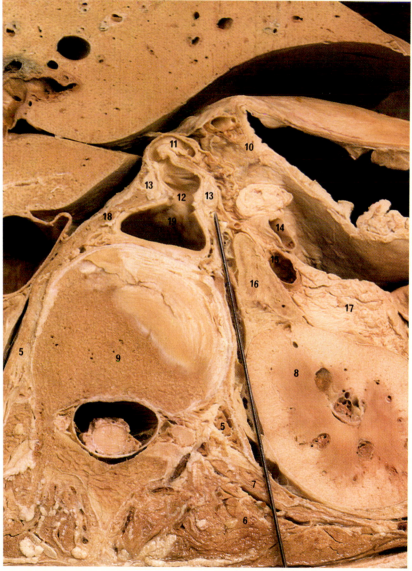

B

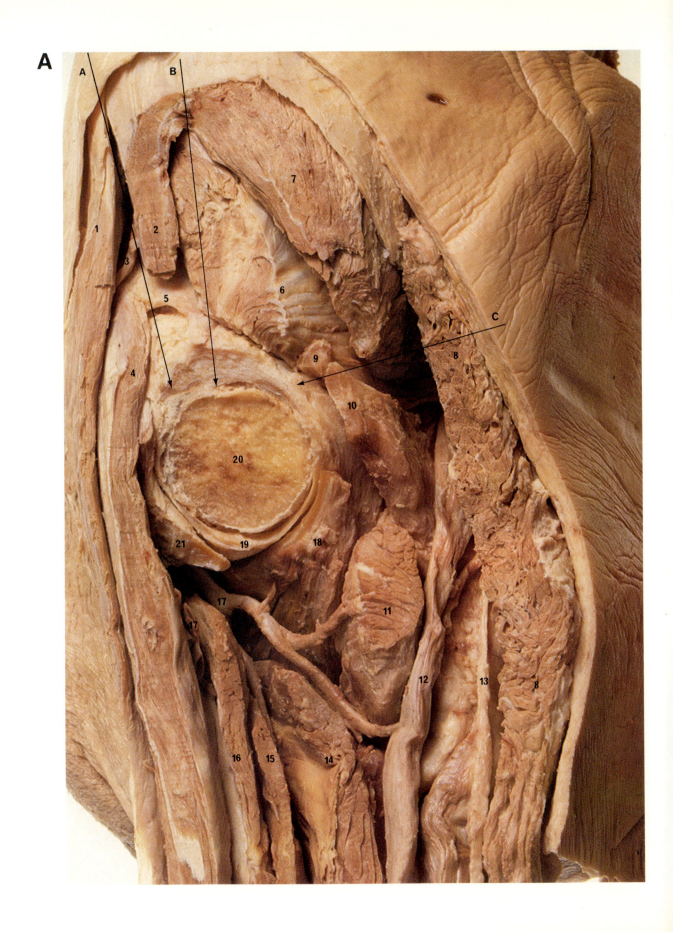

LOWER LIMB

HIP JOINT

Background

The hip joint is deeply surrounded by muscles (A). Gluteus minimus and the straight head of rectus femoris lie immediately above the joint with gluteus medius more superficially. Obturator externus spirals beneath the joint from front to back. The lower part of iliacus with the tendon of psoas major on its medial side crosses the front of the capsule, while behind it from above down are piriformis, obturator internus and the gemelli and quadratus femoris, all under cover of gluteus maximus.

The major vessels and nerves are not in immediate contact with the joint. In the femoral triangle, the femoral artery lies in front of the psoas tendon with the femoral vein medially overlying pectineus and the femoral nerve laterally overlying iliacus. The obturator nerve is more deeply placed, with its anterior and posterior divisions passing anterior and posterior to adductor brevis which is deep to pectineus and adductor longus. At the back numerous structures pass out of the greater sciatic foramen apart from piriformis: the superior gluteal nerve and vessels emerge above piriformis, and the remaining structures all emerge below the muscle – the pudendal nerve, internal pudendal vessels and the nerve to obturator internus entering the lesser sciatic foramen by crossing the ischial spine or sacrospinous ligament in that order from medial to lateral, and the inferior gluteal vessels and nerve, the sciatic nerve, nerve to quadratus femoris and the posterior femoral cutaneous nerve lying more laterally.

Access to the joint and to the extracapsular part of the neck of the femur is commonly obtained by one of four routes. The posterior involves splitting gluteus maximus in the line of its fibres and dividing piriformis, obturator internus and gemelli and quadratus femoris to expose the posterior part of the capsule. There is a variety of anterior and lateral approaches which basically open up intervals in front of, through, or behind tensor fasciae latae. The anterior approach is through the interval between the tensor and sartorius, then detaching the tensor, rectus femoris and the anterior parts of gluteus medius and iliacus from the hip bone to expose the upper and anterior parts of the capsule. The anterolateral route involves opening the gap between the tensor and gluteus medius and allowing the upper part of the capsule to be approached underneath the anterior borders of gluteus medius and minimus. In the lateral approach the iliotibial tract is incised to expose the greater trochanter whose tip together with the attachments of gluteus medius and minimus is detached and turned upwards to give access to the upper part of the capsule.

Anterolateral and posterior approaches are described here because they illustrate much of the relevant hip anatomy, and they are commonly used for total prosthetic hip replacement ('artificial hip') and other procedures.

A

Sagittal section of the left hip. The arrows indicate the lines of approach to the joint by the anterior (A), anterolateral (B) and posterior (C) routes.

1 Sartorius
2 Tensor fasciae latae
3 Ascending branch of lateral circumflex femoral artery
4 Rectus femoris
5 Reflected head of rectus femoris
6 Gluteus minimus
7 Gluteus medius
8 Gluteus maximus
9 Piriformis
10 Obturator internus and gemelli
11 Quadratus femoris
12 Sciatic nerve
13 Posterior femoral cutaneous nerve
14 Adductor magnus
15 Adductor brevis
16 Pectineus
17 Medial circumflex femoral artery
18 Obturator externus
19 Capsule
20 Head of femur
21 Iliacus

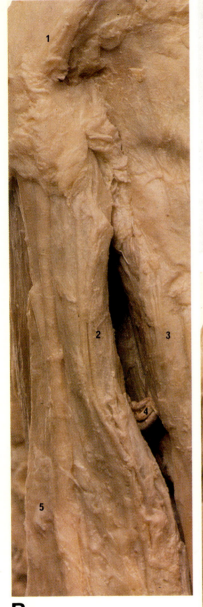

B

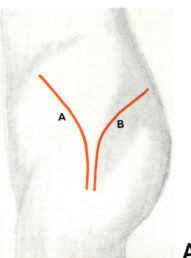

A

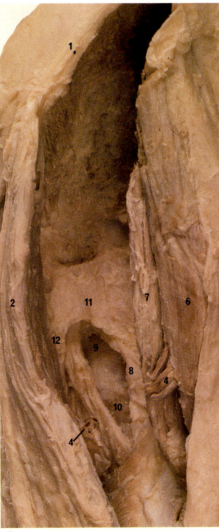

C

Anterolateral Approach

A skin incision (A) is made from a point 2.5 cm behind the anterior superior iliac spine to the tip of the greater trochanter, and then vertically down along the anterior margin of the trochanter for about 10 cm.

The interval between tensor fasciae latae and gluteus medius is identified and the overlying gluteal fascia is divided so that the muscles can be separated up to the iliac crest (B). The upper ends of the muscles may be fused, with the tensor overlapping gluteus medius, and dissection with a knife may be necessary. The ascending branch of the lateral femoral circumflex artery and its accompanying veins cross the gap deep to these muscles and must be ligated.

The anterior parts of gluteus medius and minimus are raised from the hip bone and retracted posteriorly (C).

After clearing fat, the upper part of the capsule of the hip joint will be seen, with the reflected head of rectus femoris attached to the upper part of the acetabular rim (C). This head (and if necessary the straight head also) can be detached to give greater exposure of the capsule which can be incised or removed according to the type of operation being performed.

If a hip prosthesis is being inserted, the joint is dislocated with transection of the neck of the femur and removal of the head, the acetabular cartilage and soft tissues scraped away, a new cup inserted and keyed in position, and the stem of the new femoral head inserted into the marrow cavity of the femoral shaft and articulated with the cup.

Hazards and Safeguards

The ascending branch of the lateral femoral circumflex artery and the accompanying veins are large vessels that pass deep to rectus femoris, tensor fasciae latae and gluteus medius, and require ligation as the gap between the tensor and gluteus medius is opened up (B). The nerve to the tensor also crosses the gap (at a higher level than the vessels) and should be preserved but it can be sacrificed if necessary for adequate exposure.

The sciatic nerve must not be damaged if the joint is being dislocated to remove the head for a prosthetic replacement.

Posterior Approach

A skin incision (A) is made from the posterior border of the greater trochanter to the posterior superior iliac spine and downwards below the trochanter for 8 cm in the line of the shaft of the femur.

The fascia lata is incised vertically over the upper femur and the cut continued through the gluteal bursa and then into gluteus maximus which is split in the line of its fibres along the same line as the upper part of the skin incision (D). The gap in the muscle and fascia is opened up to display the fat that overlies the short lateral rotators and the sciatic nerve, and the fat is removed with appropriate ligation of blood vessels.

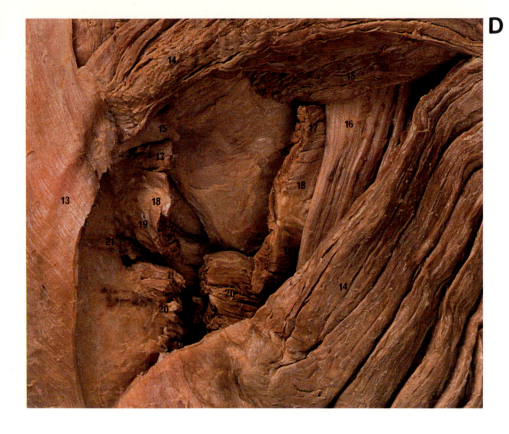

D

1 Iliac crest
2 Fascia over tensor fasciae latae
3 Fascia over gluteus medius
4 Ascending branch of lateral circumflex femoral artery
5 Tip of greater trochanter
6 Gluteus medius
7 Gluteus minimus
8 Capsule
9 Head of femur
10 Neck of femur
11 Reflected head of rectus femoris
12 Straight head of rectus femoris
13 Fascia lata
14 Gluteus maximus
15 Piriformis
16 Sciatic nerve
17 Superior gemellus
18 Obturator internus
19 Inferior gemellus
20 Quadratus femoris
21 Branch of medial circumflex femoral artery

The sciatic nerve is displaced medially and piriformis, obturator internus and the gemelli are divided at their femoral attachments to expose the posterior part of the capsule which can be incised or removed as required (D). Part or all of the attachments of gluteus medius and minimus can also be detached from the greater trochanter to provide more access to the upper part of the joint.

Hazards and Safeguards

The sciatic nerve emerges below piriformis and passes downwards superficial to obturator internus and the gemelli and quadratus femoris. Turning the medial cut ends of the muscles backwards over the nerve helps to protect it. It must not be damaged if the joint is being dislocated to remove the femoral head.

Branches of the medial circumflex femoral vessels emerge above and below quadratus femoris to anastomose with the inferior gluteal vessels and ascending branches from the profunda femoris (cruciate anastomosis) and can be ligated as required.

The inferior gluteal nerve which provides the motor supply to gluteus maximus is below the line of incision through the muscle. The superior gluteal nerve supplying gluteus medius and minimus and tensor fasciae latae is protected because it runs between the two gluteus muscles.

A
Incision lines for anterolateral (A) and posterior (B) approaches.

B
Left hip, from the lateral side. The interval between tensor fasciae latae and gluteus medius is opened up; it is crossed by branches of the lateral circumflex femoral vessels.

C
Deeper dissection of B. The anterior parts of gluteus medius and minimus are stripped from the hip bone and retracted backwards to expose the upper part of the joint capsule which is being incised. It may be necessary to detach the reflected or straight heads of rectus femoris to obtain more exposure.

D
Left hip, from behind. Gluteus maximus is split in the line of its fibres. The back of the capsule is exposed by vertical incisions through the lateral ends of piriformis, obturator internus and gemelli and if necessary the upper part of quadratus femoris. The sciatic nerve which emerges below the medial part of piriformis can be retracted medially and protected by turning the cut ends of obturator internus and gemelli backwards over the nerve.

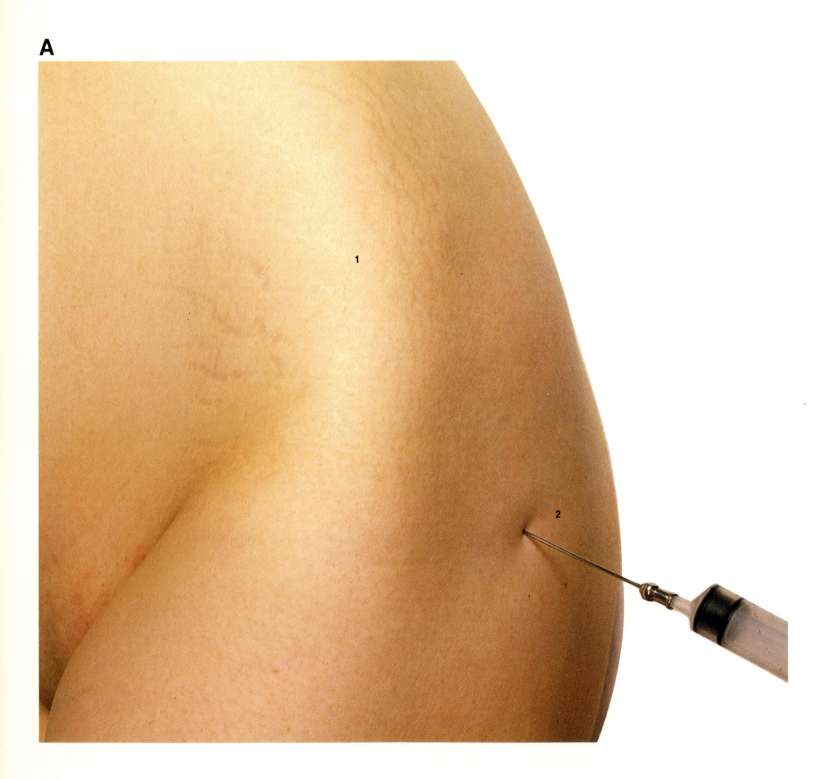

Puncture of the Hip Joint

The greater trochanter is palpated, and the needle inserted from the side, in front of its upper margin and approximately parallel to the femoral neck (A), so that the needle enters the capsule obliquely after passing through the attachments of gluteus medius and minimus (B).

An alternative approach is from the front 5 cm below the anterior inferior iliac spine, passing upwards, backwards and medially.

A

Puncture of the left hip joint, from the side at the upper anterior margin of the greater trochanter.

B

Dissection of A, from the left and front, with removal of part of gluteus medius and minimus, tensor fasciae latae and the joint capsule.

1 Anterior superior iliac spine
2 Greater trochanter
3 Tensor fasciae latae
4 Gluteus minimus
5 Gluteus medius
6 Capsule
7 Neck of femur
8 Vastus lateralis

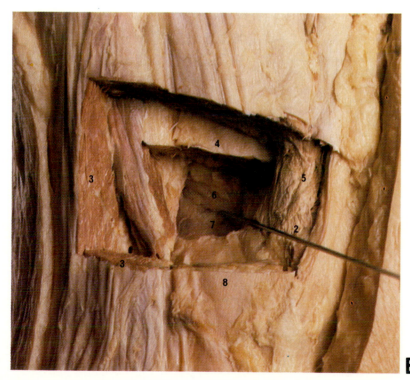

B

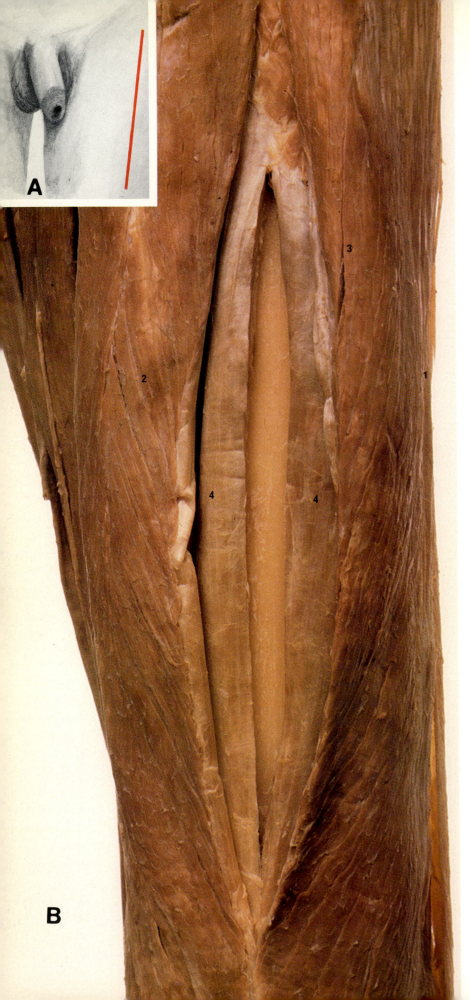

A

B

FEMUR

Background

The greater trochanter of the femur is palpable and so are the condyles at the lower end, but the shaft is deeply surrounded by muscles and not palpable. Vastus intermedius clothes much of the anterior and lateral parts of the shaft, with vastus medialis and vastus lateralis on their respective sides and rectus femoris at the front. Sartorius crosses superficially from the lateral to medial side in its course towards the knee. The hamstrings are at the back with the three adductors and gracilis on the posteromedial side. The largest vessel of the thigh, the femoral artery, is only close to the bone low down, where it passes through the opening in adductor magnus to become the popliteal artery. The major nerves are not close relations but the positions of the femoral and sciatic nerves help to determine the approach routes to the shaft.

The anterior approach passes between rectus femoris and vastus lateralis and the bone is reached through the substance of vastus intermedius.

The posterolateral approach is made behind vastus lateralis and in front of biceps and the lateral intermuscular septum, which is followed inwards to the linea aspera.

Anterior Approach

A skin incision (A) is made along the middle two thirds of a line from the anterior superior iliac spine to the lateral margin of the patella.

The deep fascia is incised and the line between the lateral border of rectus femoris and vastus lateralis is defined and opened up to expose the underlying vastus intermedius which is then incised vertically down to the bone (B and C).

Hazards and Safeguards

This approach through vastus intermedius avoids all major vessels and nerves.

A
Incision line.

B
Left thigh, from the front. The fascia lata is incised to open up the interval between the lateral edge of rectus femoris and vastus lateralis. Vastus intermedius is then split vertically down to the bone. There are no major vessels or nerves in this area.

C
Cross section of the upper third of the left thigh, showing the exposure of the anterior surface of the femur between rectus femoris and vastus lateralis and through the substance of vastus intermedius.

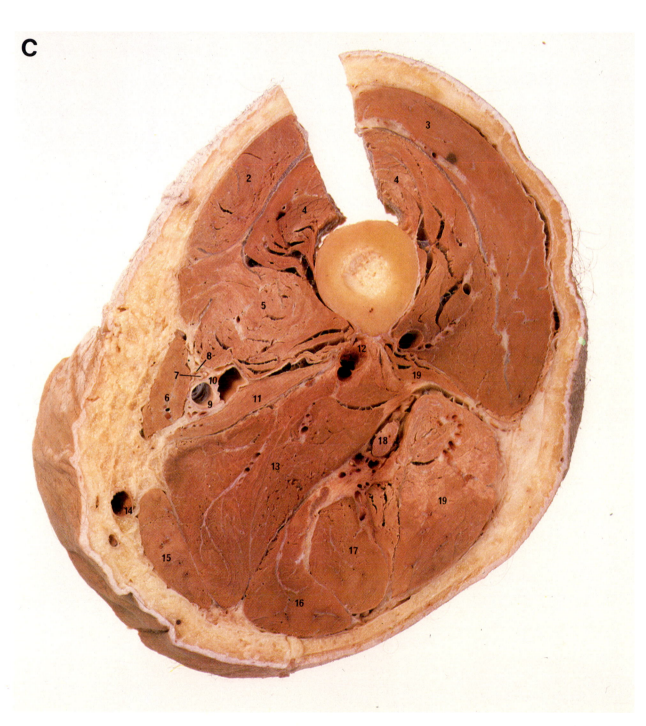

1 Fascia lata
2 Rectus femoris
3 Vastus lateralis
4 Vastus intermedius
5 Vastus medialis
6 Sartorius
7 Saphenous nerve
8 Nerve to 5
9 Femoral artery
10 Femoral vein
11 Adductor longus
12 Profunda femoris vessels
13 Adductor magnus
14 Saphenous vein
15 Gracilis
16 Semimembranosus
17 Semitendinosus
18 Sciatic nerve
19 Biceps femoris

C

Posterolateral Approach

A skin incision (A) is made along the middle third of a line from the posterior border of the greater trochanter to the biceps tendon above the knee.

The deep fascia is incised and retracted backwards so that the muscle fibres of vastus lateralis can be traced back along the lateral intermuscular septum (B, C and D) to the linea aspera (near which they become mixed with those of the short head of biceps).

Hazards and Safeguards

Some peforating branches of the profunda vessels need to be ligated as the bone is approached.

The approach lies in front of the intermuscular septum, so the sciatic nerve in the posterior compartment is not endangered.

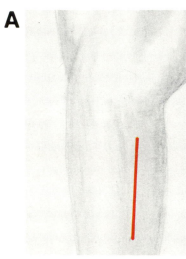

A

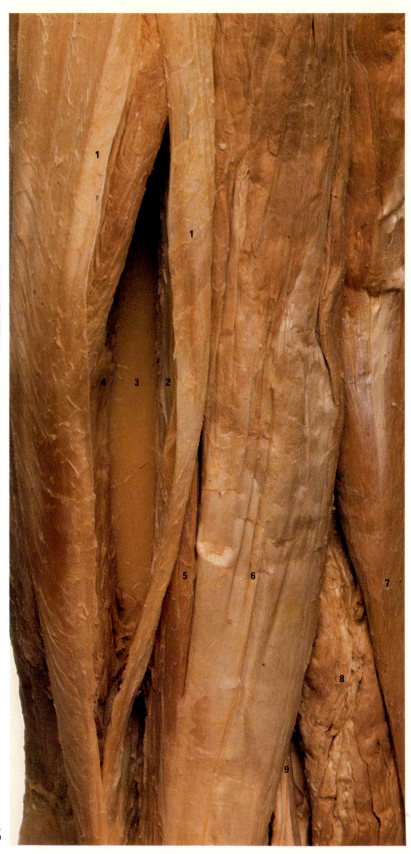

A
Incision line.

B
Left thigh, from the left and behind. The fascia lata is incised along the line of the lateral intermuscular septum, i.e. just behind the part of the fascia that constitutes the iliotibial tract and in front of biceps. Vastus lateralis is dissected off from the front of the septum and is scraped forward off the femur to expose the bone. By keeping in front of the septum, the sciatic nerve is protected.

C
Cross section of the left lower thigh (at the level of the opening in adductor magnus).

D
The same section, orientated like C for comparison with B, showing the line of detachment of vastus lateralis from the front of the lateral intermuscular septum and the side of the femur.

B

174

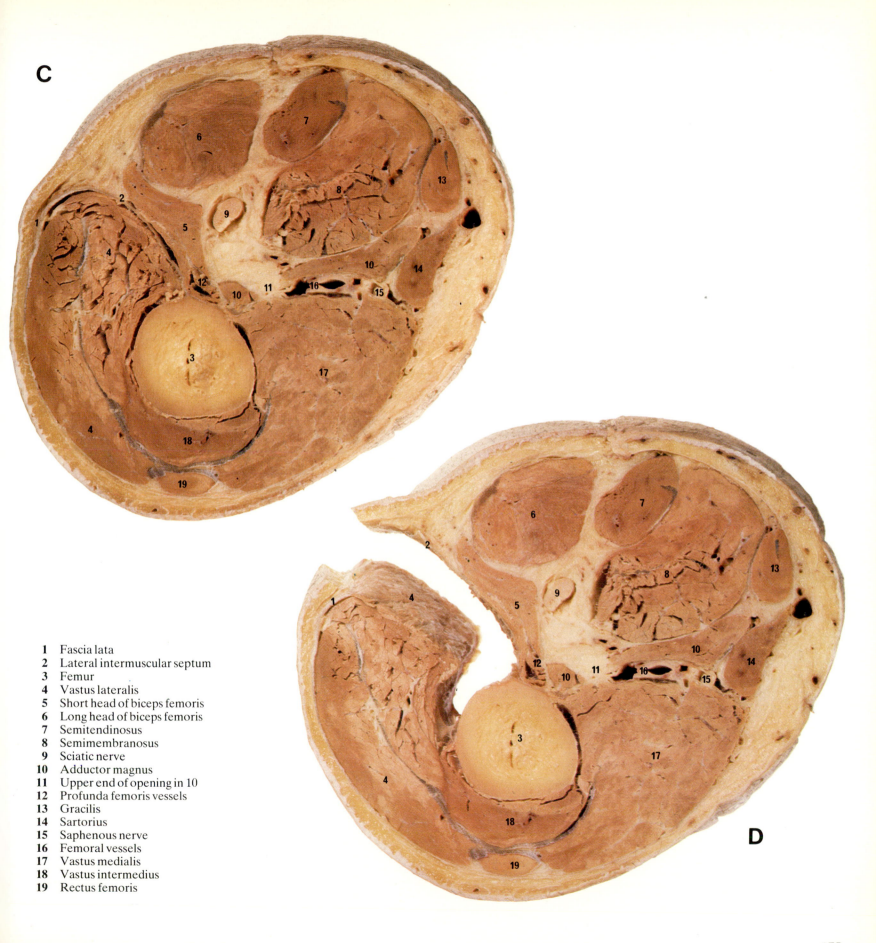

C

D

1 Fascia lata
2 Lateral intermuscular septum
3 Femur
4 Vastus lateralis
5 Short head of biceps femoris
6 Long head of biceps femoris
7 Semitendinosus
8 Semimembranosus
9 Sciatic nerve
10 Adductor magnus
11 Upper end of opening in 10
12 Profunda femoris vessels
13 Gracilis
14 Sartorius
15 Saphenous nerve
16 Femoral vessels
17 Vastus medialis
18 Vastus intermedius
19 Rectus femoris

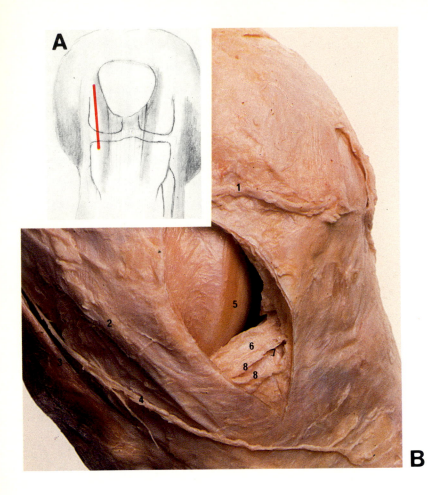

A

B

KNEE JOINT

Background

Unlike the hip, the knee joint is not deeply surrounded by muscle and a number of bony landmarks and tendons in the region of the joint are readily palpable. These include the condyles and epicondyles of the femur, the condyles and tuberosity of the tibia, the patella and the head of the fibula. The patellar ligament is in front of the lower part of the joint; on the lateral side at the back the tendon of biceps passes to the head of the fibula with the common peroneal nerve immediately behind the tendon, while on the posteromedial side the tendons of semimembranosus and semitendinosus can be felt, that of semitendinosus being the more superficial and thinner of the two. In the popliteal fossa at the back the tibial nerve is the most superficial of the major contents, with the popliteal vein underlying the nerve. The popliteal artery underlies the vein; it is thus the deepest of the major structures in the fossa and the one nearest the capsule of the joint. The horns of the menisci and the cruciate ligaments are attached to the intercondylar area of the tibia. The tibial collateral (medial) ligament is firmly fused to the medial meniscus; the fibular collateral (lateral) ligament has no union with the lateral meniscus but is attached to the popliteus tendon. The peripheral margins of the menisci are connected to the upper margin of the tibia by the coronary ligaments. The infrapatellar fat pad reflects the synovial membrane backwards below the patella. The suprapatellar bursa is an upward extension of the joint cavity behind the quadriceps and reaches for several centimetres above the patella.

The joint can be entered easily by incisions on either side of the patella (anteromedial or anterolateral approaches) or behind either collateral ligament (posteromedial or posterolateral approaches), or through the popliteal fossa (posterior approach). A short anteromedial approach is commonly used for dealing with a torn medial meniscus (the commonest knee joint injury) and is described here, together with the posterior approach.

Anteromedial Approach

A vertical skin incision (A) is made 2 cm medial to the patella (with the knee flexed to a right angle) and the incision deepened to enter the joint cavity (B).

Hazards and Safeguards

The lower part of the incision should not extend more than 1 cm below the upper margin of the tibia, to avoid damaging the infrapatellar branch of the saphenous nerve (B).

A
Incision for anteromedial approach.

B
Left knee, from the front and medial side. The capsule is opened to give access to the medial meniscus. The incision must not extend more than 1 cm below the upper margin of the tibia to avoid cutting the infrapatellar branch of the saphenous nerve; it curves forwards in front of the lower end of sartorius.

C
Incision line for posterior approach.

D
Left popliteal fossa, with fat removed. The sural nerve, identified either medial or lateral to the small saphenous vein but always close to it below the level of the joint, can be followed upwards to the centre of the fossa to lead to the tibial nerve which is the most superficial of the major neurovascular structures in the fossa. The popliteal vein is deep to the nerve, with the artery deep to the vein. The gap between semimembranosus and the tibial nerve can be opened up to expose the upper end of the medial head of gastrocnemius.

E
As B after detachment of the medial head of gastrocnemius from its femoral origin to reveal the joint capsule by turning the muscle laterally; this helps to protect the nerve to this head (seen in D) and the main neurovascular bundle.

F
Cross section of the left knee, from below, showing the approach to the joint between the tibial nerve and semimembranosus, with detachment of the medial head of gastrocnemius.

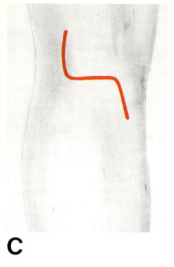

C

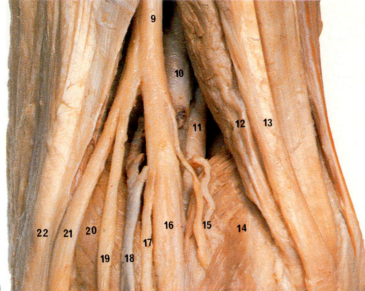

D

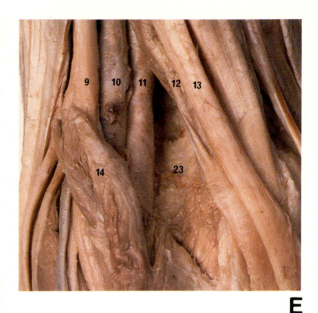

E

Posterior Approach

An S-shaped skin incision (C) is made, extending along the posterior border of biceps and its tendon on the upper lateral side of the popliteal fossa, then transversely across the fossa and finally along the lower medial side of the fossa posterior to the semitendinosus tendon.

The skin flaps are retracted and the deep fascia is incised in the midline; the small saphenous vein is ligated if necessary but the sural nerve must be preserved.

The sural nerve is followed upwards to lead to the tibial nerve which is carefully defined, together with the space between the nerve and semimembranosus so that the underlying medial head of gastrocnemius can be displayed (D).

The popliteal vessels are displaced laterally; in order to do this the middle genicular and possibly the superior medial genicular vessels are ligated.

The medial head of gastrocnemius is traced upwards, detached from its origin and retracted towards the midline, so exposing the joint capsule which can then be opened (E and F).

Hazards and Safeguards

The large vessels and nerves in the popliteal fossa are obvious hazards.

The sural nerve, which lies superficial to the deep fascia below the knee, is used as a guide to the tibial nerve – follow the sural nerve upwards to pierce the deep fascia and lead to the tibial nerve which is its parent trunk. In the popliteal fossa the tibial nerve lies superficial to the popliteal vein, with the popliteal artery deep to the vein.

The nerve and vessels to the medial head of gastrocnemius must not be damaged but as both this head of the muscle and the main neurovascular bundle are retracted laterally the risk is minimized.

1 Branch of medial femoral cutaneous nerve	20 Lateral head of gastrocnemius
2 Sartorius	21 Common peroneal nerve
3 Gracilis	22 Biceps femoris
4 Infrapatellar branch of saphenous nerve	23 Capsule
5 Medial condyle of femur	24 Plantaris
6 Medial meniscus	25 Saphenous nerve
7 Upper edge of tibia	26 Great saphenous vein
8 Cut edge of coronary ligament	27 Lateral condyle of femur
9 Sciatic nerve	
10 Popliteal vein	
11 Popliteal artery	
12 Semimembranosus	
13 Semitendinosus	
14 Medial head of gastrocnemius	
15 Nerve to 14 and sural artery	
16 Tibial nerve	
17 Sural nerve	
18 Small saphenous vein	
19 Peroneal communicating nerve	

F

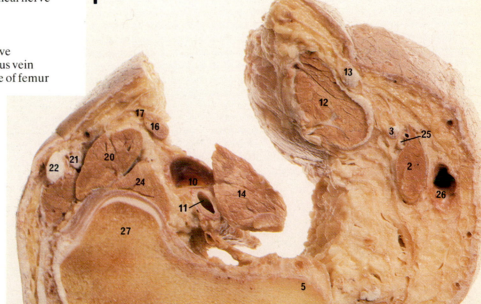

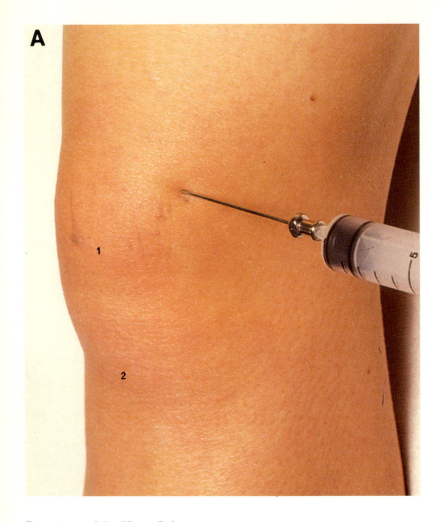

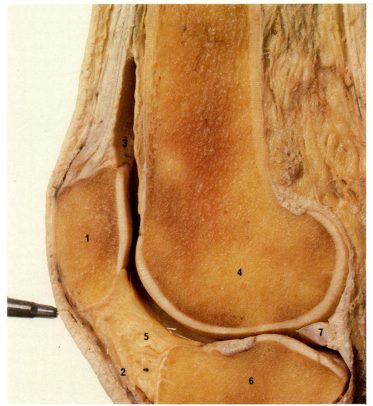

1 Patella
2 Patellar ligament
3 Suprapatellar bursa
4 Lateral condyle of femur
5 Infrapatellar fat pad
6 Lateral condyle of tibia
7 Lateral meniscus

Puncture of the Knee Joint

For aspiration the needle is inserted from the side just above the upper border of the patella and level with its lateral border (A). The needle enters the suprapatellar bursa but this is always widely continuous with the joint cavity and is the site for draining joint effusions ('water on the knee').

For injection the joint is entered at the lower border of the patella on either side of the patellar ligament. The needle passes backwards through the infrapatellar fat pad (B) to enter the cavity between the femoral condyle and meniscus. The site used for arthroscopy is on the lateral side of the patellar ligament.

With the lower approaches the cartilage of the joint surfaces and the menisci must not be damaged. Aspiration through the suprapatellar bursa avoids this possibility.

A
Site for aspiration of the left knee joint through the suprapatellar bursa, at the upper lateral margin of the patella.

B
Sagittal section of the left knee joint through the lateral condyles of the femur and tibia, showing needles inserted into the suprapatellar bursa and through the infrapatellar fat pad.

TIBIA

Background

The medial surface of the tibia is subcutaneous throughout its length but much of the rest of the bone is covered by muscle. Tibialis anterior is attached to part of the lateral surface, while posteriorly there are attachment areas for soleus, flexor digitorum longus and tibialis posterior. The great saphenous vein and saphenous nerve run obliquely across the lower part of the medial surface.

Access to the subcutaneous medial surface is obviously easy but posteromedial and posterolateral routes can also be used. It may seem odd to approach the tibia by what appears to be an unnecessarily complicated route from the *lateral* side, but diseased or scarred tissue over the medial surface may make it unsuitable for good healing.

Anterior Approach

A skin incision (C) is made over tibialis anterior just lateral to the anterior border of the tibia and a skin flap raised to expose the medial surface of the bone. The lateral surface is exposed by detaching tibialis anterior (D).

Hazards and Safeguards

The skin incision should not be made over the bone itself since one made over muscle provides better healing.

1 Medial surface of tibia
2 Anterior border
3 Lateral surface
4 Cut edge of periosteum
5 Tibialis anterior
6 Saphenous nerve and
   great saphenous vein
7 Soleus
8 Gastrocnemius
9 Flexor digitorum longus
10 Deep peroneal nerve
11 Anterior tibial artery
12 Extensor digitorum longus
13 Extensor hallucis longus
14 Interosseous membrane
15 Fibula
16 Tibialis posterior
17 Peroneal artery
18 Tibial nerve
19 Posterior tibial artery

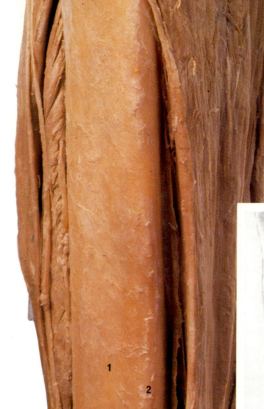

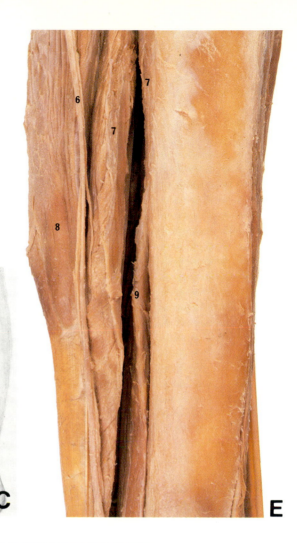

Posteromedial Approach

A skin incision (C) is made along the posterior border of the tibia.

The deep fascia is incised in the line of the skin incision to expose the medial border of soleus which is detached from the medial part of the posterior surface of the tibia (E), followed by detachment of flexor digitorum longus from the lateral part of the posterior surface.

Hazards and Safeguards

The great saphenous vein and saphenous nerve cross the posterior border of the tibia obliquely somewhere about the junction of the middle and lower thirds of the bone.

C
Incision lines for anterior (A) and posteromedial (B) approaches.

D
Left leg, from the front with deep fascia removed. Tibialis anterior is detached from the lateral surface of the tibia and the periosteum is elevated.

E
Left leg, from the posteromedial side with deep fascia removed. Soleus and flexor digitorum longus are being detached and displaced backwards from the posterior surface of the tibia.

F
Cross section of the upper left leg, from below. For approaching the tibia from the front the skin incision is made over tibialis anterior (in the line of the upper arrow), not directly over the bone. For the posteromedial approach the incision is along the posterior border of the bone (lower arrow).

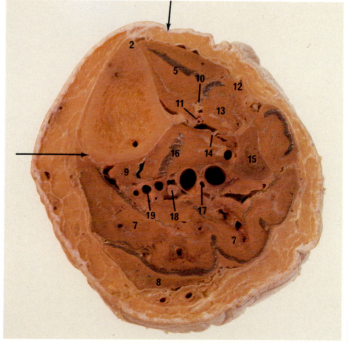

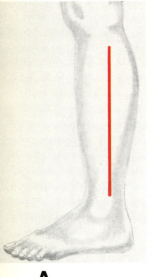

A

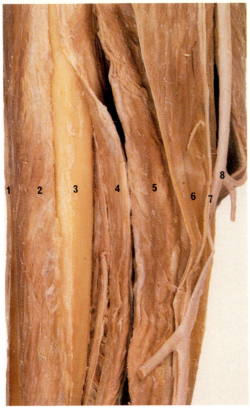

B

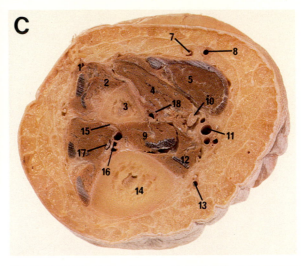

C

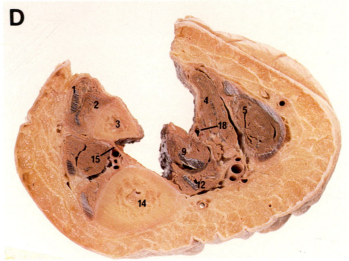

D

1	Peroneus longus
2	Peroneus brevis
3	Fibula
4	Flexor hallucis longus
5	Soleus
6	Gastrocnemius
7	Sural nerve
8	Small saphenous vein
9	Tibialis posterior
10	Tibial nerve
11	Posterior tibial artery
12	Flexor digitorum longus
13	Great saphenous vein
14	Tibia
15	Interosseous membrane
16	Anterior tibial artery
17	Deep peroneal nerve
18	Peroneal vessels

Posterolateral Approach

A skin incision (A) is made in the line of the posterior border of the fibula.

The deep fascia is incised in the line of the skin incision to expose the plane between peroneus longus and soleus. By opening up the interval between these muscles, flexor hallucis longus is stripped backwards from the posterior surface of the fibula (B).

The more deeply-placed tibialis posterior (C) is then stripped from the fibula, posterior interosseous membrane and tibia (D).

Hazards and Safeguards

At the upper end of the fibula the common peroneal nerve lies against the neck of the bone deep to peroneus longus and is the guide to the cleft between peroneus longus and soleus.

The peroneal vessels lie between flexor hallucis longus and tibialis posterior and must be carried backwards with these muscles as they are stripped off the fibula (C and D). The tibial nerve and posterior tibial vessels lie between soleus and the deeper flexor muscles and should not be liable to damage.

A
Incision line.

B
Left leg, from the lateral side, with deep fascia removed. For the lateral approach to the tibia soleus, flexor hallucis longus and tibialis posterior are detached from the fibula, and this dissection shows the first stage of this approach, with soleus and flexor hallucis longus being displaced backwards from the fibula.

C
Cross section of the left lower leg, orientated sideways.

D
The same section, for comparison with B, showing the line of approach to the tibia from the lateral side. Soleus, flexor hallucis longus and tibialis posterior are detached from the fibula, and tibialis posterior is further detached from the interosseous membrane and the back of the tibia. The peroneal vessels must be carried backwards with the muscles.

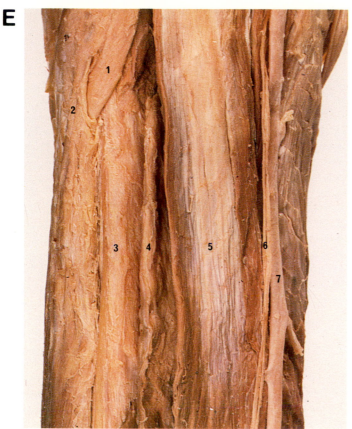

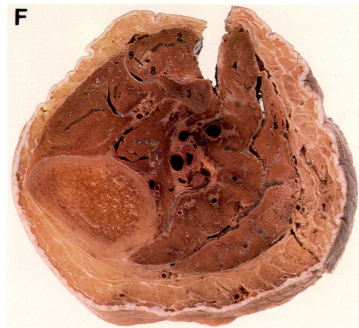

FIBULA

1 Common peroneal nerve
2 Peroneus longus
3 Fibula
4 Soleus
5 Gastrocnemius
6 Sural nerve
7 Small saphenous vein
8 Peroneus brevis
9 Superficial peroneal nerve

Background

The head of the fibula and the lower end with the lateral malleolus are subcutaneous and palpable. The very narrow anterior surface in front of the interosseous membrane gives origin to extensor hallucis longus and extensor digitorum longus, with peroneus longus and brevis on the lateral surface. Soleus is attached to the upper part of the bone at the back with flexor hallucis longus and tibialis posterior at deeper levels. The common peroneal nerve is in contact with the neck of the bone, and divides there under cover of peroneus longus into three branches – the nerve to tibialis anterior and the superficial and deep peroneal nerves.

The common peroneal nerve is used as the guide to the exposure of the fibula from the lateral side, since when followed down behind the tendon of biceps it leads to the gap between peroneus longus in front and soleus behind.

Approach

A skin incision (as in A) is made along the line of the posterior border of the fibula from behind the head to behind the lateral malleolus. The incision is extended upwards for 9 cm along the tendon of biceps.

The deep fascia is incised at the medial edge of the biceps tendon to expose the common peroneal nerve which is followed down to indicate the interval between soleus and peroneus longus (E). The slip from peroneus longus that overlies the nerve and passes to the lateral condyle of the tibia is cut so that the nerve can be moved away from the bone.

The peroneal muscles are turned forwards and soleus backwards to expose the shaft of the bone (E and F).

Hazards and Safeguards

Apart from the common peroneal nerve and its branches under cover of the upper part of peroneus longus, no other major structures are at risk. The superficial peroneal nerve is protected between the peroneal muscles.

E

Left leg, from the lateral side, with deep fascia removed. The common peroneal nerve is the guide to the interval between peroneus longus in front and soleus behind; the fibula is exposed by opening up the gap between these muscles. The part of peroneus longus that covers the nerve can be cut to move the nerve away from the bone if necessary.

F

Cross section of the left upper leg (above the origins of flexor digitorum longus and the peroneal artery), showing the line of approach to the fibula between peroneus longus and soleus.

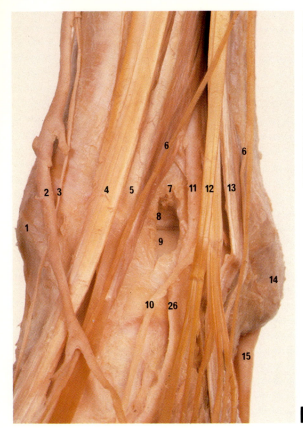

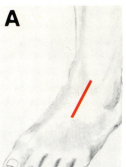

B

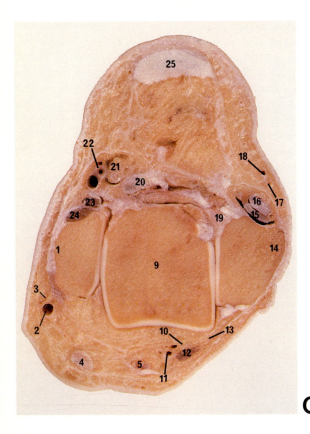

C

ANKLE JOINT

Background

The arrangement of tendons, vessels and nerves in the ankle region allows a variety of approaches to the ankle joint. Superficially the great saphenous vein and saphenous nerve lie in front of the medial malleolus, while the small saphenous vein and the sural nerve lie behind the lateral malleolus. Deep to the deep fascia the order of structures in front of the joint from medial to lateral is: tibialis anterior, extensor hallucis longus, anterior tibial vessels, deep peroneal nerve and extensor digitorum longus. Between the medial malleolus and tendo calcaneus the order of structures from front to back is: tibialis posterior, flexor digitorum longus, posterior tibial vessels, tibial nerve and flexor hallucis longus. Behind the lateral malleolus are the tendons of peroneus brevis and peroneus longus, the brevis tendon being in front of the longus.

At the front the route of approach to the joint is between the tendons of extensor hallucis longus and extensor digitorum longus. For a posteromedial approach the tendons of tibialis posterior and flexor digitorum longus are displaced forwards, while postero-laterally the tendons of peroneus brevis and peroneus longus can be similarly displaced.

Anterior Approach

A vertical skin incision (A) is made in the midline of the front of the ankle extending 4 cm above and below the joint line.

The tendons of tibialis anterior, extensor hallucis longus and extensor digitorum longus are identified and the extensor retinaculum divided to expose the anterior tibial vessels and deep peroneal nerve between the two extensor tendons (B and C). The vessels, nerve and tendons are displaced so that the joint capsule can be incised (B).

Hazards and Safeguards

At the level of the ankle joint the deep peroneal nerve lies on the lateral side of the anterior tibial vessels, the artery having a vena comitans on either side and giving off medial and lateral malleolar branches.

A

Incision line.

B

Left ankle, from the front, with the deep fascia (including the extensor retinacula) removed. The capsule of the ankle joint is opened between the tendons of extensor hallucis longus and digitorum longus, avoiding the deep peroneal nerve and anterior tibial vessels. (The anterior tibial artery becomes the dorsalis pedis artery on crossing the joint line.)

C

Cross section of the left ankle. At the front the anterior tibial vessels and deep peroneal nerve are between the tendons of extensor hallucis longus and digitorum longus. Behind the medial malleolus the posterior tibial vessels and tibial nerve are between the corresponding flexor tendons, but the hallucis tendon is the more posterior with the tendon of flexor digitorum longus lying against that of tibialis posterior.

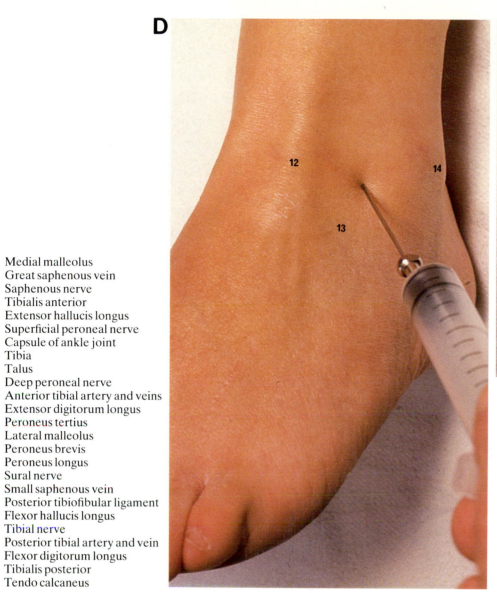

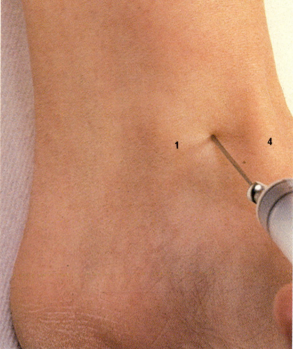

1 Medial malleolus
2 Great saphenous vein
3 Saphenous nerve
4 Tibialis anterior
5 Extensor hallucis longus
6 Superficial peroneal nerve
7 Capsule of ankle joint
8 Tibia
9 Talus
10 Deep peroneal nerve
11 Anterior tibial artery and veins
12 Extensor digitorum longus
13 Peroneus tertius
14 Lateral malleolus
15 Peroneus brevis
16 Peroneus longus
17 Sural nerve
18 Small saphenous vein
19 Posterior tibiofibular ligament
20 Flexor hallucis longus
21 Tibial nerve
22 Posterior tibial artery and vein
23 Flexor digitorum longus
24 Tibialis posterior
25 Tendo calcaneus

Puncture of the Ankle Joint

The line of the joint is palpated medial to the lateral malleolus, between the malleolus and the tendon of peroneus tertius.

The needle is introduced here (D), passing backwards and slightly downwards to enter the joint cavity between the tibia and talus.

An alternative site is in front of the medial malleolus, medial to the tibialis anterior tendon (E).

The needle must not damage the articular cartilage; moving the foot helps to define the joint line.

D
Puncture of the left ankle joint, between the lateral malleolus and peroneus tertius, and entering the joint between the tibia and talus (viewed from above; the needle in fact should pass slightly downwards).

E
Puncture of the left ankle joint, in front of the medial malleolus and medial to the tibialis anterior tendon.

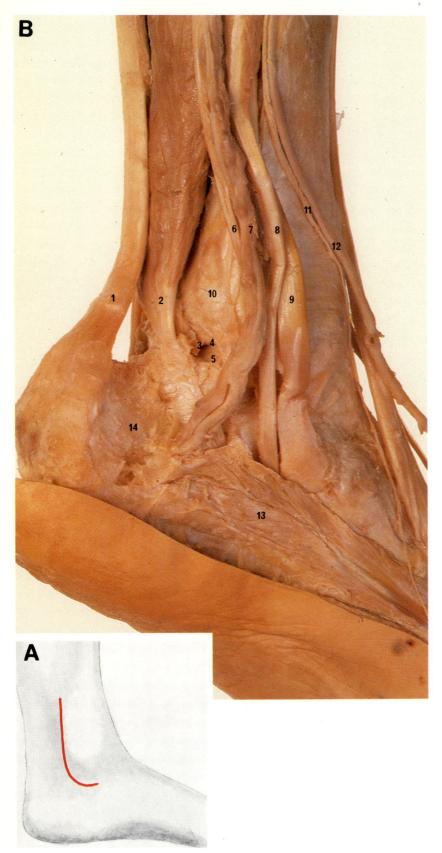

B

Posteromedial Approach

A skin incision (A) is made behind the medial malleolus extending 5 cm above the tip and curving 2.5 cm below and forwards (a 'hockey-stick' incision).

The tendons of tibialis posterior and flexor digitorum longus are freed from their compartments of the flexor retinaculum and displaced forwards (B).

The posterior tibial vessels and tibial nerve are retracted medially to expose the joint capsule, with flexor hallucis longus lying laterally (B). The communicating branch from the posterior tibial artery to the peroneal artery is divided.

Hazards and Safeguards

At the level of the ankle joint the tibial nerve lies behind the posterior tibial vessels, the artery having a vena comitans on either side.

A

Incision line for the posteromedial approach.

B

The left ankle from the posteromedial side after removal of the deep fascia and flexor retinaculum. The tendons of tibialis posterior and flexor digitorum longus have been displaced forwards on to the medial malleolus so that they lie behind the great saphenous vein and saphenous nerve. The tibial nerve and posterior tibial vessels have been retracted medially so that the joint capsule can be entered medial to flexor hallucis longus.

1	Tendo calcaneus
2	Flexor hallucis longus
3	Capsule of ankle joint
4	Tibia
5	Talus
6	Tibial nerve
7	Posterior tibial artery and veins
8	Flexor digitorum longus
9	Tibialis posterior
10	Medial malleolus
11	Saphenous nerve
12	Great saphenous vein
13	Abductor hallucis
14	Calcaneus
15	Lateral malleolus
16	Peroneus brevis
17	Peroneus longus
18	Sural nerve
19	Small saphenous vein

Posterolateral Approach

A hockey-stick incision is made behind the lateral malleolus, similar to that for the posteromedial approach (A).

The tendons of peroneus longus and brevis are freed from the superior peroneal retinaculum and displaced forwards (C). The lowest muscle fibres of peroneus brevis may need to be detached from the fibula.

The small saphenous vein and sural nerve are identified in the space between the peroneal tendons and the tendo calcaneus and displaced so that the capsule of the joint can be incised (C).

Hazards and Safeguards

The small saphenous vein and sural nerve must be preserved but there are no deeply placed vessels and nerves at risk in this approach.

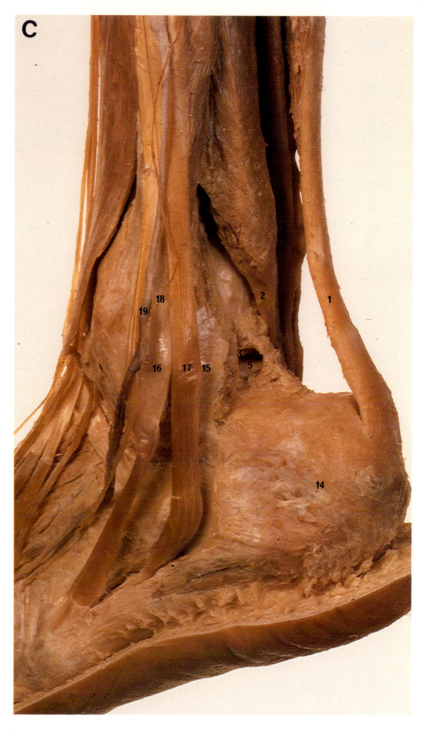

C

The left ankle from the posterolateral side after removal of the deep fascia and peroneal retinacula. The tendons of peroneus brevis and longus have been displaced forwards on to the lateral malleolus, together with the sural nerve and small saphenous vein that are normally behind the malleolus. The ankle joint capsule has been opened below and lateral to the tendon of flexor hallucis longus. (The fibrofatty tissue of the space in front of the tendo calcaneus has been removed.)

LUMBAR PLEXUS

Background

While a single injection of the brachial plexus can anaesthetize the whole of the upper limb, complete local anaesthesia of the lower limb requires the separate injection of the lumbar and sacral plexuses or of several nerves, in particular the sciatic, femoral, obturator and lateral femoral cutaneous. With the possible exception of pudendal nerve block in obstetrics, local injections of the lumbar and sacral plexuses and their branches are rarely used, especially since spinal or epidural anaesthesia produces a more convenient and effective 'local' for the lower part of the body. But approaches to these plexuses and their main branches are described below as examples of applied anatomy.

The lumbar plexus is formed by the ventral rami of the first four lumbar nerves within the substance of psoas major. It therefore lies in front of the transverse processes of lumbar vertebrae, with vessels of the external vertebral venous plexus between the muscle and the bones. The branches of the plexus emerge from different parts of psoas: the genitofemoral nerve through the anterior surface, the obturator nerve and the lumbosacral trunk (the contribution made by the lumbar plexus to the sacral plexus) from the medial margin, and the iliohypogastric, ilio-inguinal, lateral femoral cutaneous and femoral nerves from the lateral margin. In the paravertebral region it is relevant to lumbar nerve blocks to note that (1) the upper edge of a spine of one lumbar vertebra is approximately level with the upper margin of the transverse process of that vertebra (A), and (2) a needle above the transverse process of one vertebra will be adjacent to the nerve numbered one above that vertebra, e.g. L2 nerve will be above L3 transverse process.

The plexus may be blocked from behind by a paravertebral approach to individual lumbar nerves which involves introducing the needle through the gap between transverse processes into the substance of psoas as it lies adjacent to the vertebral column.

Lumbar Plexus Block

The spines of lumbar vertebrae are palpated and identified by counting from the fourth which is level with the line drawn between the highest points of the iliac crests.

A skin wheal is raised 4cm lateral to the upper edge of each chosen vertebra; this is level with the gap between adjacent transverse processes, and for the second lumbar nerve, for example, the approach would be above the third lumbar spine with the needle passing above the third transverse process (A and B).

The needle is inserted perpendicularly through the wheal (C). The transverse processes are about 5cm from the skin surface, so the tip of the needle must pass deeper than this. If the transverse process is encountered at this depth the needle is partially withdrawn and redirected slightly upwards to clear the process and slightly medially. The injection is made after aspiration to ensure that the needle is not in a vessel or in a meningeal nerve sheath.

The procedure is repeated at each required level.

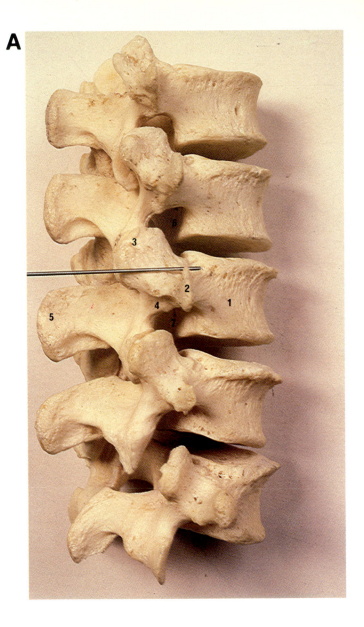

A

Hazards and Safeguards

Before the injection of anaesthetic solution a radiological check with a small amount of contrast medium should be made to ensure that the needle is depositing solution within the psoas sheath.

Aspiration is essential to ensure that the needle is not in a vessel (especially the external vertebral venous plexus) or in the subarachnoid space (through the dural sheath of a spinal nerve).

Lumbar sympathetic blockade may occur, especially if the needle is advanced too far, in which case the aorta on the left or the inferior vena cava on the right could be entered.

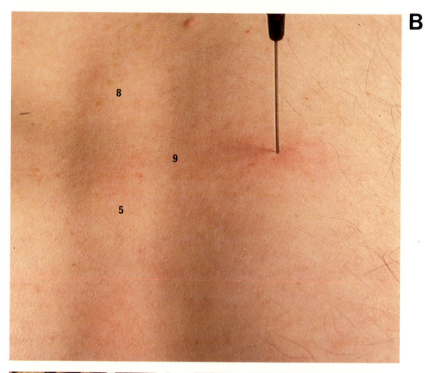

B

A

Lumbar vertebrae, from the right and slightly behind, showing how a needle above the third lumbar spine passes just above the transverse process of that vertebra, so that the ventral ramus of the *second* lumbar nerve can be anaesthetised after it has emerged from the intervertebral foramen above.

B

Flexed lumbar spine, from behind and below, showing the injection site 4 cm from the midline for the second lumbar ventral ramus above the level of the *third* lumbar spine.

C

Cross section at the level of the lower part of the third lumbar vertebra, from below, with a needle entering the right psoas sheath to anaesthetise the ventral ramus of the second lumbar nerve within the psoas sheath. Since the section is through the *lower* part of the third lumbar vertebra (see A), the third lumbar nerve is seen emerging through the intervertebral foramen and is still in front of the zygapophyseal joint.

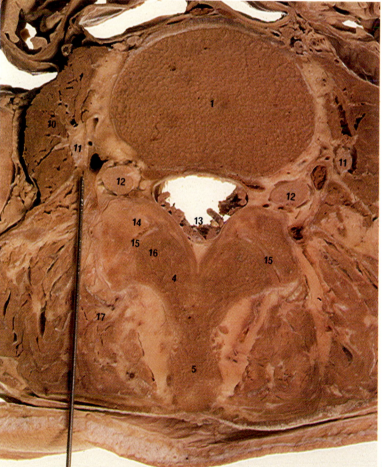

C

1 Third lumbar vertebra
2 Transverse process of 1
3 Superior articular process of 1
4 Lamina of 1
5 Spine of 1
6 Intervertebral foramen for second lumbar nerve
7 Intervertebral foramen for third lumbar nerve
8 Spine of second lumbar vertebra
9 Groove at medial border of erector spinae
10 Psoas major
11 Second lumbar ventral ramus
12 Third lumbar nerve
13 Subarachnoid space and cauda equina
14 Superior articular process of fourth lumbar vertebra
15 Zygapophyseal joint
16 Inferior articular process of 1
17 Erector spinae

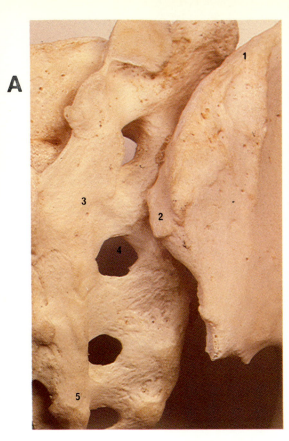

A

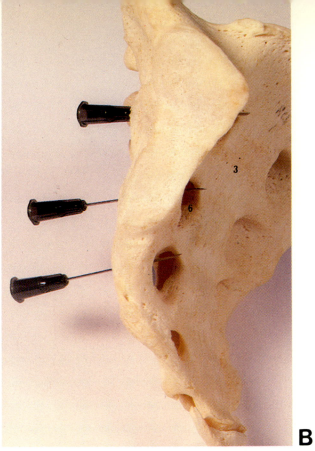

B

C

1   Iliac crest
2   Posterior superior iliac spine
3   Second piece of sacrum
4   Second posterior sacral foramen
5   Sacral cornu
6   Second anterior sacral foramen
7   Dimple over 3
8   Cut gonadal vessels
9   Ureter
10 Internal iliac artery
11 Internal iliac vein
12 Sympathetic trunk
13 First sacral ventral ramus
14 A lateral sacral artery
15 Piriformis
16 Second sacral ventral ramus
17 Third sacral ventral ramus

SACRAL PLEXUS

Background

The sacral plexus is formed in front of piriformis on the posterior pelvic wall by the union of the lumbosacral trunk (part of the fourth and the whole of the fifth lumbar ventral rami, from the lumbar plexus) with the ventral rami of the first three, and part of the fourth, sacral nerves. The ventral rami of sacral nerves emerge from the corresponding anterior sacral foramina which are in a direct backward line with the posterior sacral foramina (A and B). Because of this, sacral plexus block can be achieved by introducing solution from behind into the appropriate posterior sacral foramina.

Sacral Plexus Block

The posterior superior iliac spine and the sacral cornu are palpated (C).

The second sacral foramen is 1 cm below and medial to the posterior superior iliac spine; the first is 3.5 cm above it and the third 2.5 cm below it, with the fourth 2 cm below the third, all on a line that is not quite vertical but directed to a point 1 cm lateral to the sacral cornu.

The required foramen can be entered by a needle that is first directed rather medially to contact bone at the medial side of the foramen and then withdrawn slightly so that it can be redirected further into the foramen.

The procedure is repeated for each required nerve.

Hazards and Safeguards

There is more soft tissue overlying the upper foramina than the lower, and the distance between the openings of a pair of anterior and posterior sacral foramina is 2.5 cm in the case of the first, diminishing to 0.5 cm in the fourth (B), so that the distance the needle has to be advanced varies considerably for each level.

Excessive penetration into the pelvis may lead to puncture of pelvic vessels or viscera (D), and the subarachnoid space is at risk if dural nerve sheaths are entered.

A

Right half of the sacrum and adjacent hip bone, from behind. The second posterior sacral foramen is 1 cm below and medial to the posterior superior iliac spine.

B

Sacrum from the right, with needles of the same length introduced through the upper three posterior sacral foramina and pushed through into the anterior foramina, indicating how the sacrum becomes thinner from top to bottom.

C

Right sacro-iliac region. The iliac crest and posterior superior iliac spine are palpable and there is normally a dimple in the skin at the level of the second piece of the sacrum.

D

Right half of a median sagittal section of the pelvis, with peritoneum and viscera removed to show needle tips pushed through from the upper three posterior sacral foramina. The needles here are introduced too far for sacral nerve anaesthesia but this has been deliberate in order to indicate where in the pelvis they will appear if there is excessive penetration.

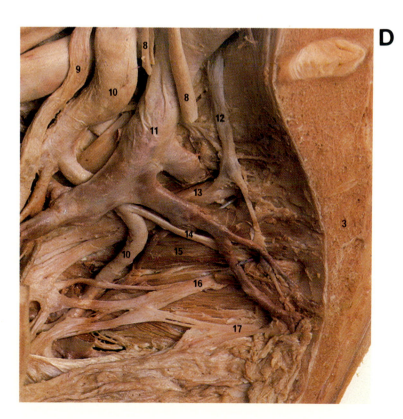

SCIATIC NERVE

Background

In the gluteal region the sciatic nerve is one of a number of structures that leave the greater sciatic foramen below piriformis and lie under cover of gluteus maximus. Passing down into the back of the thigh it runs deep to the long head of biceps and down between adductor magnus and the hamstrings supplying all these muscles. In the lower thigh above the apex of the popliteal fossa it divides into the tibial nerve which continues in the midline of the fossa and the common peroneal nerve which follows biceps along the lateral edge of the fossa.

The nerve can be exposed in the gluteal region by tracing it upwards from the lower border of gluteus maximus. In the thigh the approach begins in the popliteal fossa by finding the common peroneal nerve behind biceps and following that nerve upwards to the parent sciatic nerve which lies under cover of biceps.

Approach in the Gluteal Region

A curved skin incision (A) is made from below the middle of the iliac crest laterally towards the greater trochanter of the femur and then back towards the midline at the lower border of gluteus maximus.

The sciatic nerve is identified distal to the lower border of gluteus maximus and deep to the long head of biceps which approaches the nerve from the medial side (B).

The nerve is traced upwards. The insertion of gluteus maximus into the upper part of the fascia lata and the gluteal tuberosity of the femur can be detached as high as is necessary.

Hazards and Safeguards

The gluteal fold (fold of the buttock) does not correspond to the lower border of gluteus maximus. The sciatic nerve in this area lies a little to the medial side of the midpoint of a line between the tip of the greater trochanter and the medial side of the ischial tuberosity.

The posterior femoral cutaneous nerve runs downwards in the same line as the sciatic nerve but is superficial to biceps.

Approach in the Thigh

The upper part of the nerve can be exposed as above; for the lower part the incision is continued in the midline (A) but deviating at the upper part of the popliteal fossa towards the head of the fibula.

The common peroneal nerve is identified as it adheres to the posterior border of biceps at the lateral margin of the popliteal fossa (D). This nerve is followed upwards to lead to the sciatic nerve which itself continues upwards beneath the long head of biceps, which can be retracted medially or laterally.

Hazards and Safeguards

The posterior femoral cutaneous nerve is superficial to biceps.

Occasionally the tibial and common peroneal parts of the sciatic nerve are separate, with the common peroneal piercing piriformis instead of emerging below the muscle and running parallel with the tibial nerve to the apex of the popliteal fossa.

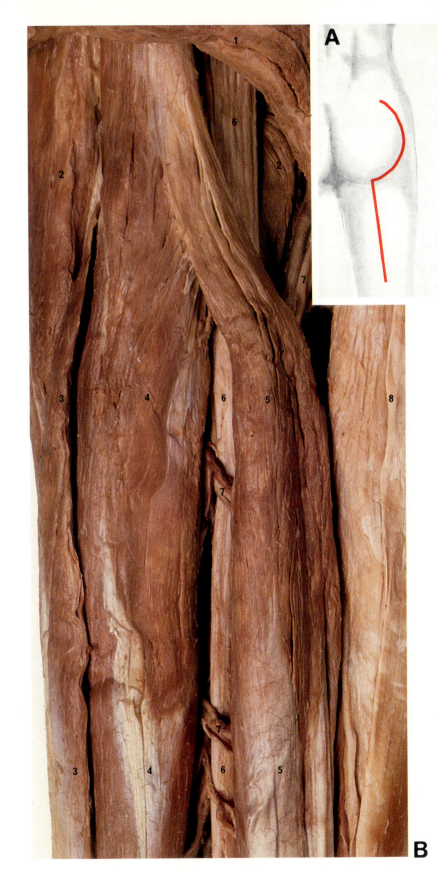

190

1 Gluteus maximus
2 Adductor magnus
3 Semimembranosus
4 Semitendinosus
5 Long head of biceps femoris
6 Sciatic nerve
7 Branches of 13
8 Deep fascia over vastus lateralis
9 Posterior femoral cutaneous nerve
10 Short head of biceps femoris
11 Lateral intermuscular septum
12 Femur
13 Profunda femoris vessels
14 Vastus intermedius
15 Vastus medialis
16 Upper end of opening in 2
17 Femoral artery
18 Femoral vein
19 Saphenous nerve
20 Sartorius
21 Gracilis
22 Great saphenous vein
23 Tendon of biceps femoris
24 Common peroneal nerve
25 Peroneal communicating nerve
26 Small saphenous vein
27 Sural nerve
28 Tibial nerve

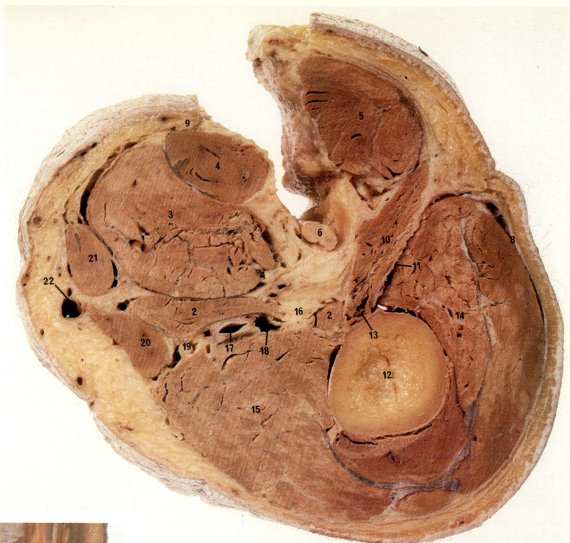

C

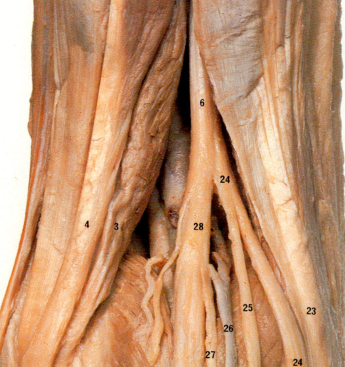

D

The muscular branches of the sciatic nerve to the hamstrings and adductor magnus all arise from the medial side of the nerve; only the branch to the short head of biceps comes off the lateral side, and these facts must be remembered when following the nerve upwards in the thigh.

A
Incision line.

B
Right upper thigh, from behind, after removal of most of the deep fascia. Above, the sciatic nerve has been displayed beneath the lower border of gluteus maximus, while lower down the long head of biceps has been retracted laterally to show the underlying nerve.

C
Cross section of the right lower thigh, showing the line of approach to the sciatic nerve, with the long head of biceps displaced laterally and semitendinosus and semimembranosus on the medial side of the approach line.

D
Right popliteal fossa, after removal of deep fascia and fat. The sciatic nerve can be found by following the common peroneal nerve upwards along the posterior border of biceps.

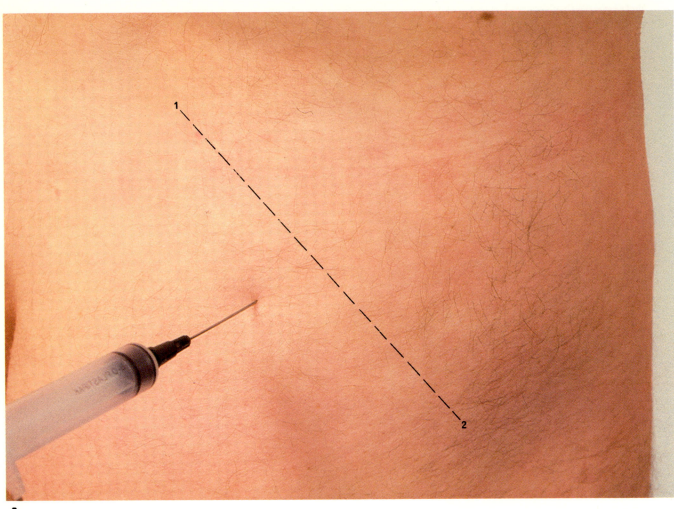

A

Sciatic Nerve Block

Sciatic nerve block can be achieved by passing a needle through gluteus maximus to infiltrate the perineural tissues after the nerve has emerged from the greater sciatic foramen below piriformis.

The tip of the greater trochanter and the posterior superior iliac spine are palpated; the line between them indicates the upper border of piriformis (A).

From the midpoint of the above line, another line is drawn down from it but perpendicular to it (i.e. slightly medially) for 3 cm. The needle is introduced at this point (A and B), perpendicular to the skin surface and through gluteus maximus for 6–8 cm. The needle should contact the hip bone below and lateral to the greater sciatic foramen, and is withdrawn slightly before injection (after aspiration to ensure it is not in a vessel).

If directed too high and too far, the needle may pass into the pelvis.

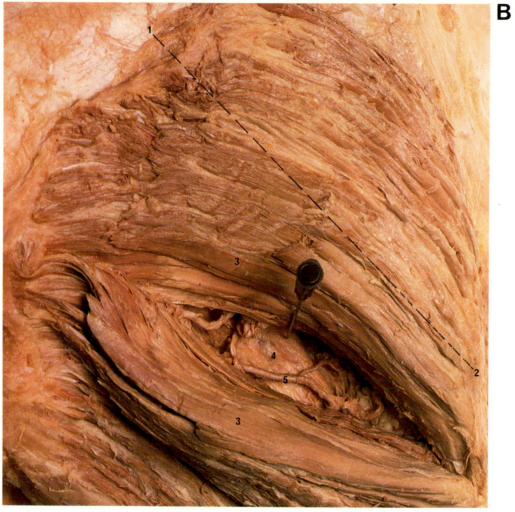

B

A

Right gluteal region, from the right and behind. The point for sciatic nerve block is 3 cm below the midpoint of a line from the posterior superior iliac spine to the tip of the greater trochanter.

B

Right gluteus maximus, from behind, split in the line of its fibres to show the sciatic nerve. The line between the posterior superior iliac spine and the tip of the greater trochanter indicates the upper border of piriformis, beneath whose lower border the nerve emerges from the pelvis.

1 Posterior superior iliac spine
2 Tip of greater trochanter
3 Gluteus maximus
4 Sciatic nerve
5 Branch of inferior gluteal artery

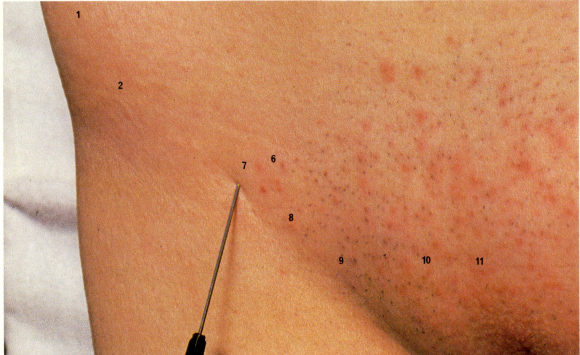

A

1	Anterior superior iliac spine
2	Lateral femoral cutaneous nerve
3	Fascia lata
4	Sartorius
5	Iliacus
6	Inguinal ligament
7	Femoral nerve
8	Femoral artery
9	Femoral vein
10	Pubic tubercle
11	Pubic symphysis
12	Cut edge of femoral sheath
13	Labium majus
14	Pectineus
15	Anterior division of obturator nerve
16	Obturator vessels
17	Branch of medial circumflex femoral artery
18	Adductor brevis
19	Adductor longus
20	Great saphenous vein

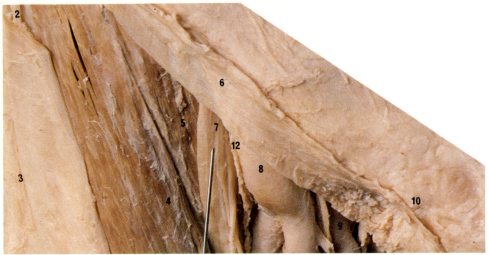

A
Right femoral nerve block. The femoral artery is palpated below the inguinal ligament and midway between the anterior superior iliac spine and the pubic symphysis, and the injection is made 1 cm lateral to the artery.

B
Right femoral triangle. The femoral nerve is lateral to the artery, deep to the fascia lata but outside the femoral sheath. The lateral femoral cutaneous nerve is 2.5 cm below and medial to the anterior superior iliac spine.

B

FEMORAL AND LATERAL FEMORAL CUTANEOUS NERVES

Background

The femoral nerve emerges from the lateral border of psoas major in the iliac fossa and runs down in the groove between psoas and iliacus to enter the thigh beneath the inguinal ligament, with the femoral artery on its medial side. The nerve is outside the femoral sheath, and just below the ligament it breaks up into a sheaf of branches with an anterior group that is mostly cutaneous and a posterior group supplying rectus femoris and the vasti.

Damage to the nerve is usually caused by stab wounds of the lower abdomen and its exposure in the leg is virtually never necessary, but nerve block can be carried out below the inguinal ligament.

The lateral femoral cutaneous nerve enters the thigh from the iliac fossa by passing deep to (but occasionally through) the inguinal ligament 1–2 cm medial to the anterior superior iliac spine. It runs downwards beneath the deep fascia for several centimetres, crossing sartorius, and then becomes subcutaneous as it divides into anterior and posterior branches.

The nerve can be blocked after it has entered the thigh, just below the inguinal ligament.

Femoral Nerve Block

The femoral artery is palpated below the inguinal ligament, midway between the anterior superior iliac spine and the pubic symphysis.

Anaesthetic solution is introduced 1 cm lateral to the artery (A and B).

Lateral Femoral Cutaneous Nerve Block

The anterior superior iliac spine is palpated.

The site of injection is 2.5 cm below and medial to the spine (B). A certain amount of 'give' should be detected as the needle penetrates the deep fascia.

Hazards and Safeguards

Although beneath the deep fascia but lateral to the femoral sheath, the femoral nerve may be very superficial in thin subjects and must not be transfixed by the needle. Superficial circumflex iliac vessels may cross the path of the needle.

The lateral femoral cutaneous nerve is also beneath the deep fascia at the injection site, and the needle must penetrate the fascia; the nerve only becomes subcutaneous several centimetres lower down.

OBTURATOR NERVE

Background

After emerging from the medial border of psoas major and running along the side wall of the pelvis, the obturator nerve passes into the thigh through the obturator canal, dividing while in the canal into anterior and posterior branches which supply the three adductor muscles, obturator externus and gracilis.

The nerve can be blocked while in the canal by a frontal approach.

Obturator Nerve Block

The pubic tubercle is palpated and a skin wheal raised 1.5 cm below and lateral to it.

The needle is inserted perpendicular to the skin (C) and advanced until contact is made with the superior ramus of the pubis. It is then partially withdrawn and redirected slightly upwards and outwards to enter the obturator canal at a level about 2 cm deeper than the original bony contact (D). The injection is made after aspiration to ensure that the needle is not in a vessel.

Hazards and Safeguards

Apart from involving obturator vessels or femoral vein tributaries, it is possible that excessively deep penetration might reach the bladder or vagina.

C

Right obturator nerve block, 1.5 cm below and lateral to the pubic tubercle.

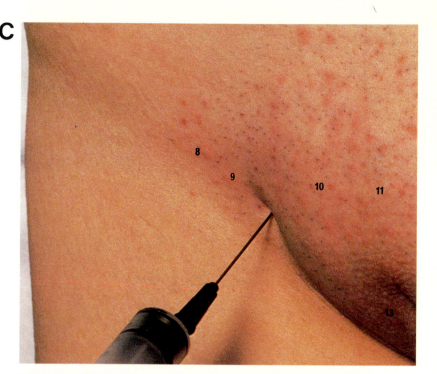

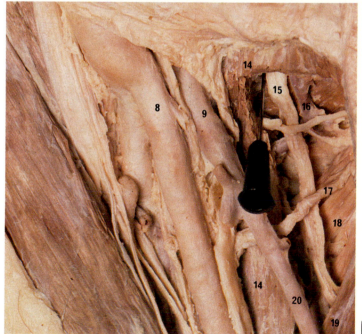

D

Right femoral triangle. Deep dissection with part of pectineus removed to show the opening of the obturator canal and the anterior division of the obturator nerve overlying adductor brevis (the posterior division passes behind adductor brevis and is not seen here). The needle is advanced through pectineus into the canal after making contact with its bony wall.

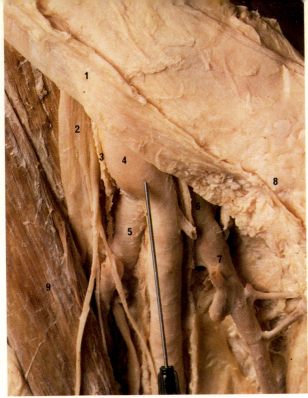

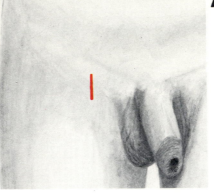

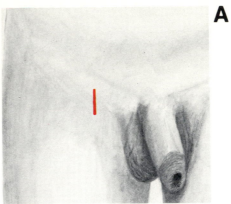

B

1 Inguinal ligament
2 Femoral nerve
3 Cut edge of femoral sheath
4 Femoral artery
5 Profunda femoris artery
6 Femoral vein
7 Great saphenous vein
8 Pubic tubercle
9 Sartorius
10 Vastus medialis
11 Nerve to 10
12 Saphenous nerve
13 Rectus femoris
14 Vastus intermedius
15 Adductor longus
16 Adductor magnus
17 Gracilis
18 Sciatic nerve
19 Femur

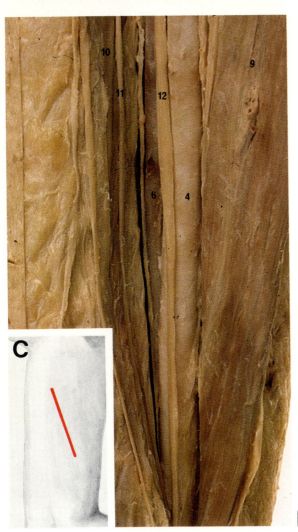

C

D

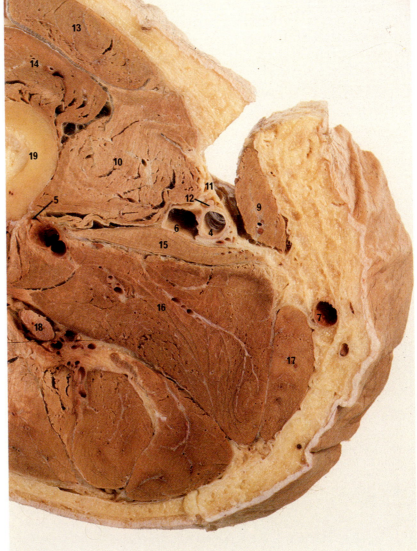

E

FEMORAL ARTERY

Background

The femoral artery is the continuation of the external iliac artery, the change of name occurring as the vessel passes beneath the inguinal ligament from the abdomen into the thigh. In the femoral triangle below the inguinal ligament the artery lies at the mid-inguinal point (midway between the anterior superior iliac spine and the pubic symphysis), with the femoral vein on the medial side of the artery and the femoral nerve on the lateral side. The two vessels are within the femoral sheath but the nerve is outside it. The profunda femoris artery arises from the posterolateral side of the femoral, usually about 3.5 cm below the inguinal ligament, and passes behind the femoral artery and vein. At the apex of the femoral triangle the femoral vessels enter the adductor canal where they lie in a trough between adductor longus and vastus medialis under cover of sartorius.

The superficial position of the artery, even in the canal, makes its exposure easy. Below the inguinal ligament it can be conveniently punctured to obtain arterial blood. It is also the site commonly used for introducing a catheter for arteriography. The catheter can be pushed up through the external and common iliac arteries into any part of the aorta; arteriograms of the aorta itself and of the renal, mesenteric, subclavian, carotid and coronary vessels and their branches can all be obtained via the femoral route with suitable positioning of the catheter. (The axillary or brachial artery is an alternative route – page 77.)

Approach in the Femoral Triangle

A vertical skin incision (A) is made over the artery which lies about 3 cm lateral to the pubic tubercle – a palpable landmark.

The great saphenous vein is retracted medially and sartorius laterally.

The deep fascia lateral to the femoral vein is incised to open the femoral sheath and expose the artery (B).

Hazards and Safeguards

The artery lies between the vein and nerve, and any venous tributaries that interfere with the exposure can be ligated.

The profunda femoris artery should be identified; it normally arises from the posterolateral aspect of the femoral artery but it occasionally has a double origin.

Approach in the Adductor Canal

A skin incision (C) is made along the line of the anterior border of sartorius.

Sartorius is retracted backwards and the fascia that forms the roof of the canal is incised to exposure the artery (D and E).

Hazards and Safeguards

In the canal the saphenous nerve (D and E) runs on the front of the femoral artery obliquely from the lateral to medial side and is dissected off it; the nerve to vastus medialis is on the medial side of the artery. The femoral vein lies behind the artery.

Puncture of the Femoral Artery

The artery is identified by palpation below the inguinal ligament and needle inserted into it here (B).

The femoral nerve is lateral to the artery and the vein medial to it.

A
Incision line in the femoral triangle.

B
Right femoral triangle, with deep fascia removed. The femoral sheath is opened to display the femoral artery with the vein on its medial side and the nerve outside the sheath laterally. The position of the needle for puncture is also shown. Compare with A on page 194.

C
Incision line over the adductor canal.

D
Right adductor canal. Sartorius is reflected backwards and the femoral artery dissected out from its fascial sheath. The saphenous nerve is on the front of the artery and the nerve to vastus medialis medial to it.

E
Cross section of the middle of the right thigh, with the incision over the adductor canal. Sartorius is reflected backwards to expose the artery.

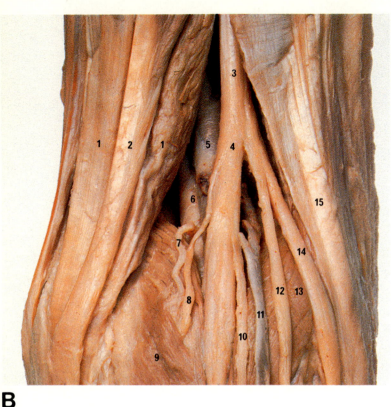

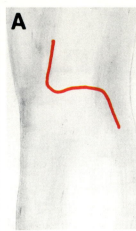

1	Semimembranosus
2	Semitendinosus
3	Sciatic nerve
4	Tibial nerve
5	Popliteal vein
6	Popliteal artery
7	Sural artery
8	Nerve to 9
9	Medial head of gastrocnemius
10	Sural nerve
11	Small saphenous vein
12	Peroneal communicating nerve
13	Lateral head of gastrocnemius
14	Common peroneal nerve
15	Biceps femoris
16	Iliotibial tract
17	Lateral intermuscular septum
18	Vastus lateralis
19	Femur
20	Vastus medialis

B

POPLITEAL ARTERY

Background

The popliteal artery is the continuation of the femoral artery, the change of name occurring as the vessel passes through the opening in adductor magnus to enter the popliteal fossa. In the fossa it is the deepest of the main neurovascular structures, being under cover of its companion vein which in turn is deep to the tibial nerve. The artery runs downwards and slightly laterally in the fossa to end at the lower border of popliteus by dividing into the anterior and posterior tibial arteries.

Apart from a posterior midline approach, the popliteal artery can also be exposed from either side. Laterally the route is between the lower part of biceps and the lateral intermuscular septum; on the medial side the opening in adductor magnus can be displayed deep to sartorius, while lower down the artery is exposed by retracting the medial head of gastrocnemius via a path lateral to semitendinosus and semimembranosus.

Posterior Approach

A Z-shaped skin incision (A) is made with the upper end medially over the lower part of semitendinosus and semimembranosus, the horizontal part in a skin crease in the popliteal fossa and the lower part laterally over the biceps tendon.

The small saphenous vein is traced through the deep fascia to its union with the popliteal vein and the fascia incised vertically.

The tibial and common peroneal nerves are identified (B) and dissected free from surrounding fat.

The popliteal vein, deep to the tibial nerve, is cleared with ligation of any tributaries necessary (especially veins from gastrocnemius), and the popliteal artery is then found deep to the vein (B).

Hazards and Safeguards

The tibial nerve and its branches must not be damaged as dissection proceeds deeper.

Ligation of various tributaries of the popliteal vein will be necessary to give adequate exposure of the artery.

Lateral Approach

A skin incision (C) is made along the lower part of the posterior border of the iliotibial tract (where the lateral intermuscular septum fuses with the tract).

The deep fascia is divided just behind the tract, and the space between the tract and septum in front and biceps behind is opened up (D and E).

The space can be enlarged upwards by detaching the lower part of the short head of biceps from the lateral supracondylar line.

Biceps is displaced backwards, and dissection in the popliteal fat reveals the popliteal vessels, the vein at this level being lateral to the artery.

Hazards and Safeguards

As it crosses the lateral condyle of the femur, biceps is in contact with a small part of the capsule of the knee joint which must not be damaged.

The tibial and common peroneal nerves are displaced backwards as biceps is retracted backwards.

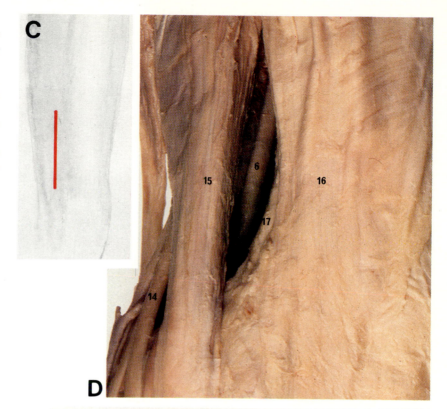

A

Incision line in the popliteal fossa.

B

The right popliteal fossa after removal of deep fascia and fat. The sural nerve when followed upwards leads to the tibial nerve. The small saphenous vein when followed upwards leads to the popliteal vein. The popliteal artery is deep to the vein. Of the motor branches of the tibial nerve, only the nerve to the medial head of gastrocnemius is visible here without displacing the main nerve.

C

Incision line for the lateral approach.

D

Right lower thigh, from the lateral side. The deep fascia has been incised in front of biceps. Note that the popliteal vein is seen first on this approach; the artery is deeper, medial to the vein.

E

Cross section of the upper part of the right popliteal fossa, viewed sideways for easier comparison with D, showing the line of approach to the popliteal vessels through the deep fascia behind the lateral intermuscular septum and in front of biceps. The artery lies medial to the vein and is collapsed in this specimen.

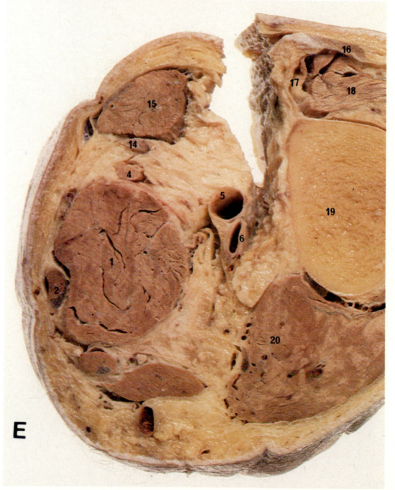

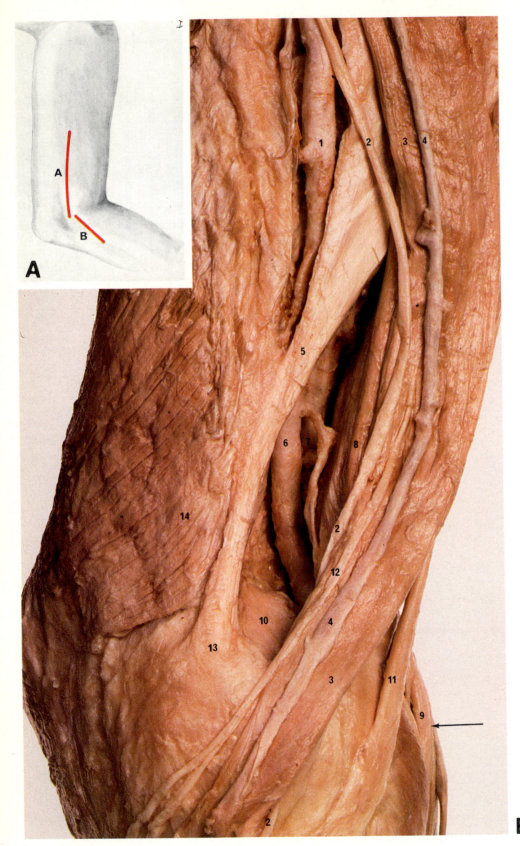

1 Femoral artery
2 Saphenous nerve
3 Sartorius
4 Great saphenous vein
5 Tendon of adductor magnus
6 Popliteal artery
7 Popliteal vein
8 Semimembranosus
9 Semitendinosus
10 Medial head of gastrocnemius
11 Gracilis
12 Infrapatellar branch of 2
13 Adductor tubercle
14 Vastus medialis
15 Medial condyle of femur
16 Lateral condyle of femur
17 Popliteus tendon
18 Biceps femoris
19 Common peroneal nerve
20 Peroneal communicating nerve
21 Lateral head of gastrocnemius
22 Plantaris
23 Tibial nerve
24 Sural nerve
25 Small saphenous vein

Medial Approach (Upper)

With the thigh laterally rotated and the knee slightly flexed, a skin incision (A) is made along the lower part of a line from the pubic tubercle to the adductor tubercle, and continued down over the medial condyle of the femur.

The deep fascia is divided along the anterior border of sartorius, which is displaced backwards (B).

The saphenous nerve is identified at the medial side of the knee as it emerges from the subsartorial canal between sartorius and gracilis (B), and when followed upwards leads to the femoral artery. This vessel can then be followed down, cutting through the adductor magnus tendon that forms the boundary of the opening for the artery to enter the popliteal fossa.

Hazards and Safeguards

The skin incision must avoid the great saphenous vein and saphenous nerve which at the level of the knee joint lie one handsbreadth behind the medial border of the patella. As it leaves the adductor canal the nerve is accompanied by the saphenous branch of the descending genicular artery.

Medial Approach (Lower)

A vertical skin incision (A) is made from the lower end of the medial condyle of the tibia along the posterior border of the bone.

The deep fascia is incised and the plane between semimembranosus and semitendinosus medially and the medial head of gastrocnemius laterally is defined.

The medial head of gastrocnemius is displaced backwards (C), and dissection laterally through the popliteal fat reveals the popliteal vein with the artery slightly deeper and more anterior.

Hazards and Safeguards

Tributaries of the popliteal vein may need to be divided to give good exposure of the artery.

A

Incision line for upper (A) and lower (B) approaches.

B

Right lower thigh, from the medial side, with deep fascia removed. Sartorius, the saphenous nerve and the great saphenous vein are retracted backwards. The tendon of adductor magnus forms the boundary of the opening in the muscle through which the femoral artery passes from the adductor canal to become the popliteal artery. In the medial exposure sartorius is first retracted backwards, the saphenous nerve is identified where it emerges between sartorius and gracilis at the side of the knee and followed upwards to lead to the femoral artery in the lower part of the adductor canal, and the artery is then followed down through the gap in adductor magnus. The tendon of adductor magnus can be cut if necessary.

C

Cross section of the lower part of the right popliteal fossa (at the level of the arrow in B and orientated sideways), showing the line of approach to the lower part of the popliteal artery passing medial to the medial head of gastrocnemius which is displaced backwards. Semitendinosus and semimembranosus remain on the medial side of the approach line. There are large veins at the deep surface of gastrocnemius.

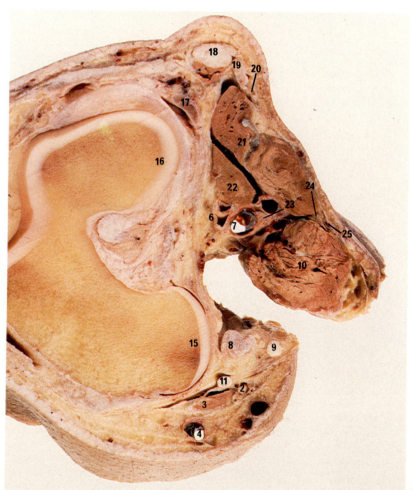

C

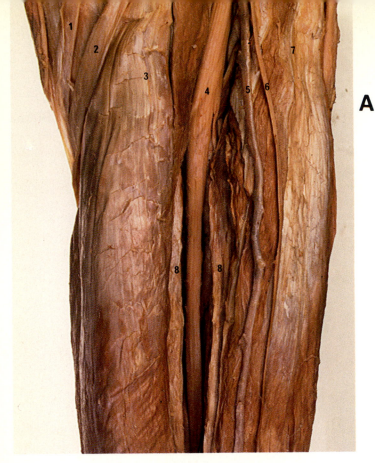

A

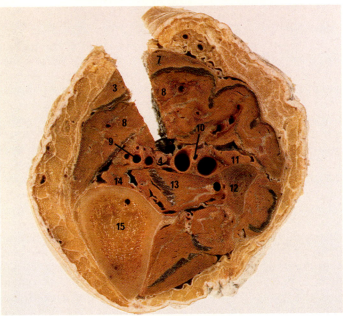

B

A

Right upper leg, from behind, with deep fascia removed. Gastrocnemius and soleus are split vertically to display the tibial nerve. The small saphenous vein and sural nerve are retracted laterally.

B

Cross section of the middle of the right leg, with gastrocnemius and soleus incised to approach the tibial nerve. Note the profusion of veins associated with soleus; these are the ones in which thrombosis occurs.

COMMON PERONEAL, TIBIAL AND DEEP PERONEAL NERVES

Background

At or near the apex of the popliteal fossa the sciatic nerve divides into the tibial and common peroneal nerves. The common peroneal runs downwards and laterally adhering to the posterior border of biceps and giving off the peroneal (sural) communicating branch. Below the attachment of biceps to the head of the fibula, the common peroneal lies against the neck of the bone, under cover of the uppermost fibres of peroneus longus, where it divides into superficial and deep peroneal branches. The superficial positions of the common peroneal nerve behind biceps at the lateral margin of the popliteal fossa, and of the tibial nerve in the centre of the fossa, make their exposure here easy, and they are illustrated on page 191, D. To expose the tibial nerve in the leg, gastrocnemius and soleus are split vertically down the centre (this page, A and B).

The superficial peroneal nerve passes down between peroneus longus and brevis, supplying them and then becoming cutaneous, and the need to expose this nerve rarely arises. The deep peroneal is more important, supplying the extensor muscles in the anterior compartment of the leg. It runs down in front of the interosseous membrane with the anterior tibial vessels, at first lying lateral to tibialis anterior. At the ankle it lies between extensor hallucis longus and digitorum longus and divides into superficial and deep terminal branches. The deeply placed upper part of the nerve can be exposed by incising lateral to tibialis anterior, while at the ankle it is found between the two extensor muscles.

Approach to Deep Peroneal Nerve

A vertical skin incision (C) is made 1cm lateral to the anterior border of the tibia.

The deep fascia is incised and the gap between tibialis anterior medially and extensor digitorum and hallucis longus laterally is opened up to reveal the nerve (D and E) which from above downwards lies lateral to, then in front of, and again lateral to, the anterior tibial vessels.

Hazards and Safeguards

The anterior tibial artery in the upper part of the leg lies in front of the interosseous membrane but lower down it lies against the tibia; the deep peroneal nerve approaches the upper part of the artery from the lateral side. At the ankle the nerve and vessels are between the two extensor tendons (F and G).

C

Incision line for deep peroneal nerve.

D

Right leg, from the front. The gap between tibialis anterior medially and extensor digitorum longus and extensor hallucis longus laterally is opened up to display the deep peroneal nerve and anterior tibial artery in front of the interosseous membrane. The nerve at first lies lateral to the artery, and here two nerve branches to tibialis anterior cross in front of the artery.

1 Gracilis
2 Semitendinosus
3 Medial head of gastrocnemius
4 Tibial nerve
5 Small saphenous vein
6 Sural nerve
7 Lateral head of gastrocnemius
8 Soleus
9 Posterior tibial artery
10 Peroneal artery
11 Flexor hallucis longus
12 Fibula
13 Tibialis posterior
14 Flexor digitorum longus
15 Tibia
16 Extensor digitorum longus
17 Interosseous membrane
18 Deep peroneal nerve
19 Anterior tibial artery
20 Tibialis anterior
21 Anterior border of 15
22 Extensor hallucis longus
23 Peroneus brevis
24 Superficial peroneal nerve
25 Peroneus longus
26 Great saphenous vein
27 Saphenous nerve
28 Medial malleolus
29 Capsule
30 Medial malleolar artery
31 Lateral malleolar artery
32 Peroneus tertius
33 Lateral malleolus
34 Talus (beneath capsule in F)
35 Dorsalis pedis artery
36 Posterior tibial artery

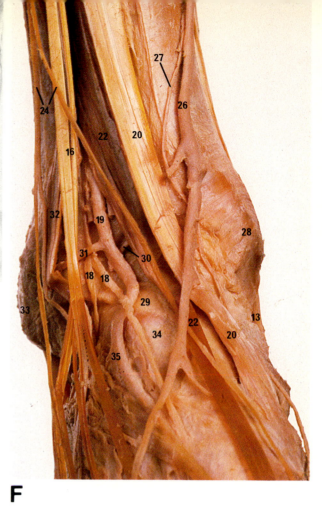

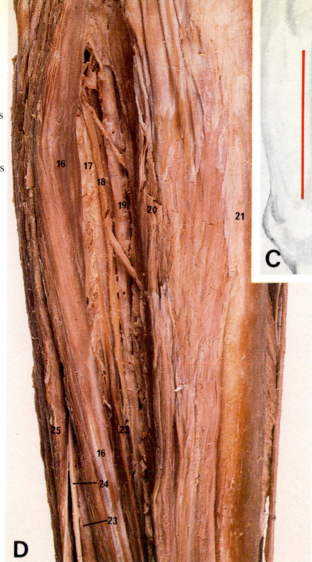

D

E
Cross section of the lower right leg, showing the line of approach to the deep peroneal nerve.

F
Right ankle, from the front, with deep fascia and extensor retinacula removed. Extensor digitorum longus is retracted slightly laterally to give a clearer view of the artery and nerve in front of the ankle joint. The artery is here somewhat tortuous as it crosses the joint line to become the dorsalis pedis artery, and the medial terminal branch of the nerve usually stays lateral to the artery, not crossing it as it does here.

G
Cross section of the right ankle, for comparison with F.

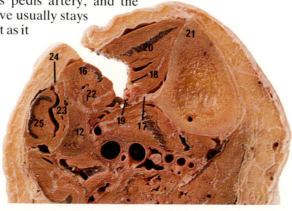

E

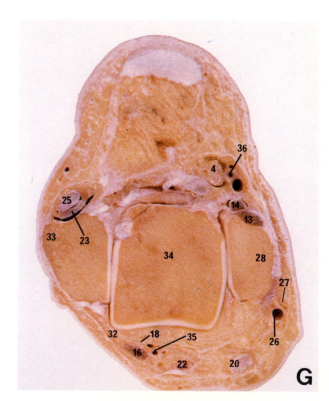

G

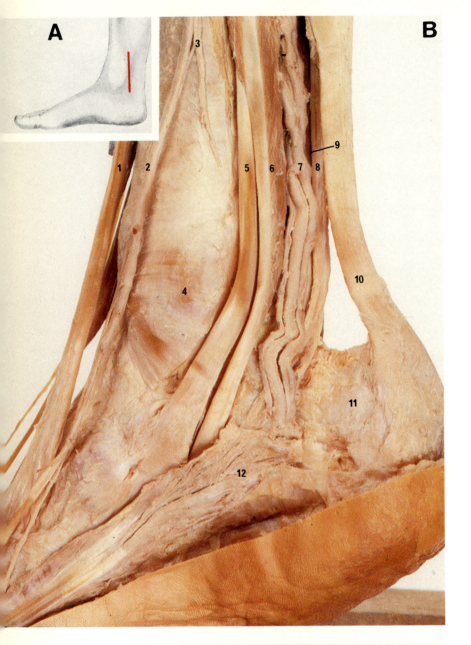

POSTERIOR TIBIAL ARTERY

Background

The posterior tibial artery begins at the lower border of popliteus as the continuation of the popliteal artery. It runs down the back of the leg on the tibial side, at first under cover of gastrocnemius and soleus but above the ankle it is covered only by skin and deep fascia. It can be exposed here for making an arteriovenous shunt with the great saphenous vein for haemodialysis.

Approach

A vertical skin incision (A) is made behind and above the medial malleolus.

The posterior tibial vessels lie 2.5 cm medial to the medial border of the tendo calcaneus and can be exposed by incising the deep fascia here (B).

Hazards and Safeguards

At and above the medial malleolus the tibial nerve lies immediately behind the posterior tibial vessels (C); the tendon of flexor digitorum longus is in front of the vessels.

If the incision is extended upwards the great saphenous vein will be encountered as it passes obliquely backwards off the medial surface of the tibia. It can be dissected out and joined by a cannula to the posterior tibial artery for haemodialysis.

A
Incision line for posterior tibial artery.

B
Right lower leg and ankle, from the medial side, with deep fascia and flexor retinaculum removed. Behind the medial malleolus the posterior tibial artery and its venae comitantes lie between the flexor digitorum longus tendon in front and the tibial nerve behind.

C
Cross section of the right leg above the medial malleolus, for comparison with B and E, orientated sideways.

D
Incision line for sural nerve.

E
Right lower leg and ankle, from the posterolateral side, with the deep fascia intact showing superficial veins and nerves. The sural nerve may lie on either side of the small saphenous vein; the vein is the guide to the nerve.

SURAL NERVE

Background

The sural nerve arises from the tibial nerve in the middle of the popliteal fossa and runs down the leg to the back of the lateral malleolus and then along the lateral side of the foot. It is only cutaneous in distribution with no muscle supply, and for this reason can be used as a nerve graft.

Approach

A skin incision (D) is made along a line from the middle of the popliteal fossa to the midpoint between the lateral malleolus and the tendo calcaneus; the length of nerve required for grafting determines the length of the incision, measured from below upwards.

The nerve is identified behind the lateral malleolus and adjacent to the small saphenous vein (E), and is followed upwards as far as necessary.

Hazards and Safeguards

The nerve may lie lateral or medial to the small saphenous vein but always close to it; the vein serves as a guide. The nerve in most of its course is superficial to the deep fascia which it pierces some distance below the popliteal fossa (the vein piercing the fascia of the roof of the fossa).

1 Tibialis anterior
2 Great saphenous vein
3 Saphenous nerve
4 Medial malleolus
5 Tibialis posterior
6 Flexor digitorum longus
7 Posterior tibial artery and veins
8 Tibial nerve
9 Flexor hallucis longus
10 Tendo calcaneus
11 Calcaneus
12 Abductor hallucis
13 Tibia
14 Small saphenous vein
15 Sural nerve
16 Peroneal artery and veins
17 Fibula
18 Peroneus brevis
19 Peroneus longus
20 Superficial peroneal nerve
21 Extensor digitorum longus and peroneus tertius
22 Extensor hallucis longus
23 Anterior tibial artery and veins
24 Deep peroneal nerve
25 Lateral malleolus

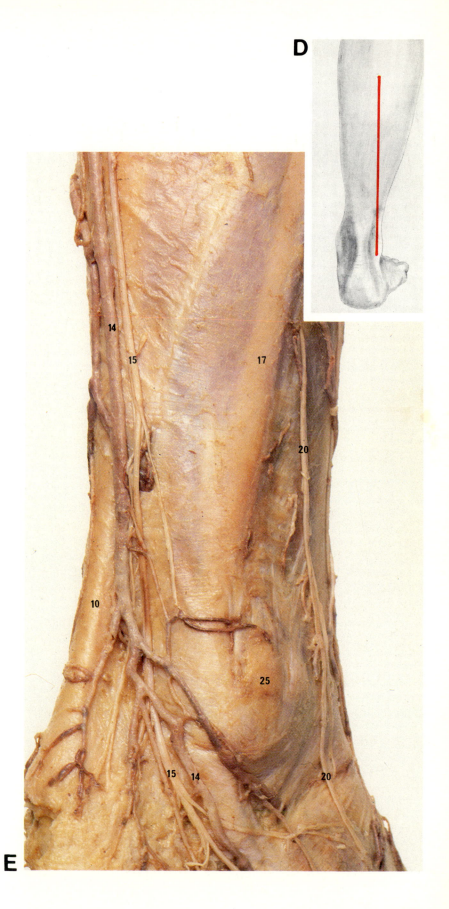

205

GREAT SAPHENOUS VEIN

Background

The great saphenous vein, the longest in the body, is the continuation of the medial marginal vein of the foot. It runs upwards in front of the medial malleolus and slowly passes backwards off the medial surface of the tibia, coming to lie at the level of the knee joint a handsbreadth behind the medial border of the patella. From there it runs upwards to a point 3.5 cm below and lateral to the pubic tubercle where it pierces the cribriform fascia to enter the femoral vein. From the knee and below it is accompanied by the saphenous nerve which at first is immediately behind the vein but lower down the nerve may cross deep to the vein to lie immediately in front of the vein. About 7.5 cm above the medial malleolus the nerve bifurcates into two branches that run in front of and behind the vein; one of the branches may cross the vein superficially. The vein has numerous communications with the small saphenous vein (which runs upwards behind the lateral malleolus in close association with the sural nerve – page 205 – and joins the popliteal vein in the popliteal fossa), and with numerous perforating veins which connect deep leg veins (deep to the deep fascia) with the superficial veins (superficial to the deep fascia). Several perforating veins behind the lower tibia may drain into a posterior arch vein which in turn joins the great saphenous some way below the knee. The great saphenous vein contains about 20 valves, more of them in the part below the knee than above it (the small saphenous has up to 12 valves).

A number of tributaries enter the great saphenous vein just before it joins the femoral vein. Although the exact number is variable there are usually five or six which approach the vein from various directions and which are useful guides leading to it. The superficial circumflex iliac, superficial epigastric and superficial external pudendal veins run into the great saphenous from the lateral side, from above and from the medial side respectively; the deep external pudendal runs in posteromedially on a deeper level (but occasionally it drains directly into the femoral vein); and posteromedial (accessory saphenous) and anterolateral tributaries are often present.

It is the upper and lower ends of the great saphenous vein that commonly require to be exposed in the operative treatment of varicose veins, and these approaches are described. The vein at the ankle was formerly a frequent site for 'cutting down' for transfusion, but its use for this purpose has fallen out of favour because of the frequency of thrombosis, and arm veins are now chosen in preference where possible.

Approach

A skin incision (A) 5–7 cm long is made below and parallel to the inguinal ligament and centred on the saphenous opening which is 3.5 cm below and lateral to the pubic tubercle which is a palpable landmark.

The superficial fascia is divided to expose the great saphenous vein at the saphenous opening (B).

All the tributaries of the vein in this area are dissected out, and the great saphenous itself is traced to its union with the femoral

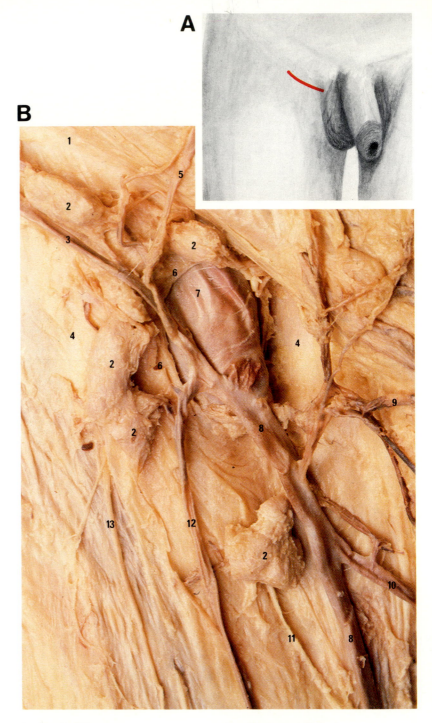

1	Inguinal ligament	**10**	Posteromedial vein
2	Lymph nodes	**11**	Medial femoral cutaneous nerve
3	Superficial circumflex iliac vein	**12**	Anterolateral vein
4	Fascia lata	**13**	Intermediate femoral cutaneous nerve
5	Superficial epigastric vein		
6	Margin of saphenous opening	**14**	Medial surface of tibia
7	Femoral vein	**15**	Medial malleolus
8	Great saphenous vein	**16**	Saphenous nerve
9	Superficial external pudendal vein	**17**	Perforating vein

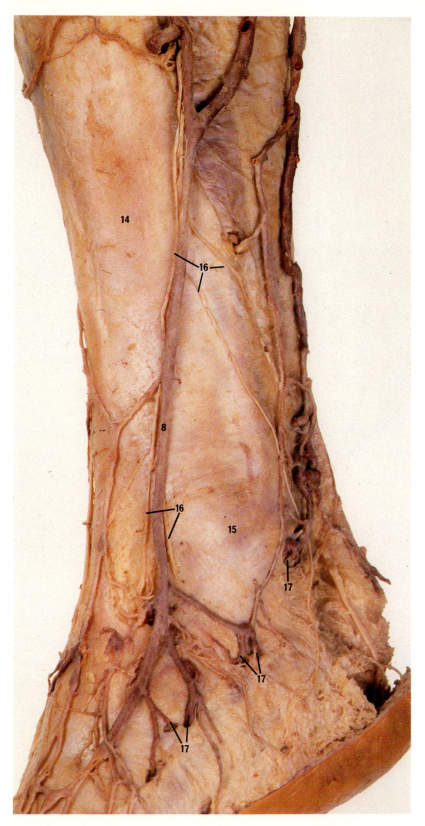

C

vein by dissecting away the cribriform fascia that overlies the saphenous opening.

In varicose vein operations all tributaries and the great saphenous vein itself are ligated and divided. If the stripping method is being used the stripper is introduced down the great saphenous vein, advancing it past the valves and side tributaries by gentle up-and-down manoeuvring until it reaches the level of the medial malleolus (C) where it is exposed by a transverse skin incision. (If the stripper cannot be passed to this level, the skin incision is made over wherever the end of the stripper lies.) With the ends of the vein appropriately tied to the stripper, the stripping procedure is frequently carried out in a downwards direction from groin to ankle, although stripping in the opposite direction is also possible (but see below).

Hazards and Safeguards

Correct identification of the great saphenous and femoral veins is obviously essential. In thin patients the femoral vein may be surprisingly near the surface, but the number of tributaries converging on the great saphenous identifies it from the femoral which is deep to the falciform margin of the saphenous opening. The femoral artery is lateral to the femoral vein and can be distinguished by its pulsation. The profunda femoris artery usually arises from the posterolateral side of the femoral and runs deep to the parent vessel but rarely it crosses to run in front of the femoral vein.

At the medial malleolus branches of the saphenous nerve may lie both in front of and behind the great saphenous vein (C). The nerves are usually deep to the vein but may be superficial. They are liable to injury when cutting down on to the vein or when ligating it. They may also be damaged by stripping, especially when branching of the nerve is superficial to the vein and the stripping is carried out from the ankle towards the groin, catching the bifurcating nerve by the up-going stripper and so avulsing it upwards with the vein.

A
Incision line.

B
Right inguinal region and upper thigh. The cribriform fascia of the saphenous opening is removed to show the great saphenous vein entering an unusually large femoral vein. In this specimen the superficial circumflex iliac, superficial epigastric and anterolateral tributaries join to form a common trunk that enters the great saphenous just as it joins the femoral vein.

C
Right ankle and lower leg, from the medial side. The great saphenous vein lies in front of the medial malleolus, with branches of the saphenous nerve in front of and behind the vein. They are at risk when the vein is being exposed here.

207

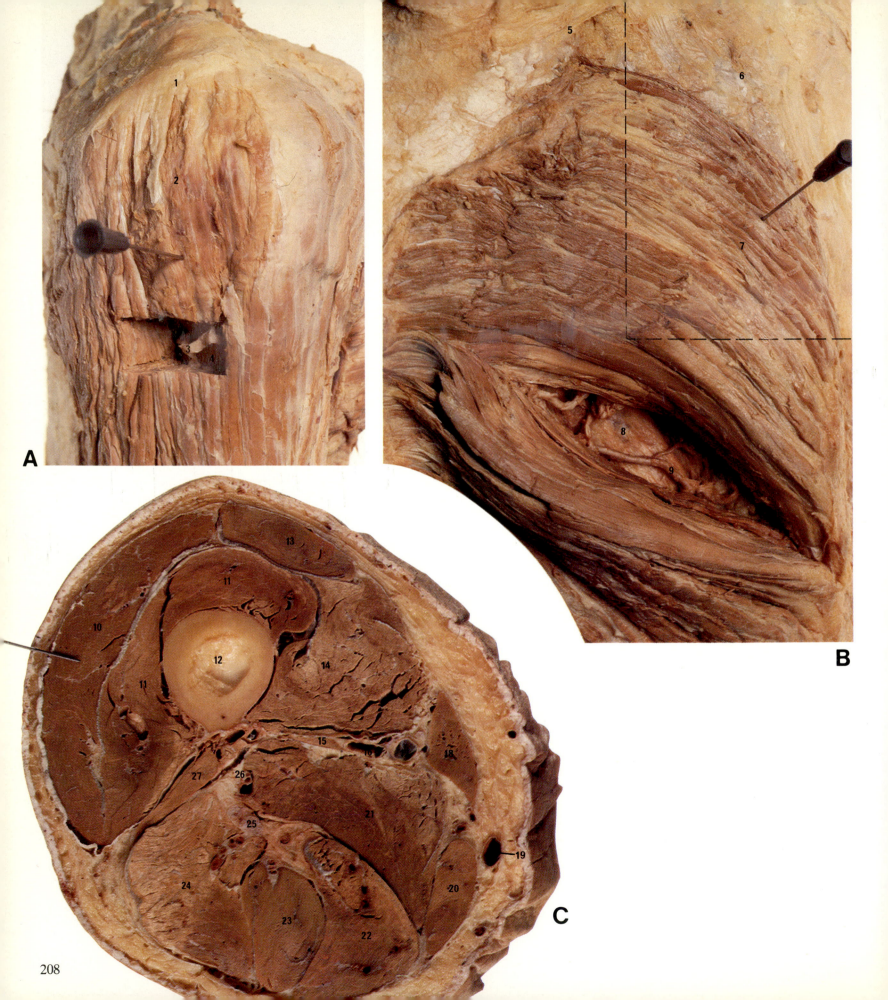

A

B

C

INTRAMUSCULAR INJECTIONS

Background

The common sites for intramuscular injection are the deltoid muscle at the shoulder, the gluteal region at the back of the hip, and vastus lateralis in the thigh. These provide readily accessible muscle masses which can be injected with safety, but particular care must be taken in the gluteal region to define the injection site correctly because of the presence of the sciatic nerve.

Deltoid Injection

The site is on the lateral side of the bulge at the shoulder, no more than 4 cm below the lower border of the acromion (A).

Hazards and Safeguards

The axillary nerve curls forwards from behind the humerus into deltoid about 5–6 cm below the acromion.

Gluteal Injection

It is essential to understand the correct definition of the buttock, which is the back of the gluteal region and extends *from the iliac crest* to the gluteal fold (fold of the buttock).

The safe injection site is the *upper outer quadrant* of the buttock. Depending on the exact position chosen, the needle passes into gluteus medius or the upper part of gluteus maximus (B).

Hazards and Safeguards

The upper outer quadrant of the buttock is an area higher and more lateral than many people imagine, especially if a sun-tanned bikini line is erroneously taken as the upper boundary of the buttock instead of the iliac crest. Unless the properly defined upper outer quadrant is used the sciatic nerve is in great danger.

To illustrate the safe area on yourself, place the tip of the left thumb on the left anterior superior iliac spine and the rest of the thumb and thenar eminence along the iliac crest; the rest of the outstretched hand lies over the safe area.

Vastus Lateralis Injection

The site is on the lateral side of the thigh a handsbreadth or more below the greater trochanter.

Hazards and Safeguards

This is a safe site well away from all major vessels and nerves (C).

A
Injection into the right deltoid, between the acromion and the axillary nerve.

B
Injection into the right gluteal region, in the buttock's upper outer quadrant as demarcated by the interrupted lines and well above the level of the sciatic nerve.

C
Injection into the right vastus lateralis, demonstrated in a cross section of the upper thigh.

1	Lower edge of acromion
2	Deltoid
3	Axillary nerve
4	Humerus
5	Iliac crest
6	Fascia over gluteus medius
7	Gluteus maximus
8	Sciatic nerve
9	Branch of inferior gluteal artery
10	Vastus lateralis
11	Vastus intermedius
12	Femur
13	Rectus femoris
14	Vastus medialis
15	Adductor longus
16	Femoral vein
17	Femoral artery
18	Sartorius
19	Great saphenous vein
20	Gracilis
21	Adductor magnus
22	Semimembranosus
23	Semitendinosus
24	Long head of biceps
25	Sciatic nerve
26	Profunda femoris vessels
27	Short head of biceps

INDEX

Abdomen and pelvis 110–165
Abortion 159
Acromion 54, 59, 209
Adam's apple 21
Adenoidectomy 25
Adenoids 24
Ampulla, hepatopancreatic 130
Anaesthesia, see also Nerve block
  epidural 49
  infiltration of teeth 37
  spinal 48
Anal canal 152
Anteflexion 160
Anteversion 160
Appendectomy 144
Appendicectomy 144
Appendices epiploices 146
Appendix (vermiform) 144
Arch, palmar, superficial 88
  zygomatic 32, 45
Artery, see also Vessels
  alveolar, inferior 40, 43
    posterior superior 29
  aorta 51, 98, 142, 164
  appendicular 144
  axillary 73
  basilar 46
  brachial 58, 77
  brachiocephalic 18, 100
  caecal, anterior 145
    posterior 144
  carotid, common 12, 17, 19
    external 12, 17, 26
    internal 12, 17, 24, 47
  cervical, superficial 15, 70
  circumflex femoral 166, 168
  coeliac trunk 133, 164
  colic, left 146, 149
    middle 119, 146
    right 144, 146
  coronary 98, 101
  cystic 130
  digital 91
  epigastric, inferior 110
    superior 110
  facial 20, 24, 36
  femoral 197
  gastric 119
    short 119, 132
  gastroduodenal 118, 122
  gastro-epiploic 119, 122, 147
  gluteal, inferior 163, 167, 193, 209
    superior 167
  hepatic 122, 126, 130
  ileocolic 144, 146

iliac, common 142
  deep circumflex 110
  external 142, 151, 160, 163
  internal 140, 142, 151, 161, 163
infra-orbital 29
intercostal 96
labial, superior 36
laryngeal, superior 18
lingual 20
malleolar 202
marginal 146
maxillary 28, 35, 40
meningeal, middle 35, 40, 45
mesenteric, inferior 143, 146, 152
  superior 123, 146
obturator, abnormal 117, 161
palatine, greater 29, 39
palmar arch, superficial 88
pancreaticoduodenal 122
peroneal 179, 204
popliteal 198
profunda brachii 80
  femoris 196
pudendal, internal 163
pulmonary 98
  trunk 98
radial 68, 83
  recurrent 81
rectal, middle 152, 161, 163
  superior 152
renal 136
sacral, lateral 150
  median 152
sigmoid 146
sphenopalatine 28
splenic 118, 132, 134, 164
subclavian 73, 108
suprarenal 134
suprascapular 15, 17, 70
temporal, superficial 27
testicular 116
thoracic, internal 97
thoraco-acromial 75
thyrocervical trunk 12, 74
thyroid, inferior 12, 19, 22, 106
  superior 13, 18, 22
tibial, anterior 179, 180, 182, 202, 204
  posterior 179, 180, 182, 202, 204
tonsillar 24
ulnar 84
umbilical, obliterated 155, 158
uterine 158
vaginal 161, 163

vertebral 19, 48
vesical, inferior 155
  superior 155
Axilla 72, 74, 96, 109

Bile duct 119, 122, 129, 130
Biopsy, kidney 139
  liver 128
  testis 158
Bladder, female 158
  male 155
Block, see Nerve block
Breast 96
Bronchi 104
Burr holes 44
Bursa, radial 91
  subdeltoid (subacromial) 52, 54
  ulnar 90

Caecum 144
Calcaneus 184, 204
Caldwell-Luc procedure 28
Canal, adductor 197
  anal 152
  femoral 117
  inguinal 110, 116
  lumbrical 89
  palatine, greater 34
  pterygoid 28
  pudendal 162
Capsule, see also Joints
  parotid 26
  prostate 155
  submandibular 20
  thyroid 22
Cardiopulmonary bypass 100
Carpal bones 70
  tunnel 87
Cartilage, cricoid 21
  of external acoustic meatus 26
  thyroid 18, 21
Catheterisation, urethral 155, 158
  venous 14
Cauda equina 48
Cerebral hemisphere 46
Cerebrospinal fluid 46, 48
Cholangiography 130
Cholecystectomy 130
Cholecystostomy 130
Choledochotomy 130
Cisterna magna 48
Clavicle 11–18, 52, 70–74, 108
Clitoris 158
Colectomy 146
Colliculus, seminal 155
Colon 146
Colostomy 152

Compartments of peritoneum 123
Condyles of femur 176, 178
  of tibia 176
Convulsions 19
Cornu, sacral 49
Cranial cavity 44
Craniotomy 44
Crest, iliac 168, 186, 189, 209
Cystostomy 156

Dacryocystorrhinostomy (DCR) 30
D and C 159
Dialysis 83, 204
Diaphragm 100, 107
  pelvic 152
Diaphragma sellae 47
Diploë 44
Drainage, intercostal 94
  pericardial 100
  peritoneal 110
Duct, bile 119, 122, 129, 130
  cystic 130
  ejaculatory 117, 155
  hepatic 130
  lymphatic, right 11, 12
  nasolacrimal 30
  pancreatic 122
  submandibular 20, 42
  thoracic 11, 12, 22, 71, 106, 108
Ductus arteriosus 102
  deferens (vas) 116, 118
Duodenum 122

Embolectomy 101
Endarterectomy 18
Epicondyle, lateral of humerus 60, 63, 78, 81, 82
  medial of humerus 58, 60, 63, 77, 84
Epididymis 117, 158
Epistaxis 28
Examination, rectal 152
  vaginal 159
Eye 30

Fascia, axillary 72
  cervical, deep 11, 18, 20, 26, 74
  clavipectoral 16, 52, 74
  investing 11, 18, 20, 26, 74
  lata 169, 173, 206
  pelvic 155
  pretracheal 21, 22
  prevertebral 11, 12, 19, 71, 72, 108
  rectovesical (Denonvilliers') 152, 155
  renal 134

Sibson's 19
Waldeyer's 152
Femur 172
Fibula 181
Fissure, orbital, inferior 30, 34
    superior 30
    pterygomaxillary 34
Flexure, colic 145
    duodenojejunal 122, 143
Fold, palatoglossal 24
    palatopharyngeal 24
Foramen, epiploic 122, 130
    incisive 39
    infra-orbital 28, 36
    intervertebral 50
    magnum 48
    mandibular 42
    mental 43
    ovale 32, 40, 42
    palatine, greater 34, 39
    rotundum 28, 34
    sphenopalatine 29, 39
    spinosum 40, 45
Foreskin 156
Fossa, cranial, anterior 46
    middle 45
    cubital 60, 64, 77, 86, 93
    iliac 140
    incisive 39
    infratemporal 34, 40
    ischiorectal 154
    for lacrimal sac 30
    navicular 155
    pituitary 46
    pterygopalatine 28, 34, 38
    tonsillar 24

Gall bladder 130
Gallstones 130
Ganglion, cervicothoracic 19
    coeliac 165
    pterygopalatine 28, 39
    stellate 19, 108
    sympathetic 19, 108, 164
    trigeminal 32
Gastrectomy 119
Genital organs, female 158
    male 155
Gland, bulbo-urethral (Cowper's)
    155
    of Littré 155
    parathyroid 22, 23
    parotid 11, 12, 26, 42
    pituitary 46
    prostate 155
    of Skene 158
    submandibular 11, 12, 20
    suprarenal 134
    thyroid 11, 12, 21, 22
    vestibular, greater (Bartholin's)
    154
Goitre 22

Hand spaces 88
Head, neck and spine 10–51
Haemorrhage, extradural 44
Haemothorax 16, 72, 109
Heart 98–103
Hemicolectomy 146, 149
Hemiplegia 12
Hernia, femoral 117
    inguinal 116
Hiatus, sacral 49
Hodgkin's disease 132
Horner's syndrome 12, 19, 72, 108
Humerus 58
Hydrocoele 158
Hyoid bone 18
Hyperparathyroidism 23
Hypophysectomy 47
Hysterectomy 160

Impression, trigeminal 32
Incision, abdominal 110
    Battle's 111
    gridiron 114
    iliac 112
    Kocher's 112
    lumbar 138
    McBurney's 114
    midline 110
    muscle-cutting 112, 113
    paramedian 111
    pararectal 111
    Pfannenstiel's 114
    rooftop 112
    Rutherford Morison's 112
    subcostal 112
    thoraco-abdominal 95
    transverse 112, 115
Intervertebral disc 50
Intramuscular injections 208
Ischaemia, cerebral 12
    hepatic 126
Isthmus of thyroid gland 21, 22

Joint, acromioclavicular 55
    ankle 182
    elbow 60
    hip 167
    knee 176
    shoulder 52
    sternoclavicular 19
    wrist 68
    zygapophyseal (facet) 50

Kidney 136
Kocher's incision 112
    manoeuvre 123

Laminectomy 50
Laminotomy 50
Laryngotomy 21
Larynx 21
Ligament, arcuate, median 142
    of Berry 22

broad 158
cervical (cardinal, Mackenrodt's)
    158
coraco-acromial 52
coronary of knee joint 176
    of liver 136
gastrosplenic 132
inguinal 116, 196, 207
interspinous 49
lacunar 116
lienorenal 132
of liver 126
of ovary 158
palpebral, medial 30
pectineal 117
round 158
sphenomandibular 42
supraspinous 49
suspensory of duodenum 122
    of ovary 158
triangular 126
umbilical, medial 155
    median 155
uterosacral 158
Ligamentum arteriosum 102
    flavum 49, 50
    nuchae 48
Linea alba 110, 115
Lingula 42
Liver 126
Lobe, liver 126
    lung 104
    thymus 97
    thyroid 11, 12, 22
Lobectomy, liver 126
    lung 104
Lower limb 166–207
Lung 104
Lymph and lymph nodes, breast 96
    cervical 11
    colon 146
    inguinal 152, 206
    oesophagus 106
    ovary 160
    rectum and anal canal 152
    stomach 119
    uterus 160

Mandible 20, 26, 33, 34, 38, 40, 42
Massage, cardiac 99
Mastectomy 96
Maxilla 28, 37, 38
Medulla oblongata 48
Membrane, atlanto-occipital 48
    cricothyroid 21
    interosseous of leg 179, 181, 202
    perineal 155
    suprapleural 16, 19, 108
Meniscus, medial 176
Mesentery 122
Meso-appendix 144
Mesocolon, sigmoid 145
    transverse 122, 145

Mesosalpinx 158
Mesovarium 158
Mobilisation of duodenum 124
Muscle
    abductor digiti minimi 91
        hallucis 204
        pollicis brevis 86
        pollicis longus 69
    adductor brevis 166, 195
        longus 173, 195
        magnus 166, 172, 198
        pollicis 89
    anconeus 60, 67
    biceps brachii 52, 58, 76
        femoris 172, 181, 191, 198, 202
    brachialis 58, 62, 82
    brachioradialis 58, 80
    buccinator 32, 42
    bulbospongiosus 154, 157
    constrictor, inferior 22
        superior 24
    coracobrachialis 52, 75
    cricothyroid 21, 22
    deltoid 52, 209
    depressor anguli oris 43
        labii inferioris 43
    diaphragm 100, 107
    digastric 12, 26
    erector spinae 51, 138
    extensor carpi radialis brevis 87
        carpi radialis longus 81
        carpi ulnaris 60, 67
        digiti minimi 69
        digitorum 68
        digitorum longus 182, 202
        hallucis longus 182, 202
        indicis 67
        pollicis brevis 69
        pollicis longus 68
    flexor carpi radialis 68, 82, 86
        carpi ulnaris 67, 84
        digiti minimi brevis 91
        digitorum longus 178, 182, 204
        digitorum profundus 67
        digitorum superficialis 86
        hallucis longus 180, 182
        pollicis brevis 86
        pollicis longus 68
    gastrocnemius 176, 199, 200, 202
    gemelli 167
    gluteus maximus 167, 190, 209
        medius 167, 209
        minimus 167
    gracilis 172, 201
    hamstring 172
    hyoglossus 20
    iliacus 166, 194
    infraspinatus 54
    intercostal 94
    interossei, hand 89
    latissimus dorsi 80, 95, 108
    levator anguli oris 36
        ani 152, 155

labii superioris 36
   palpebrae superioris 30
lumbrical, hand 89
masseter 34, 40
mylohyoid 20
oblique, external 110
   inferior 31
   internal 110
omohyoid 12, 14, 108
opponens digiti minimi 91
   pollicis 86
orbicularis oculi 30
palmaris brevis 88
   longus 68, 86
pectineus 166, 195
pectoralis major 52, 74, 96
   minor 52, 71, 74, 96
peroneus brevis 182
   longus 181, 182
   tertius 182
piriformis 162, 167
plantaris 176
platysma 20
pronator quadratus 64
   teres 61, 64
psoas major 164, 167, 186
pterygoid, lateral 34, 38, 40, 42
   medial 42
puborectalis 152, 155
pyramidalis 110
rectus abdominis 110
   femoris 167, 172
   inferior 31
   lateral 31
   medial 47
   superior 31
sartorius 167, 172, 194, 196, 198
scalenus anterior 11, 71, 74, 108
   medius 71
semimembranosus 173, 177, 198
semitendinosus 173, 177, 198
serratus anterior 94, 96, 109
soleus 178, 181, 202
sphincter, external anal 152
   internal anal 152
   urethrae 155
sternocleidomastoid 11, 12, 14,
   18, 22, 26, 107, 108
sternohyoid 21, 22
sternothyroid 21, 22
stylohyoid 26
subclavius 71
subscapularis 52
supinator 60, 81
supraspinatus 54
suspensory of duodenum 122
temporalis 34, 40, 44
tensor fasciae latae 167
teres major 54
   minor 54
thyrohyoid 13
tibialis anterior 178, 182
   posterior 178, 184

transversus abdominis 110
trapezius 11, 12, 52, 54
triceps 58, 61, 81
vastus intermedius 172
   lateralis 172, 175, 209
   medialis 196
zygomaticus major 36
   minor 36

Nasopharynx 24
Neck, radical dissection 12
Nephrectomy 138
Nerve
   abducent 32
   accessory 11, 12
   alveolar, inferior 42
      posterior superior 38
   ansa cervicalis 18, 22
   auricular, great 11, 20, 26
   auriculotemporal 44
   axillary 54, 209
   brachial plexus 11, 12, 70
   cervical plexus 11, 12
   cutaneous of arm, medial 71
   cutaneous of forearm, lateral 58,
      71, 75
      medial 61, 71
   digital 92
   facial 11, 12, 20, 26, 42
   femoral 194
      lateral cutaneous 194
      medial cutaneous 206
      posterior cutaneous 190
   frontal 30
   genitofemoral 142, 162, 164
   glossopharyngeal 11, 12, 24
   gluteal, inferior 167
      superior 167
   hypoglossal 11, 12, 18, 20
   iliohypogastric 110
   ilio-inguinal 110, 116, 162
   incisive 43
   infra-orbital 28, 36
   intercostal 94, 110
   interosseous, posterior 60, 64, 80
   lacrimal 30
   laryngeal, external 18, 22
      internal 18
      recurrent 12, 19, 22, 72, 102,
         106
      superior 18
   of Latarjet 119
   to lateral pterygoid 35, 40
   lingual 20, 42
   lumbar plexus 186
   lumbosacral trunk 186, 188
   mandibular 40
   masseteric 35, 40
   maxillary 32, 34
   median 58, 68, 77, 86
   mental 43
   musculocutaneous 52, 75
   nasopalatine 39

obturator 195
occipital, greater 44
oculomotor 46
ophthalmic 30
optic 31, 34, 36, 47
palatine, greater 39
pectoral, lateral 17, 52, 71, 75, 96
   medial 71, 96
peroneal, common 202
   communicating 176, 202
   deep 182, 202
   superficial 202
petrosal, greater 32
   lesser 32
phrenic 11, 12, 71, 74, 94, 97, 99,
   102, 108
to pronator teres 61
of pterygoid canal 28
pudendal 162
radial 58, 80
rectal, inferior 162
roots 48, 50
sacral plexus 189
saphenous 176, 179, 182, 197,
   201, 204, 206
sciatic 190, 209
subcostal 138
supra-orbital 31, 44
suprascapular 54
supratrochlear 31
sural 177, 205
temporal, deep 35, 40
thoracic, long 94, 96, 108
thoracodorsal 96, 108
tibial 202
trochlear 32
ulnar 60, 77, 84
vagus 11, 12, 18, 102, 106, 119,
   121
Vidian 28
Nerve block
   alveolar, inferior 42
      posterior superior 38
   brachial plexus 72
   coeliac plexus 165
   digital 92
   femoral 194
      lateral cutaneous 194
   incisive 43
   infra-orbital 36
   lingual 42
   lumbar plexus 186
   lumbar sympathetic 164
   mandibular 40
   maxillary 34
   median 78, 87
   mental 43
   nasopalatine 39
   obturator 195
   palatine, greater 39
   pudendal 162
   radial 82
   sacral plexus 189

sciatic 192
stellate ganglion 19
supra-orbital and supratrochlear
   31
trigeminal ganglion 32
ulnar 78, 84
Neuralgia, trigeminal 32
Neurectomy, Vidian 28
Node, see also Lymph
   sinuatrial 101
Notch, coronoid 42
   frontal 30
   jugular 16
   mandibular 34, 40
   supra-orbital 30

Oesophagus 106
Olecranon 59, 63
Omentum, greater 119, 145
   lesser 119, 130, 145
Orbit 30, 46
Ovariectomy (oophorectomy) 160
Ovary 158

Pancreas 122
Pancreatoduodenectomy 123
Paracentesis 110
Parotid gland 26
Parotidectomy 26
Patella 176, 178, 206
Pelvis 150–163, 189
   renal 136
Penis 155
Pericardium 101, 107
Peritoneum 94, 110, 112, 122, 126,
   142, 152, 155, 158
Pisiform bone 84
Pituitary gland 46
Plate, lateral pterygoid 34, 40
Pleura 16, 94, 104, 107, 138
Plexus, brachial 11, 12, 70
   cervical 11
   choroid 48
   coeliac 165
   dental, superior 37
   lumbar 186
   pterygoid 34, 38, 41
   sacral 189
Pneumonectomy 104
Pneumothorax 16, 19, 72, 108, 128
Potassium 129
Portacaval anastomosis 130
Pouch, hepatorenal (Morison's)
   136
   recto-uterine (of Douglas) 152,
      159
   rectovesical 152, 155
   vesico-uterine 158
Pressure, central venous 16
Process, coracoid 52
   mastoid 11, 26, 48
   styloid of radius 64, 68, 83
      of skull 26

of ulna 67, 68, 86
Processus vaginalis 116
Prostate gland 155
Pterion 45
Pulse 68
Puncture, ankle joint 183
  brachial artery 78
  brachiocephalic vein 14, 15
  cisternal 48
  elbow joint 63
  femoral artery 197
  hip joint 171
  internal jugular vein 14
  knee joint 178
  lumbar 49
  radial artery 83
  shoulder joint 57
  subclavian artery 16
  ulnar artery 84
  wrist joint 69
Pupil 32, 36
Pylorus 122

Radius 64
Raphe, pterygomandibular 42
Rectum 152
Resection, abdominoperineal 153
  anterior 153
Retinaculum, extensor of ankle 182
  of wrist 68, 91
  flexor of ankle 184
    of wrist 68, 90
  peroneal, superior 184
Retrobulbar injection 31
Rhinorrhoea 28
Ring, femoral 117
  inguinal 116
Root of mesentery 122
Rotator cuff 52

Sac, greater 134
  lacrimal 30
  lesser 122, 132
Scalp 44
Scaphoid bone 70
Scapula 52
Seminal vesicle 117
Septum, atrial 101
  of hand spaces 89
  intermuscular, lateral of arm 81
    lateral of thigh 172, 175, 199
    medial of arm 60, 77
  ventricular 101
Sheath, axillary 75
  carotid 11, 12, 18, 106
  rectus 110
  synovial 91
Sinus, carotid 12
  cavernous 32, 34
  ethmoidal 46
  frontal 44
  intercavernous 46

maxillary 28
  sagittal, superior 44
  sphenoidal 46
  tonsillar 24
Spine, iliac, anterior superior 168,
    172, 194, 196, 209
    posterior inferior 188
    posterior superior 188
  ischial 162
  of scapula 54
  of vertebra 48, 165, 186
Snuffbox 69, 83, 93
Space, epidural 48
  extradural 48
  hand 88
  intercostal 94, 128
  midpalmar 89
  pterygomandibular 41
  pulp 91
  quadrilateral 54
  subaponeurotic 88
  subarachnoid 48
  subcutaneous 88
  subungual 92
  thenar 89
  web 89
Spermatic cord 116, 118
Spinal cord 48
Spleen 132
Splenectomy 132
Sternotomy, median 94
Sternum 94
Stomach 119
Stones, renal 142
Submandibular gland 20
Suprarenal gland 134
Sympathectomy 108, 164
Sympathetic trunk 18, 108, 164
Symphysis, pubic 155, 194, 196

Taeniae coli 144, 146
Talus 182, 203
Tears 30
Teeth 34–43
Tendo calcaneus 185, 204
Tendon, adductor magnus 200
  ankle 182
  biceps brachii 60, 77, 93
    femoris 172, 177, 190, 198, 202
  extensor pollicis brevis 70
    pollicis longus 69
  flexor carpi radialis
    carpi ulnaris 82, 86
  palmaris longus 86
  psoas major 167
  supraspinatus 55
  wrist 68
Testis 158
Thoracotomy 94
Thorax 94–109
Thymectomy 97
Thymus 97
Thyroid gland 12, 22

Thyroidectomy 22
Tibia 178
Tonsillectomy 24
Tonsils 24
Trachea 19, 21, 22
Tracheostomy 21
Tracheotomy 21
Tract, biliary 130
  iliotibial 175, 199
  olfactory 47
Transplantation, cardiac 103
  kidney 140
  liver 129
Trapezium bone 70
Trephine 44
Triangle, anterior 11
  digastric 11, 20
  femoral 197
  posterior 11, 12, 74
Trochanter, greater 168, 170, 172,
    192
Trunk, of brachial plexus 71
  coeliac 165
  pulmonary 98, 101
  thyrocervical 12, 74
  vagal 106, 119
Tubal ligation 160
Tube, auditory 25
  uterine 158
Tubercle, adductor 198, 200
  pubic 195, 196, 198, 207
Tuberosity, ischial 162, 190
  tibial 176
Tunica albuginea 158
  vaginalis 158

Ulna 66
Upper limb 52–93
Ureter 140, 142, 155, 160
Urethra 154, 158
Uterus 158

Vagina 158
Vagotomy 119, 121
Valve, aortic 101
  mitral 101, 102
  venous 206
Valvotomy, mitral 101, 102
Varices, oesophageal 130
Vas (ductus) deferens 116, 118
Vasectomy 118
Vein, see also Vessels
  angular 30
  axillary 75
  azygos 105
  basilic 77, 93
  brachiocephalic 15
  cephalic 52, 93
  duodenal 122
  facial 18
  femoral 117
  gastric 119
  gonadal 140

hepatic 126
  iliac 140, 142
  jugular, anterior 11, 21
    external 11, 12, 16, 26, 108
    internal 11, 12, 14
  lumbar 142
  meningeal, middle 45
  mesenteric, inferior 143
    superior 122
  obturator 161
  oesophageal 106
  pancreatic 122
  paratonsillar 24
  portal 122, 125, 126, 130
  pulmonary 104
  rectal 152
  renal 138, 140, 143
  retromandibular 26
  saphenous, great 206
    small 198, 206
  splenic 122
  subclavian 16
  superficial of lower limb 206
    of upper limb 93
  suprarenal 134
  thyroid, inferior 21
    middle 22, 106
    superior 22
  tonsillar 24
  varicose 206
  vena cava, inferior 51, 98, 101,
    122, 126, 130, 142, 164
    superior 14, 98, 101
  vesicoprostatic 155
Venepuncture, brachiocephalic 14
  internal jugular 14
  subclavian 16
  upper limb 93
Vertebrae, lumbar 48, 186
Verumontanum 155
Vessels, see also Artery and Vein
  cervical, superficial 52, 55
  circumflex humeral 52
    iliac 94
  colic, middle 119
  ethmoidal, anterior 46
  facial 20
  femoral 175
  gastric, short 132
  gonadal 142
  intercostal 94, 110
  interosseous, anterior 87
  meningeal, middle 40
  mesenteric, superior 123
  obturator 195
  occipital 44
  ovarian 158
  peroneal 180
  profunda brachii 81
    femoris 173, 175, 191, 209
  pudendal, internal 162
  rectal, inferior 152
  splenic 132

subcostal 138
supra-orbital 30, 44
temporal, superficial 44
thoraco-acromial 17, 75
thyroid, superior 19
tibial, anterior 182, 202
   posterior 182
Vocal cord 22
Vulva 162

Wall, abdominal 110
  thoracic 94

Xiphoid process 100